OXFORD MEDICAL PUBLICATIONS

Clinical Dermatology

Oxford Core Texts

Palliative Care
Health and Illness in the Community
Clinical Dermatology
Endocrinology
Human Physiology
Paediatrics
Psychiatry
Medical Imaging
Neurology
Oncology

CLINICAL DERMATOLOGY

Rona M. MacKie MD DSc FRCP FRC Path

Leverhulme Research Fellow
Emeritus Professor of Dermatology
University of Glasgow;
Consultant Dermatologist,
Greater Glasgow Health Board,
North Glasgow University NHS Trust,

FIFTH EDITION

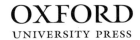

OXFORD

UNIVERSITY PRESS

OXFORD
UNIVERSITY PRESS

Great Clarendon Street, Oxford OX2 6DP

Oxford University Press is a department of the University of Oxford.
If furthers the University's objective of excellence in research, scholarship,
and education by publishing worldwide in

Oxford New York

Auckland Bangkok Buenos Aires Cape Town Chennai
Dar es Salaam Delhi Florence Hong Kong Istanbul Karachi Kolkata
Kuala Lumpur Madrid Melbourne Mexico City Mumbai Nairobi
Sao Paolo Shanghai Taipei Tokyo Toronto

Oxford is a registered trade mark of Oxford University Press
in the UK and in certain other countries

Published in the United States
by Oxford University Press Inc., New York

© Rona MacKie, 2003

The moral rights of the author have been asserted

Database right Oxford University Press (maker)

First edition published 1981 (Pbk)
Second edition published 1986 (Pbk)
Third edition published 1991 (Pbk)
Fourth edition published 1996 (Pbk)
Fifth edition published 2003 (Pbk)

A catalogue record for this title is available from the British Library.

Library of Congress Cataloging in Publication Data
(Data available)

ISBN 0 19 852580 X

10 9 8 7 6 5 4 3 2 1

Typeset by EXPO Holdings, Malaysia

Printed in Italy
by Giunti Industrie Grafiche

Preface to 5th edition

Since the last edition of this book was published in 1997, there have been exciting advances in dermatology, both in treatment and in our understanding of the molecular biology of disease. However, these two developments have not been as closely linked as one might have hoped, a phenomenon not peculiar to dermatology. In the important areas of severe psoriasis and atopic eczema, we now have a new and potent range of immunosuppressives and cytokine modifying agents, which have undoubted efficacy. Safety issues are not yet entirely established and post-marketing surveillance will require to be stringent

Molecular genetics has contributed to our knowledge of the exact genetic mechanisms responsible for some of the rare, but devastating genetically-determined blistering diseases and dyskeratoses. These advances are academically satisfying, but whether or not they will need to more effective therapy in these areas remains to be seen.

Dermatological teaching has undergone a major change in many parts of the world. Here in Glasgow, we have moved from a traditionally taught medical undergraduate curriculum to a problem-based learning approach. Our first students from this new course graduated in 2001. They have been lively and inquiring during their time in dermatology, but dedicated time in dermatology has been reduced to accommodate other areas of the curriculum and new opportunistic slots for dermatological experience have appeared in the context of problem-based learning approaches. A number of dermatologically relevant problem cases have been prepared for group problem-based learning in Glasgow, and some of these are included in Chapter 1 in the hope that they will be used and adapted in other medical schools around the world. There are also a number of suggested topics for either individual or group special study modules at the end of individual chapters.

The web becomes an ever more extensive source of information for both the medical and nursing professions, and their patients. I have included a reasonable number of currently reliable web sites. They are worth visiting and, particularly in the case of patient association websites, remember that your patients may well have been there first.

As always it has been a pleasure to work with my colleagues at Oxford University Press. I am grateful particularly to Catherine Barnes for her friendly support and encouragement.

Rona M MacKie
Glasgow October 2002.

Contents

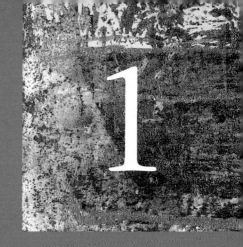

Problem-based learning scenarios

- Scenario 1: the problem of atopic eczema prognosis and management in childhood

- Scenario 2: the management of possible occupational dermatitis in a young man

- Scenario 3: the management of a patient with moderately severe psoriasis

- Scenario 4: leg ulcers

- Scenario 5: cutaneous malignancy

- Scenario 6: cutaneous malignancy

- Scenario 7: bullous disorders

- Scenario 8: acne vulgaris

- Scenario 9: infection in an immunocompromised patient

- Scenario 10: connective tissue disorder

- Scenario 11: scabies

Problem-based learning scenarios

The object of these case histories is to form a realistic scenario around which problem based learning can take place. It is suggested that these scenarios are discussed with a group of students or with students individually, and a list made of the facts needed to respond to the questions. Students can then use both this book and the wider world of journals, larger textbooks, and a computer search to gather together the knowledge needed. This can then be presented to a group of fellow students 2–3 weeks later.

A teaching facilitator is valuable to guide the knowledge search if it appears to be going off course, or if the facilitator perceives that the information which the students perceive they require is far beyond the scope needed. The facilitator is there to point out sources of information which the students may have missed, but not to collect the data for them.

Scenario 1: the problem of atopic eczema prognosis and management in childhood

Catriona Ross is a 35-year-old Member of Parliament. She has been married for 3 years and has a baby boy aged 18 months, who has had mild eczema since the age of 6 months. Recently, this eczema has become very much more active. Both Catriona and her husband have a family history of asthma.

Catriona has been given a number of topical preparations by her general practitioner, but she does not feel that these have made any difference to her son's skin. She wishes to discuss with you the alternative treatments that may be available for her child and asks for an explanation as to why this eczema cannot be completely cured. She is also interested in the possible outlook for any further children that she and her husband may want to have.

Aims

To explore the genetic background, clinical features, and management of atopic dermatitis in a young child.

Learning objectives

By the end of this scenario:

1. You should be able to make a diagnosis or suspect a diagnosis of atopic dermatitis in both children and adults.

2. You should have some understanding of the relationship between asthma and atopic dermatitis.

3. You should be able to describe a simple treatment plan for different degrees of severity of atopic dermatitis in both children and adults.

4. You should have some idea of the features that may influence the prognosis of dermatitis in young children.

Scenario 2: the management of possible occupational dermatitis in a young man

Donald Nicolson is a 20-year-old chef working in one of Scotland's award-winning restaurants. He has done this job since the age of 16 and is hoping to develop his career in the catering industry as a professional chef. In the past year he has developed a problem with hand dermatitis and has red scaly lesions, mainly on the fingers. This clears when he is on holiday.

Donald wants further investigations undertaken. He feels that he may be developing problems as a result of the materials he handles in his regular employment and is concerned about the future outlook.

Aims

To explore the problem of occupational dermatitis.

Learning objectives

By the end of this scenario:

1. You should have some thoughts on how to differentiate an irritant from allergic contact dermatitis.
2. You should understand the technique of patch testing, and be able to explain to a patient what will be done to them and why.
3. You should have some understanding of the dermatological hazards of working in the catering industry.
4. You should be able to give a patient sensible advice on hand care aimed at preventing or improving hand dermatitis.

Scenario 3: the management of a patient with moderately severe psoriasis

Malcolm Brown is a 28-year-old lawyer working in a large office in Sydney. He has had psoriasis since the age of 15. This has been managed with various topical preparations and occasional treatments with ultraviolet light given at the local hospital.

Over the last 6 months, concomitant with a heavy increase in workload, his psoriasis has become very much more active and difficult to control. Because of court appearances, he is particularly concerned that lesions are now developing on his face and hands. An additional complication is the fact that Malcolm has recently become engaged and is concerned about any future children being at increased risk of psoriasis.

Malcolm therefore wishes to know more about treatments available for psoriasis and about the risk of inheriting psoriasis in families who already have the disease.

Aims

To explore the range of treatments available for psoriasis and its genetic background.

Learning objectives

By the end of working with this patient:

1. You should have learned how to make a clinical diagnosis of psoriasis.

2. You should have learned how to describe some of the abnormalities found in the epidermal keratinocyte and psoriatic plaques.

3. You should have developed a list of treatments for psoriasis of varying grades of severity. While compiling this, list the complications of these treatments alongside the treatments themselves.

4. You should have developed some understanding about the contribution of inherited and environmental influences on the development and severity of psoriasis.

Scenario 4: leg ulcers

Annie Graham is aged 63 and has a family history of diabetes. She is overweight and has, for several years, had painful itchy areas around both ankles. After a recent fall while trying to run for a bus 3 months ago, she developed a raw area on the inner surface of the right ankle, which has not yet healed.

1. What is the differential diagnosis here?

2. What investigations are appropriate and how would you carry them out?

3. What is the best management of this lady at the present time?

4. What general and what specific advice would you give Mrs Graham for the future?

Learning objectives

At the end of this case you should have:

1. Developed some understanding of the different types of leg ulcers.

2. Developed an understanding of factors predisposing to these different types of leg ulcers.

3. Learned when to do ABPIs and what their significance is in managing your patient.

4. Understand the principles of leg ulcer bandaging.

5. Have some understanding of how guidelines for the profession are currently being prepared and used.

Scenario 5: cutaneous malignancy

John McLaren is 53 and was born in South Africa, but came to Scotland as an undergraduate. He is an architect and spends a lot of time on building sites. He is also a keen sailor.

John's general practitioner is concerned about several raised scaling lesions on his rapidly balding scalp and also about a solitary crusted lesion on his hand.

1. What is the differential diagnosis here?

2. What investigations are appropriate?

3. What advice would you give John for the future?

Learning objectives

By the end of learning about this patient you should have:

1. Acquired some understanding of dermatological conditions aggravated by excessive sun exposure.
2. Learned the differential diagnosis of non-melanoma skin cancer.
3. Understood the management of actinic keratosis and squamous cell carcinoma.
4. Have some ideas about advice on sun protection for different sections of the population.

Scenario 6: cutaneous malignancy

You are carrying out a general practitioner's surgery on a sunny afternoon in June in the UK. The previous week has been sun awareness week in the media and, during this time, there has been a programme shown on television about the problems of skin cancer in Australia. Your third and fourth patients of the clinic are Jenny and Anne Brown, two elderly widows aged 65 and 72 who are keen overseas travellers. These ladies watched the programme on skin cancer, have looked at each other's skin, and have found large numbers of greyish brown lesions, mainly on their backs.

The two sisters are very anxious about the possibility of skin cancer particularly melanoma.

1. What is the differential diagnosis of pigmented lesions of this type?
2. What risk factors for melanoma would you enquire about of these sisters?
3. Given the scenario you have just received, what is the most likely diagnosis?
4. How would you treat these lesions, and how would you reassure and advise your patients?

Learning objectives

By the end of learning about these two ladies you should have:

1. Developed an understanding of the range of pigmented lesions that may present in the skin.
2. Understand the presenting clinical features of benign and malignant cutaneous pigmented lesions, and have some idea of how to differentiate between the two.
3. Know how to manage seborrhoeic keratosis.
4. Developed appropriate advice for elderly patients who travel a lot on sensible sun exposure.

Scenario 7: bullous disorders

You are the medical officer at a home for the elderly. Mrs Jane MacKenzie, aged 92, has been admitted from her own home for assessment because of increasing confusion. In addition, she has had itchy red skin for the past 3 months according to her daughter.

On examination she has erythema on her trunk, thighs, and upper arms. The possibility of an adverse drug reaction is suspected. She appears to be on a multi-plicity of medications including digoxin, bendrofluazide, voltarol, and cimetidine. Three days after admission she develops blisters on the previously red skin of her upper arms.

1. What is the differential diagnosis of this lady's cutaneous lesions?

2. What investigations might be helpful here?

3. What is the appropriate management of the condition?

4. What will you tell her daughter about the prognosis?

Learning objectives

By the end of this scenario:

1. You should understand the common causes of blisters in the elderly.

2. You should be able to describe the presentation and investigation of patients with bullous pemphigoid.

3. You should have some idea about the management and prognosis of bullous pemphigoid.

4. You should have some understanding of the presentation of drug eruptions in the skin and their management.

Scenario 8: acne vulgaris

You are a family practice trainee. Jennifer MacLaren is aged 16 and comes to your evening surgery with her mother. She has had acne since she was 13 and has had several repeat prescriptions for systemic antibiotics. At present Jennifer has a large number of pustules on her nose and chin, and according to her mother is very reluctant to go to school some mornings because of her appearance.

Her mother is very distressed about the situation and demands that something is done. She asks for referral to a specialist. How would you manage this patient and her mother?

Learning objectives

By the end of this scenario you should be able:

1. To understand the differential diagnosis of facial erythema, pustules, and papules in a teenager.

2. To have understanding of the management of acne vulgaris.

3. To understand the differential diagnosis of facial eruptions in older individuals.

4. To understand the range of topical and systemic treatment available for care, and when to use them.

Scenario 9: infection in an immunocompromised patient

You are a junior doctor rotating through the renal unit. Oliver Jones, a 23-year-old renal transplant recipient, attends your outpatient clinic for review of his immunosuppressive drug therapy. His only complaint is of a painful left heel, which has prevented him from training for the half marathon that he hopes to run in order to raise funds for the renal unit. On examination you find several large hyperkeratotic warty lesions on his heel.

1. What is the diagnosis here?

2. Is there a differential diagnosis?

3. What factors may have contributed to the development of these lesions?

4. What is the appropriate management?

5. What other cutaneous problems are more common in transplant recipients?

Learning objectives

By the end of this scenario you should be able:

1. To understand the range of dermatological problems more common in transplant recipients.

2. To understand the management of warts.

3. To understand the specific management of resistant warts in immunosuppressed individuals.

4. To understand other situations in which immunosuppression may alter presentation or management of dermatological disease.

Scenario 10: connective tissue disorder

As a general practitioner you are visited during a surgery by Christine Johnson, who is 23 and recently married. Her problem is that on her honeymoon in Minorca she developed a red prickly rash on her face and shoulders. She also complains of feeling vaguely tired and has joint pains.

Three months before her wedding she started on the oral contraceptive, but is on no other medication.

1. What is the differential diagnosis in this case?

2. What investigations would be helpful?

3. How would you advise Christine for the future?

Learning objectives

By the end of this scenario you should be able:

1. To understand the differential diagnosis of facial rashes in males and females at any age.

2. To understand presenting features in varying modes of presentation of lupus erythematosus.

3. To have some knowledge of the drugs that may induce or aggravate lupus erythematosus.

4. To have some understanding of the advice that needs to be given to young women who have lupus erythematosus concerning the use of oral contraceptives and pregnancy.

Scenario 11: scabies

You are working in a general practice that looks after a local old people's home. Your are phoned by the manager of the home, in some distress, because a high proportion of her catering and nursing staff have skin problems, and are complaining of intractable itch. You visit the home and find that a number of the elderly residents have fine scaling on their skin, together with large numbers of excoriations.

1. What conditions would you consider possible causes of this?

2. How would you go about investigating the situation?

3. What appropriate treatments are you aware of?

4. How could you prevent this happening in the future?

Learning objectives

By the end of this scenario you should be able:

1. To compile a list of the causes of pruritus in the elderly and appropriate investigations.

2. To understand the situations in which the scabies mite proliferates.

3. To have some knowledge of the currently available therapies for scabies and how to use them.

4. To have an understanding of how to investigate an outbreak of infectious disease in any institution.

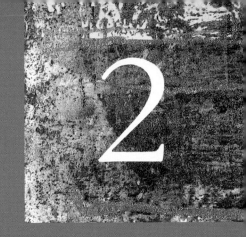

Dermatological disability: incidence, prevalence, and classification of skin disease

- Dermatological disability

- The quantity of the problem

- Classification of skin disease

- Glossary of useful terms used in dermatology and skin pathology

- Projects that could be used in a special study module

Dermatological disability: incidence, prevalence, and classification of skin disease

Introduction

Dermatologists always firmly claim that the skin is the largest organ in the body, and therefore merits more time and attention than it is allocated in most medical school undergraduate programmes. Table 2.1 lists some of its important functions. These include protection from external injury, control of fluid balance and electrolytes, temperature control, an important outpost of the nervous system, immunological functions, interaction with ultraviolet radiation, synthesizing Vitamin D, and lipid synthesis.

From the contents of Table 2.1, it will be no surprise to read that 10–15% of consultations in primary care in the UK concern a dermatological disorder. For non-fatal diseases, which includes most dermatological conditions, this may well represent only the tip of the iceberg, as many people in the community may be living with, for example, their chronic psoriasis, recurrent hand dermatitis, or other problems, either because they have in the past sought help and been unsatisfied with the response from the medical profession, or because they are not aware that anything can be done for their problem. Population- rather than hospital-based surveys suggest that this is, indeed, the case and that people with milder forms of many skin diseases either do not consult their primary care doctor or treat it themselves with over-the-counter remedies.

The quantity of physical and psychological disability, which this unmet need for dermatological care causes, cannot be estimated, but must be considerable. Even when the more severe skin diseases, such as epidermolysis bullosa, are reviewed

Key points

Dermatological disorders account for 10–15% of primary care consultations. In addition, there is considerable unmet need in the community, though this is difficult to quantify.

Table 2.1 Important functional properties of the skin

Protects from external injury
Literally holds all other organs together
Plays a part in fluid balance. Mainly excretes, but can also absorb fluid
Temperature control
An important organ of sensation
Interacts with ultraviolet radiation
Metabolizes vitamin D
Synthesizes epidermal lipids that are an important protective barrier
Cosmetic function

(p. 279), any attempt to carry out a community-based survey of prevalence reveals many previously unrecognized sufferers. It is therefore highly likely that this unmet need may be considerably greater in commoner, but less severe problems.

Dermatological disability

Quantitating dermatological disability has been assisted by the recent development and validation of a number of questionnaires. For example, the psoriasis disability index (p. 68) is a series of simple questions, which have been derived after talking to large numbers of patients with psoriasis and are designed to identify the level of disruption caused by the patient's skin problem with regard to domestic life, employment, and social activities. It may be instructive to you and useful for the patient to ask these questions both before and after a course of treatment to see whether or not **your** assessment of the value of your chosen treatment coincides with the patient's views. These scoring systems are particularly important in trials of new therapies. There are now similar questionnaires available even for relatively young children with eczema. Once again, they give useful insight into what the patient thinks and feels.

Remember also that dermatological disability may affect a whole family not just the patient. This is very obvious in the case of children with atopic eczema. The affected child may keep the whole family awake at night, and take up a large proportion of his or her mother's time by day as she applies ointments, bandages the child, and tries to distract him from persistent scratching, which will give rise to further problems.

The quantity of dermatological disease

All diseases can be measured by their incidence and prevalence. The incidence of any disease is the number of new cases identified over a period of time, usually a calendar year. A striking example of the rising incidence of a particular skin disease is the situation with cutaneous malignant melanoma where the incidence has risen rapidly over the past 30 years.

The prevalence of a disease is the term used to describe the numbers of cases of any condition in the population at a given time. Thus, long-lasting chronic conditions, such as psoriasis or eczema, are likely to have a high prevalence, whereas conditions that tend to affect individuals for only a short period of time, and either burn out or cause the patient's death will have a lower prevalence. Over the past 20 years, the prevalence of atopic disorders—asthma, allergic rhinitis, and atopic eczema— have all increased steeply. Theories to explain this include the idea that, in the so-called developed world, we have created a hyper-clean environment for young children such that they no longer have exposure to a range of minor infective agents, which in turn stimulate development of a normal immune system.

Table 2.2 lists the 10 dermatological conditions most commonly diagnosed in a busy outpatient service in Northern Europe Over the past 20 years there has been a steep rise in the dermatological workload in cutaneous malignancy and possible pre-cancerous lesions. This reflects a real rise in the incidence of these conditions related both to an increased life expectancy and also to greater opportunities for exposure to the sun in people born since 1930. This has, in turn, led

Table 2.2 The commonest causes for dermatological
referral to a northern European teaching hospital 2002

Psoriasis

Acne

Dermatitis

Seborrhoeic keratoses

Basal cell carcinoma

Actinic keratosis

Alopecia areata

Fungal infections

Melanocytic naevi

Warts

Key points

Numbers of cases of a disease are
measured by their incidence
(number of new cases identified in
a time period) and prevalence
(number of cases in a population at
a given time).

to the development of dermatological surgery as a major subspeciality. In the US
in particular, many dermatologists now spend a large part of their working week
carrying out minor surgical procedures.

Classification of skin disease

There is no entirely satisfactory method of classification of skin diseases.
Traditionally, dermatologists have used a morphological classification, using a
description of the disease in Latin as the name of the disorder, e.g. lichen planus
(see p. 78), and then grouping together conditions that were clinically similar, e.g.
the lichenoid disorders. At the present time, modern dermatologists are doing
their best to classify skin disease according to biochemically-defined functional or
genetic abnormalities. This is proceeding slowly, but there are still areas where the
old and the new terminology do not quite equate. Thus, it would be logical to
assume that all skin diseases called epidermolysis bullosa were associated with **blisters** and **lysis** of cells in the epidermis. In fact, only one subset of the epidermolysis bullosa collection of disorders does have these characteristics, while some of the
others have clearly identified abnormalities of collagen genes or of keratin genes.

Age-related skin disease

A further method of thinking about skin disease in terms of classification is to
consider the various ages of life at which the diseases are most prevalent. Thus,
a chronological classification can divide the speciality into paediatric, adoles-
cent, adult, and geriatric dermatology, with perhaps a subset of occupational
dermatology for those in employment. Again, this is not entirely satisfactory as,
although some conditions such as angiomas and atopic dermatitis are very much
commoner in early infancy, they may continue to be problems throughout adult
life.

The most useful classification is likely to be that based on the aetiology of
the disease. Once this is established for the majority of skin conditions, a new
classification should follow automatically.

Glossary of useful terms used in dermatology and skin pathology

Acantholysis: A rounding up of epidermal cells resulting from a loss of adhesion between these cells. Seen in association with benign blistering disease (pemphigus) and in epidermal malignancy.

Acanthosis: Histological term used to describe epidermal thickening due to an increase in the number of cells in the prickle cell layer of the epidermis.

Apoptosis: Non-inflammatory individual cell death. The opposite of necrosis. Seen, for example, in the epidermis in graft versus host disease.

Atopy: Literally 'strange disease'. The triad of atopic dermatitis, asthma, and allergic rhinitis (hay fever).

Balloon degeneration: Gross swelling of keratinocytes seen in epidermal viral infection, such as herpes simplex. Both the nucleus and cytoplasm are affected.

Basement membrane: A multi-layered structure between epidermis and dermis.

Bowen's carcinoma *in situ* (Bowen's disease): A form of intra-epidermal carcinoma *in situ* characterized by the presence of atypical giant cells with grossly abnormal mitotic figures.

Cheiropompholyx: An intensely itchy eruption of the sides of the fingers and palms of the hands composed of multiple small blisters.

Civatte bodies (colloid bodies): Amorphous pink globules seen at the dermo-epidermal junction in certain diseases characterized by damage to and death of basal cells (for example, lichen planus).

Comedo (blackhead): A plug of oxidized sebaceous material obstructing the surface opening of pilosebaceous follicle. Seen mainly in acne vulgaris.

Connexins: The major proteins of gap junctions that are intercellular channels allowing passage of low molecular weight material between cells.

Desmosomes: Specialized areas of intra-epidermal adhesion between keratinocytes.

Dyskeratosis: Premature and atypical keratinization of epidermal keratinocytes.

Ecthyma: A pyogenic skin infection characterized by superficial crusting and underlying ulceration.

Ephelis (freckle): A localized area of increased pigment synthesis by melanocytes.

Gap junctions: Intercellular channels that permit passage of low molecular weight material between cells. Important in the keratinocytes of the epidermis for maintaining homeostasis.

Hirsuties: Excessive growth of male-pattern hair.

Hyperkeratosis: Excessive formation of normal keratin for the body site in question.

Hypertrichosis: Excessive growth of non-androgen dependent hair.

Ichthyosis ('fish skin'): Excessively dry and scaly skin.

Inclusion bodies: Eosinophilic bodies with a clear surrounding halo. Seen in cutaneous viral infections.

Intertrigo: Dermatitis on apposing areas of skin in flexural body sites (groins, axillae).

Kerion: A severe pustular reaction on the scalp in children. Caused by animal ringworm.

Koebner or isomorphic phenomenon: The tendency for certain skin diseases, e.g. psoriasis to develop on sites of trauma.

Lichenification: Thickening (acanthosis) of the epidermis resulting in accentuation of normal skin markings.

Liquefaction degeneration: Damage to the epidermal basal layer, seen principally in lichen planus and lupus erythematosus.

Miliaria: Vesicular lesions resulting from occlusion of eccrine sweat ducts. Common in hot, humid environments.

Nikolsky's sign: The shearing of epidermis from dermis produced by lateral pressure on the epidermal surface. Positive in pemphigus vulgaris.

Parakeratosis: Abnormal or incomplete keratinization resulting in the presence of nucleated, flattened squamous cells in the stratum corneum.

Reticular degeneration (*see also* balloon degeneration): An intra-epidermal blister resulting from balloon degenerations of virally-infected epidermal cells. Some cell walls are retained and the blister thus has a multi-loculated reticular framework.

Rhinophyma: Gross hypertrophy of sebaceous gland tissue resulting in increase in volume of nasal soft tissue. A complication of rosacea.

Spongiosis: Oedema of the epidermis, mainly intracellular.

Wickham's striae: White linear markings on the surface of the violaceous papules of lichen planus.

Projects that could be used in a special study module

1. Ask the centre in which you are working (hospital, health centre, general practice, or other setting) for the disease index relating to dermatological referrals and attendances, both first attendance and return visits, over the last 6–12 months.

   Do you think that the conditions that have been diagnosed in the setting in which you are currently working reflect either the prevalence or the incidence of these conditions in the community? If not, why not? Do you think the numbers of patients seen and their diagnoses relates to severity of the disease, desire to improve employment prospects, or desire to improve cosmetic appearance? What other reasons might prompt patients to seek treatment for a chronic skin condition?

2. You are part of a public health forward planning team, predicting dermatological demand in a UK setting in the year 2005. What conditions would you predict will have become less of a burden on the health care system and which will have become a larger burden. Divide your response by age cohorts in the population, and consider the future health care needs to be met both in primary care and in a hospital setting. Include possible future needs for in-patient care, out-patient assessment, day care treatments including surgery, and care in the community from medical nursing and other relevant professions.

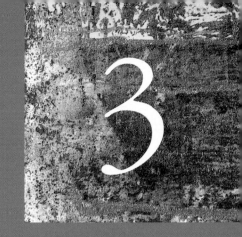

3

Essential skin biology: structure, function, and immunology

- Anatomy of the normal skin
- The epidermis
- The dermis
- The skin appendages
- Special study module project

Essential skin biology: structure, function, and immunology

The skin is a large and complex structure. An understanding of basic structure and function should help make your approach to skin disease more logical and increase your interest in the skin as a major organ of the body with a wide range of physiological functions.

Anatomy of the normal skin

The skin can be divided into three main functional areas. These are the:

- **epidermis**: the major protective layer derived from the foetal ectoderm.
- **dermis**: the major support layer of mesodermal origin.
- **skin appendages**: composed of cells derived from both ectoderm and mesoderm
  - hair follicle;
  - sebaceous gland;
  - apocrine sweat gland;
  - eccrine sweat gland;
  - nails.

In addition a fourth area, the subcutaneous **fat**, may be involved in deeply situated skin lesions such as erythema nodosum (p. 213).

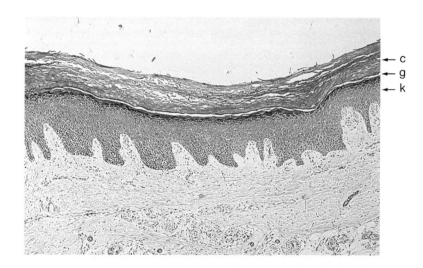

Fig. 3.1 Skin from palm of hand. The cornified layer (c), the granular layer (g), and the keratinocytes in the germinative layer (k) are all easily seen.

Key points

The epidermis consists of four layers—the cornified layer (an outer, non-nucleated barrier), granular (nuclei disintegrating), germinative or prickle cell (bulk of living keratinocytes), and basal layer (normally the only site of epidermal mitosis).

The epidermis

Beginning at the outer surface and working inwards, four distinct layers of epidermis can be observed using the light microscope (Fig. 3.1). These are the:

- **cornified or horny layer:** outer non-nucleated barrier layer;
- **granular layer:** the zone where epidermal nuclei disintegrate;
- **spinous or prickle cell layer:** the bulk of the living epidermal keratinocytes;
- **basal layer:** the only keratinocytes in **normal** epidermis, which undergo cell division.

These layers are best seen if a piece of thick, weight-bearing skin from the sole of the foot, is examined under the microscope. In this thick skin, a fifth layer can sometimes be seen just above the granular layer—the **stratum lucidum**. It is not certain whether or not this is really a functionally distinct layer or an artefact of preparation.

It is useful to become familiar with the appearance of normal skin by using the microscope to examine areas at the normal margins of excision biopsies to build up experience of the normal physiological variations in appearance of healthy skin in different body sites at different ages. For example, non-weight-bearing skin, such as that on the inner upper arm, has a thin cornified layer, and only three or four underlying layers of keratinocytes, whereas the keratinocyte layer of the sole of the foot is 20–30 cells thick.

On chronically sun-exposed sites, chiefly the face, both the epidermis and the underlying dermis may show very marked changes due to accumulated exposure to natural sunlight. This is photo-ageing and is seen clinically as thickened, wrinkled, furrowed yellowish skin. Many of the alterations in the skin that we think of as ageing are, in fact, due to ultraviolet induced damage, and distinction should be made between **photo-ageing**, which is at least partially preventable, and chronological or **biological** ageing. Figures 3.2 and 3.3 show the exposed facial skin and non-exposed trunk skin of the same 84-year-old to emphasize this point. You could also illustrate the difference between chronological ageing and photo-ageing by examining the facial skin of identical twins who had been separated at birth, one being brought up in a temperate climate, such as the UK, and one in a sunny country, such as Australia. The skin of the sun-exposed twin will look older from the age of about 20 onwards.

Cell types seen in the epidermis

These are the:

- **keratinocyte:** the main cell type;
- **melanocyte:** found in the basal layer, the pigment-producing cell;
- **Langerhans cell:** found in the mid-dermis—an important immunologically competent cell;
- **Merkel cell:** found in and around the basal layer. A member of the amine precursor uptake and decarboxylation (APUD) system.

Key points

The epidermis is an immunologically active organ.

The keratinocyte

The keratinocytes are about 95% of the cells in the epidermis. In normal skin, keratinocyte division takes place only in the basal layer, so mitotic figures should not

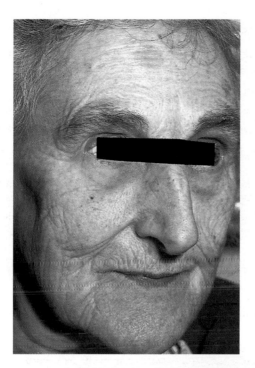

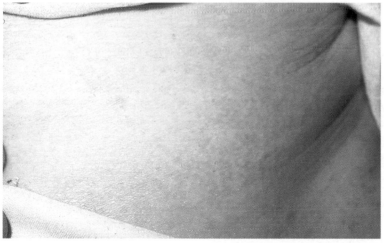

Figs 3.2 and 3.3 Skin of the face and trunk on an 84-year-old female who has lived all her life in Scotland. The wrinkling and pigment variation of the chronically exposed facial skin are not seen on the normally covered skin. The contrast would be much greater had she lived in a sunnier climate such as Australia.

normally be seen above this level. After cell division, one daughter keratinocyte remains in the basal layer and the other moves upwards through the epidermis. About 10% of the basal cells are long-lived stem cells with the major responsibility for repopulating the upper layers of the epidermis. The keratinocyte which leaves the basal layer is committed to terminal differentiation and death.

Within the spinous cell layer, the keratinocytes are connected to each other by highly specialized cellular bridges, called **desmosomes**, and these can frequently be seen under the light microscope at high power. They may be particularly easy

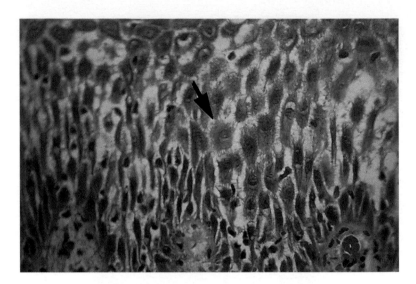

Fig. 3.4 Skin biopsy from a patient with contact dermatitis in the early acute state. There is a lot of oedema in the epidermis and this shows the desmosomes stretched between adjacent keratinocytes (arrow). In some cases the desmosomes have become ruptured.

to see in a biopsy from early dermatitis, where there is a lot of epidermal oedema (Fig. 3.4). There are no desmosomes between keratinocytes and melanocytes, or Langerhans cells, or Merkel cells. There are **hemidesmosomes** between the basal layer keratinocytes and the underlying basement membrane. Hemidesmosomes are responsible for connecting the basal cells to the basement membrane area. **Laminin** 5 is an important component of hemidesmosomes, and mutations in laminin 5 are associated with a rare, but serious congenital blistering disease, junctional epidermolysis bullosa.

At the ultrastructural level there are also intercellular channels between keratinocytes called **gap junctions**. These channels, which are made up of proteins called **connexins**, are important in maintaining epidermal homeostasis and in allowing low molecular weight material to move between cells. There are several human connexin molecules, and connexins 26, 31, and 43 appear to be particularly well represented in the epidermis. Connexin gene mutations have been identified that are associated with skin diseases, for example, connexin 26 mutations that are found in palmoplantar keratoderma and deafness.

In the **granular layer** (Fig. 3.5) the living keratinocytes are involved in a complex series of biochemical changes during which the cell nuclei disintegrate, forming the granules seen in the cytoplasm. Above this level there is the non-nucleated stratum corneum or cornified layer. The normal transit time of a differentiating keratinocyte from basal layer to the outer surface of the stratum corneum is around 28 days. In inflammation or conditions in which keratinization is abnormal, such as psoriasis, this may be very much shorter.

Development and maturation of normal healthy epidermis in this pattern is called **orthokeratosis** and produces an outer layer of non-nucleated, dead, flat keratinocytes. In some mucosal sites the normal maturation pattern is different and there is no granular layer, but an outer layer of nucleated squamous cells. The term for this pattern is **physiological parakeratosis** (Fig. 3.6).

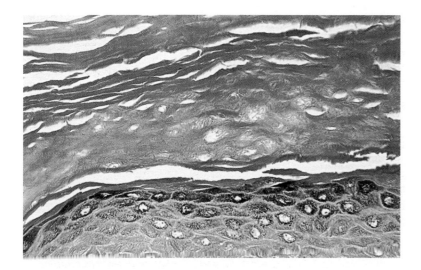

Fig. 3.5 High-power view of granular layer, showing sharp transition from the living, but non-dividing epidermal cells and the dead anucleate cornified layer.

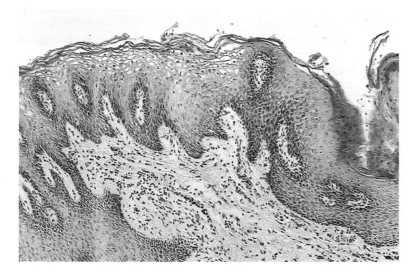

Fig. 3.6 Mucous membrane showing normal physiological parakeratosis seen in this site. Nuclei are present in the upper layers and, thus, there is no granular layer.

Pathological parakeratosis is seen in some diseases of the epidermis, psoriasis being the most common example. In this situation, the normal differentiation signals are either lacking or overridden, and there is accelerated and imperfect development of the stratum corneum. If keratinocytes are grown in tissue culture, they will come together and form interconnecting desmosomes, but the outer layer is parakeratotic as in psoriasis, rather than orthokeratototic as in normal skin.

The strength of the epidermis depends on the cohesion of the keratinocytes. They produce a structural protein, alpha-keratin, which aggregates to form tonofilaments. These tonofilaments are continuous with the desmosomes and are easily seen in the electron microscope as large cytoplasmic bundles. Another communication channel between keratinocytes are gap junctions, tiny channels that connect the cytoplasm of neighbouring cells to each other.

Genetic abnormalities of keratinization and resulting disease states

Keratins are synthesized by the keratinocytes in pairs, one basic and one acidic keratin. Genes for basic keratins have been mapped to chromosome 12 q11–q13 and those for acidic keratins to chromosome 17 q12–q13.

The basal layer of the epidermis expresses keratins 5 and 14, and genetic disturbances in the genes coding for these keratins causes the disease epidermolysis bullosa simplex (p. 280) in which the basal cells separate from each other and disintegrate, while the suprabasal keratinocytes synthesize keratins 1 and 10, and abnormalities give rise to bullous ichthyosiform erythroderma or epidermolytic hyperkeratosis. A number of other rare scaling skin disorders have been identified as being due to a genetic abnormality of other keratins, including those involved in the hair and nails.

Integrins

The integrin family are another group of important cell surface proteins associated with adhesion. LFA is a member of this family, and different integrins are characterized by expression of a wide range of alpha and beta chains. Alpha-6-beta-4-integrin appears to be particularly important in adhesion of the basal cells to the basement membrane. It is important in diseases characterized by blisters at this level, such as bullous pemphigoid (p. 273).

Cadherins

The cadherin family of adhesion molecules play a major part in adhesion of suprabasal keratinocytes to each other in association with the desmosomes. Desmoglein is a member of this family and faulty adhesion between keratinocytes due to abnormalities of these molecules is associated with the pemphigus group of blistering disorders (p. 270).

Cells expressing MHC class 2 antigens

In the normal epidermis, the only cells that normally express the MHC class 2 antigens HLA-DR, -DP, and -DQ are the Langerhans cells (see below). In a wide range of skin diseases, MHC class 2 molecule expression is induced on keratinocytes. HLA-DR, HLA-DP, and HLA-DQ expression are all markers of immunologically activated and competent cells, indicating that, in some circumstances, the keratinocytes can actively contribute to immunological reactions, not just respond as innocent bystanders.

The melanocyte

The melanocyte is the epidermal cell responsible for producing pigment in the skin. Melanocytes can be seen with H&E staining as small cells mainly in the basal layer, often with a clear halo around them, because of the absence of desmosomes to link them to adjacent basal keratinocytes. In Fig. 3.7 a silver stain has been used to show that melanocytes have dendritic processes, which stretch between adjacent keratinocytes, bringing melanocytes into surface contact with a relatively large number of keratinocytes. This cluster of keratinocytes, which all receive pigment from one melanocyte, is referred to as the **epidermal melanin unit**. On facial skin, there may be as many as one melanocyte for every five basal layer keratinocytes, but in the lower back skin this ratio is usually closer to one in 20.

Key points

Melanin is synthesized by melanocytes and moved to surrounding keratinocytes, and thus these cell types should be distinguished biochemically, not by presence of the pigment.

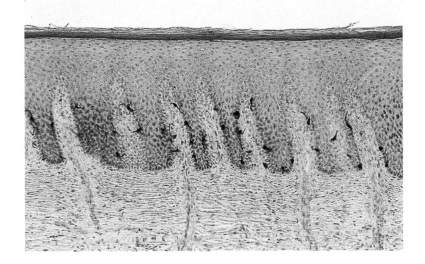

Fig. 3.7 Melanocytes in the epidermis stained with silver. Note the dendritic shape of the cells.

Chronic light exposure increases the number of melanocytes relative to keratinocytes, so that there are more, for example, in the skin of the outer upper arm than in the skin of the inner upper arm. Numbers of melanocytes are the same in equivalent body sites in white and black skin, but the rate of production of melanin pigment and its distribution is different. Darker skinned races have more active melanocytes and distribute melanin pigment to surrounding keratinocytes in smaller packages than is the case in paler skinned individuals.

Melanocytes synthesize the pigment melanin. Melanin granules are seen on ultrastructural examination as small, black, electron-dense, intracytoplasmic structures—the melanosomes. The pigment is formed from DOPA on pre-melanosomes, and this biochemical reaction is catalysed by the presence in the melanocyte of the enzymes dopa-oxidase and tyrosinase, which are not present in surrounding keratinocytes or other non-melanocytic cells.

Once the melanin granules are formed, they are distributed along the dendrites of the melanocytes and from there to adjacent keratinocytes. Melanocytes are found in man in greatest quantities in the epidermis, the hair bulb, the eye, the brain, and in very small numbers in other organs. Their function in normal skin is thought to be to provide protection from ultraviolet radiation. This appears to be reasonably effective in that sunlight-induced skin cancers of all types are much rarer on black skin than on white, although it could be argued that, in evolutionary terms, the melanocyte should be situated in the superficial, rather than the deeper part of the epidermis. This would offer greater protection to epidermal keratinocytes.

The Langerhans cell

This cell was discovered in 1860 by Paul Langerhans when he was a medical student and, until the 1970s, it had no clearly defined function. In the last 30 years there has been a dramatic advance in our knowledge of this cell, which is now recognized as an important immunologically competent cell. The Langerhans cell is derived from the bone marrow and is found on all epidermal surfaces, usually situated in the middle of the spinous layer of the epidermis. On H&E stained sections, the Langerhans cell

Key points

Langerhans cells are immunologically competent and may act as antigen presenting cells.

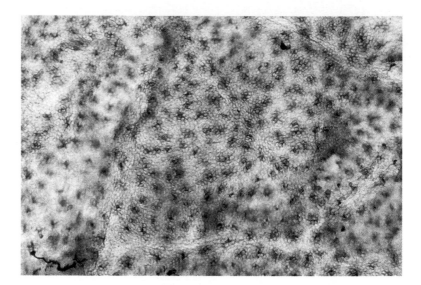

Fig. 3.8 Horizontal 'spread preparation' of the epidermis stained with an antibody specific for Langerhans cells. Note how the cells come into contact with each other by their dendritic processes and form a network.

may be seen as a slightly larger cell than those around it, with a clear halo, due to the lack of desmosomes. To see the Langerhans cell clearly, immunocytochemistry is necessary using one of the antibodies that recognizes Langerhans cells on formalin-fixed, paraffin-processed material, for example, antibody to S100 protein . With this approach it will be seen that the Langerhans cell is a dendritic cell and that, in most body sites, it is present in the epidermis in relatively large numbers, with the dendrites of one Langerhans cell in close contact with those of the next, forming a network-like structure This is best seen if the epidermis is cut parallel to the skin surface, not in the usual vertical approach (Fig. 3.8). Langerhans cells are recognized under the electron microscope by the presence of highly specific intracytoplasmic structures, the Birbeck granules. These look rather like tennis or squash racquets (Fig. 3.9) and their function is not yet understood.

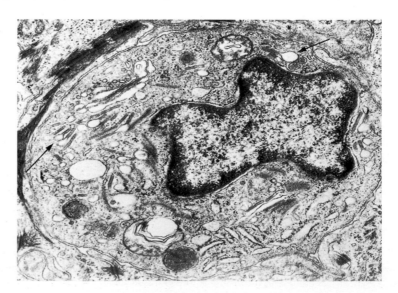

Fig. 3.9 Ultrastructure of Langerhans cell, showing the characteristic and specific tennis racquet-shaped Birbeck granule in the cytoplasm. (Arrow)

Langerhans cells in normal skin are the only cells to express MHC class 2 antigens and carry receptors for complement. They are currently believed to be members of the family of immunologically important dendritic cells found in a number of body sites including the lymph nodes and spleen. The immunological profile of these dendritic cells suggests that they have the capacity to act as antigen presenting cells. Antigen adheres very readily to their surface, but in contrast to classical macrophages, Langerhans cells do not phagocytose efficiently. In the epidermis, which obviously comes into contact with more foreign material than any other part of the body, this antigen-presenting function may be of very great importance in, for example, allergic contact dermatitis (see p. 118).

Abnormal Langerhans cell proliferation is seen in histiocytosis X, a rare condition on the borderline between proliferation and malignancy (p. 351).

The Merkel cell

These cells require immunocytochemistry or electron microscopy to be identified. Their cytoplasm is packed with electron dense granules, and the cells are found in large numbers in touch sensitive sites such as the fingertips and around the lips. They appear to be concentrated around the basement membrane area and in association with nerve endings. Their granules contain large quantities of catecholamines and because of this they are thought to be part of the APUD (amine precursor uptake and decarboxylation) system. Their exact normal function is not known, but it is thought to be related to cutaneous sensation.

A rare, but aggressive tumour, the Merkel cell tumour, may arise from these cells, usually in sun-damaged skin (p. 351).

The skin immune system

The skin is an immunologically competent organ. The individual components of this system can be called the skin immune system (SIS) or skin associated lymphoid system (SALT). As the cells involved are more than just lymphocytes, SIS is more accurate. The SIS includes Langerhans cells, which can be considered modified macrophages and are a part of the reticuloepithelial dendritic cell system, which is also found in organs such as the spleen and the lymph nodes. Lymphocytes may be seen trafficking through the epidermis and are most commonly T-lymphocytes, both of the TH1 and the TH2 subsets. In diseases such as graft-versus-host disease these lymphocytes may be seen in close apposition to necrotic keratinocytes, which appears to be undergoing a type of programmed cell death described as apoptosis, or satellite cell necrosis.

Keratinocytes are also part of the cutaneous immune system in that they express MHC class 2 antigens when activated, and both secrete and respond to immunologically active cytokines. Tumour necrosis factor alpha (TNF-alpha) is of particular current interest in view of the response of psoriasis and disease associated with major abnormalities of keratinocyte maturation to TNF-alpha inhibitors.

Key points

The effect of TNF-alpha inhibitors in psoriasis tells us that this cytokine may be deregulated in psoriasis

Growth factors

A number of these are found in the epidermis and dermis in both healthy and diseased skin. Epidermal growth factor has a structure very similar to transforming growth factor alpha and is synthesized by epidermal keratinocytes. Expression of TGF alpha is abnormal in psoriasis and is also associated with apparent over-activity of dermal fibroblasts in dermal hyperproliferative conditions, such as keloid scarring and scleroderma.

Fibroblast growth factor is a very important growth factor for normal melanocytes in culture and appears to be released in intact human skin after exposure to ultraviolet light. The significance of this, in relation to ultraviolet light exposure and subsequent risk of skin cancer, is not yet established.

Interleukins

The family of interleukins is steadily increasing, and their relevance to the epidermis in normal and diseased states is complex. However, interleukin 1 is elevated in the epidermis during sunburn, and IL10 is over-expressed in non-melanoma skin cancer and atopic dermatitis. IL 10 has been used in trials as a treatment for psoriasis with some encouraging results.

Interferons

The interferon family comprise alpha, beta, and gamma interferons. Abnormal amounts of gamma interferon are seen in allergic contact dermatitis, and are secreted from lymphocytes trafficking through the epidermis and possibly also by activated keratinocytes. Gamma interferon has been used as a treatment in trials of atopic dermatitis with variable results.

The basement membrane

The basement membrane divides the epidermis from the dermis, and is shown diagrammatically in Fig. 3.10 and ultrastructurally in Fig. 3.11. This shows that the basement membrane zone is a complex multi-layered structure and, as different diseases result from abnormalities of each of these layers, some understanding of this area is of practical, as well as academic interest. Hemidesmosomes attach the basal layer keratinocytes to the lamina lucida area and contain laminin 5.

Mutations of laminin 5 are seen in some variants of the genetically determined blistering disease epidermolysis bullosa, (p. 279).

Autoantibodies to components of the lamina lucida are found in the acquired autoimmune blistering disease, bullous pemphigoid (p. 273).

Below the basement membrane zone is the subbasal dense plate through which anchoring filaments connect the lamina lucida to the lamina densa. This is an area

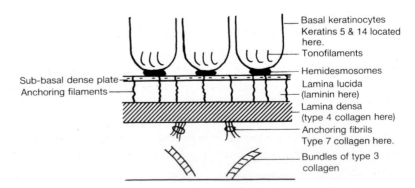

Fig. 3.10 Diagram of basement membrane zone to show its multi-layered structure.

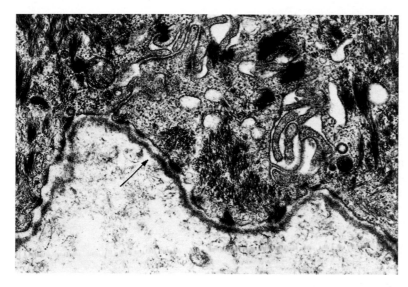

Fig. 3.11 Ultrastructure of basement membrane zone. Compare this with Fig. 3.10.

that is rich in type 4 collagen. Collagen type 7 is also found in this area, but situated a little deeper and is deficient in the dystrophic type of epidermolysis bullosa. (p. 281)

In spite of the multiple layers of which the basement membrane is composed, it is not a rigid impervious structure, but one through which cells such as lymphocytes and Langerhans cells can, and do, pass with relative ease.

Also, the basement membrane is not a flat layer dividing epidermis above from dermis below like the filling in a sandwich, but is heavily convoluted, with most convolution being seen in areas of weight-bearing skin, obviously the soles of the feet. Here, the dermal papillae, the superficial layer of the dermis, sticks up into the dermis like small pegs. These dermal papillae are also present, but less obvious, in thinner skinned sites; this is an arrangement that maximizes the surface area of contact between dermis and epidermis, and minimizes the chance of discohesion due to loss of contact between the two layers.

The dermis

The outer layer of the dermis is called the papillary dermis and contains finer collagen fibres than the deeper reticular dermis. This is easily seen if polarized light is used to examine sections of normal skin in the light microscope.

There are three main cell types in the dermis:

- the **fibroblast** produces collagen;
- the **macrophage** acts as a general scavenger;
- the **mast cell**, an important cell in type 1 immunological reactions and in interactions with the eosinophil; may have additional functions, e.g. in dermal sclerosis.

The bulk of the dermis is composed of type 3 collagen and running through this collagen there is a fine network of elastic fibres. Dermal proteoglycans surround this fibrous material and embedded within the dermis are the:

- **vasculature;**

- **lymphatics**;
- **nerves**;
- small quantities of **smooth and striated muscle**.

The blood supply

The blood supply to the dermis is through a very rich anastomosing superficial and deep plexus of small blood vessels. There is a very large reserve capacity in the dermal vasculature, which is normally only operating at 10–20% of potential capacity. After vigorous physical exercise, heat loss through the skin may be required, and the vasculature dilates to allow for this. In a number of skin diseases the blood supply to the skin is greatly increased, causing total body redness or erythroderma. The volume of blood flowing through the dilated dermal vessels in this situation can be so great that high output cardiac failure can be induced.

Figure 3.12 shows the profuse network of small vessels in the papillary dermis and the scattered larger, deeper vessels, with a network of vessels around skin appendages.

In normal skin the lymphatic drainage system is not visible, but this is also a profuse network, running from the reticular dermis to the local lymph nodes. It is often visible if dermis from lower leg of an individual over the age of 50 is examined, due to the cumulative affects of gravity over the years.

Cutaneous nerves

Both free nerve endings and specialized nerve receptors will be seen in the dermis. These nerve endings are important for the sense of touch, heat, cold, and proprioception. Nerve endings are best seen on light microscopy with a silver stain and

> **Key points**
>
> All the blood supply to the epidermis is obtained from the papillary layer of the dermis.

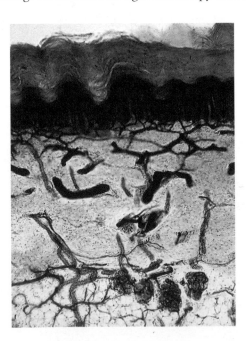

Fig. 3.12 Injected post-mortem specimen showing the abundance of the dermal vasculature.

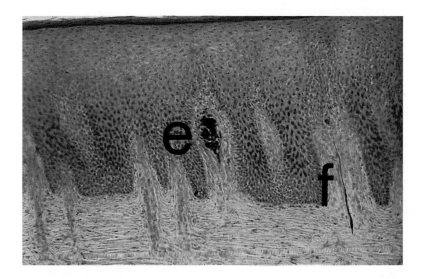

Fig. 3.13 Nerve endings demonstrated by a silver stain. Note the free nerve ending (f) and the encapsulated ending (e).

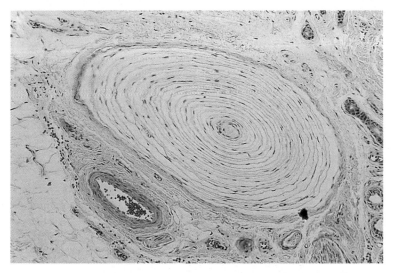

Fig. 3.14 Another type of nerve ending, the Pacinian corpuscle. This is responsible for the sensation of deep pressure.

are numerous in the papillary dermis (Fig. 3.13). Specialized receptors such as the Pacinian and Meissner corpuscles are also present (Fig. 3.14).

The skin appendages

These are the pilosebaceous unit, the eccrine sweat glands, and the nails. The pilosebaceous unit includes the:

- hair follicle;
- sebaceous gland;
- arrector pili muscle;

and in some sites, for example, axilla, the

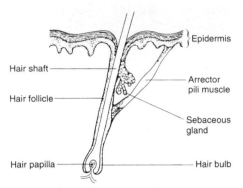

Fig. 3.15 Diagram of the pilosebaceous unit.

- **apocrine gland**.

The pilosebaceous unit is shown diagrammatically in Fig. 3.15 and histologically in Fig. 3.16. On the scalp, the predominant structure is the hair follicle with the sebaceous gland seen as a small insignificant attachment. A small strip of smooth muscle, the arrector pili muscle, may be seen, often around a lobule of sebaceous gland, and in the axilla the apocrine glands may also be seen draining into the duct leading to the surface.

The **hair follicle** is the result of interaction between down growth of foetal ectoderm, which will form the hair shaft, and the vascular hair bulb papilla, which is derived from foetal mesoderm (Fig. 3.17).

The hair shaft itself is a complex multi-layered structure with an outer cortex and an inner medulla. There are three recognizable types of hair. These are the coarse terminal hair of the scalp, the androgen-dependent terminal hair on the male chin, in the axilla, and the pubic region, and a fine growth of downy vellous hair on all body sites.

The control of growth of scalp hair is poorly understood. At any one time 80% of scalp hair is growing in **anagen**, and the remaining 20% is either resting—in

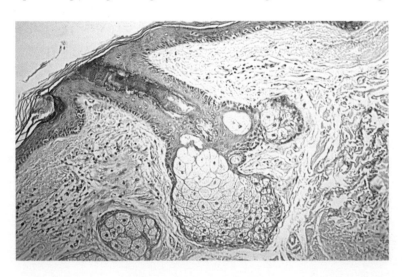

Fig. 3.16 The pilosebaceous unit, showing the sebaceous gland draining into the hair follicle canal.

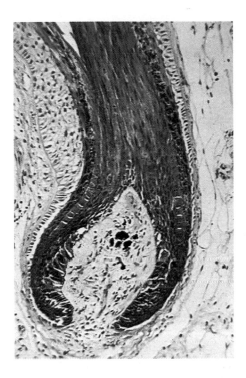

Fig. 3.17 High-power view of hair root, showing the root of the hair derived from the epidermis stretched around the dermal papilla.

catagen—or being shed—in **telogen** (Fig. 3.18). Normally, this programmed replacement of hair is scattered randomly over the scalp so that no single area is totally depleted at one time, but in **alopecia areata** (p. 254) all the hair in one scalp area is shed simultaneously.

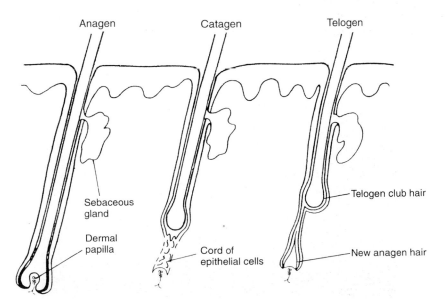

Fig. 3.18 Growth cycle of scalp hair.

The **sebaceous glands** are clusters of cells with a small dark nucleus and a foamy cytoplasm, which are well illustrated in Fig. 3.16. They cluster around the hair shafts and their secretion is formed by total destruction of the cells, a mechanism called holocrine secretion. This secretion drains into the hair follicle and is discharged on the surface through the hair follicle opening. Sebaceous glands are seen in large numbers on the face, chest, and upper back. They may be obvious as small raised pearly nodules on the face of neonates, when their enlargement is due to carry-over of maternal hormones. They rapidly shrink and become vestigial until puberty when, in response to the individual's own hormones, they become large and active—sometimes over active. This is present in acne vulgaris (p. 243).

The **apocrine sweat glands** are found predominantly in the axilla, with a few seen also in the skin of the groin. They have a secretory component seen in the deeper dermis. This secretory section has a very wide lumen, and the cells lining this lumen will be seen to be composed of columnar epithelium, which appears to form glandular secretion, by a 'nipping off' of the tops of the cells, a process known as **decapitation secretion** (Figs 3.19 and 3.20). The excretory channels of the apocrine glands most commonly drain into the canal of the hair shaft and sebum passes from here out on to the surface of the epidermis.

The **eccrine sweat glands** are seen on all body sites and are anatomically independent from the other appendages. Their secretory components are much smaller than those of the apocrine gland, with a smaller lumen (Fig. 3.21). The excretory duct of these glands winds upwards in a spiral pattern through the dermis and the epidermis to the surface.

The **nails** are very highly modified skin appendages. The nail itself or nail plate grows out from the nail matrix and rests on the underlying nail bed. The pale halo at the proximal end of the nail is called the lunula and around the edge of this there is a protective rim of cuticle (Fig. 3.22). Nails may become involved in a number of skin diseases, such as psoriasis and fungal infection. The average time for a fingernail to grow out completely from base to outer edge is approximately

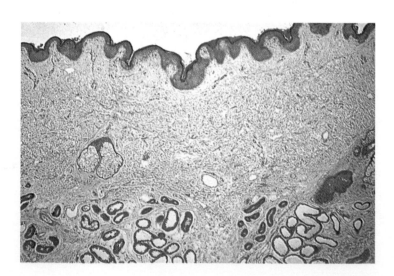

Fig. 3.19 Axillary skin showing large numbers of apocrine glands in the lower third of the section. Apocrine glands are rare in other body sites.

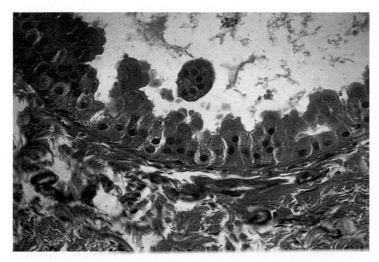

Fig. 3.20 High-power view of secretory cells in apocrine glands showing decapitation pattern of secretion.

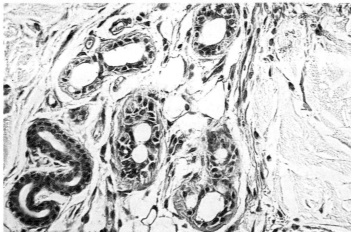

Fig. 3.21 Eccrine sweat glands—these will be seen in the deeper dermis in skin from all body sites.

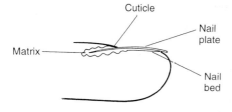

Cuticle

Nail plate

Matrix

Nail bed

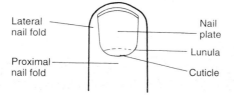

Lateral nail fold

Nail plate

Lunula

Proximal nail fold

Cuticle

Fig. 3.22 Diagram of the nail and associated structures.

6 months, and for toenails the time is 6–18 months or even longer. Thus, therapy of diseased nails requires both time and patience.

Special study module project

Carry out a literature search on the keratin family. Identify keratins that are associated with the epidermis, hair, and nails.

Now carry out a further search to identify those keratins in which mutations have been detected associated with human disease. Try to see some patients with these disease in the clinic.

How much have our advances in understanding the molecular genetics of these diseases benefited patients who currently have these disease and how much might it benefit potential future patients?

Further reading

Berker, D., Baran, R., and Dawber, R. (2001). *Disease of the nails and their management. 3rd edition.* Blackwell Scientific Publications, Oxford.

Freinkel, R.K. and Woodley, D.T. (eds) (2001) *The biology of the skin.* Parthenon Press, New York.

Sinclair, R.D., Banfield, C.C., and Dawber, R. (1999) *A handbook of diseases of the hair and scalp.* Blackwell Science, Oxford.

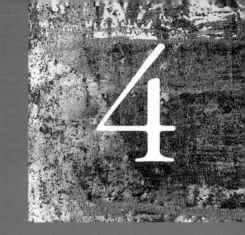

4

The dermatological history, examination, and investigations frequently used in dermatology

- History-taking

- Examination

- Investigations commonly used in dermatology

- Special study module

The dermatological history, examination, and investigations frequently used in dermatology

History-taking

Most patients with skin disease are first seen and treatment prescribed in a primary care setting or in a hospital out-patient department. A very small number require in-patient care and nowadays, in many parts of the world, this may not be in dedicated dermatology beds. It is therefore even more important than in other specialties to ask the patient all the possibly important questions in an orderly and logical framework in the primary care setting or in the out-patient clinic.

A general outline of useful points to remember in dermatological history-taking include:

1. **How long have any skin lesions been present?** Patients will often only tell you how long they have had the lesions that are currently worrying them and will not begin at the beginning of their problem.
2. **Where did the problem first appear?** It is normal to be much more concerned about socially visible skin disease than about that on normally covered sites. Therefore, patients will often ask you for help only with the patch of psoriasis on their scalp and will not, unless prompted, tell you about the large plaque on their back. Table 4.1 lists certain common dermatological problems and the likely sites of involvement.
3. **Are there any symptoms?** These are usually itch and/or pain.
   Severe itch is associated with:
   • scabies;
   • atopic eczema;

Key points

History taking should include: where and when the problem started; symptoms (severe itch, mild itch, pain); medicaments, general medical history; occupation and recreation; travel; family and household contacts; and the patient's own views of the likely cause.

Table 4.1 Frequent associations between some commoner skin diseases and body sites

Scalp	Psoriasis, seborrhoeic dermatitis, and fungal infections
Face	Atopic dermatitis, acne, rosacea, seborrhoeic dermatitis, lupus erythematosus, and other photosensitive problems
Body flexures	Seborrhoeic dermatitis, psoriasis, fungal infection, and candida infection
Feet	Toe webs—fungal infection
	Soles—juvenile plantar dermatosis
	Dorsa—contact dermatitis

- contact dermatitis;
- dermatitis herpetiformis.

Mild itch is associated with many skin conditions including:

- psoriasis
- drug eruptions
- bullous pemphigoid.

Pain is a symptom of:

- vasculitis;
- pemphigus.

4. **Topical and oral medicament history**. Ask the patient carefully about these. To many elderly patients, 'medicines' are not drugs and the question 'What drugs are you on?' does not always result in an accurate response. Begin by asking about any topical or systemic medication supplied on prescription, then move on to preparations bought over the counter in the chemist or health food shop. An increasing number of patients are using alternative therapy in the form of herbal and homeopathic preparations, and may be reluctant to reveal this in a 'conventional medicine' setting without some coaxing.

Ask specifically about sleeping pills, tablets for headaches or other aches and pains, and laxatives. Ask also about topical preparations, and even systemic medication prescribed for a relative or friend, but used by your patient—such behaviour is commoner than you might imagine.

In general hospitals, the commonest reason for a request for a dermatologist to see a patient in another ward is because of a suspected adverse drug reaction. Be very sure you have access to a full list of everything the patient has received in the past 2–3 weeks, not just the treatment being used on the day you see the patient.

5. **General medical history**. Remember that there are many skin signs that may be the first marker of serious systemic disease (see Chapter 14). Ask about general medical problems such as breathlessness, weight loss, bowel disturbance. Diabetes, Crohn's disease, and sarcoidosis can all be first recognized by their dermatological signs, provided you know what to look for.

6. **Occupational and recreational history**. Ask about the patient's environment. This may be particularly important in contact dermatitis. If the patient is working, an occupational history with brief details of materials handled in a normal working day is useful. For all patients, information about hobbies, recreation, sporting activities, and contact with animals may give a clue to the problem. Table 4.2 gives a brief list of possible problems.

Ask also about reaction to sunlight exposure. A number of skin disorders, such as lupus erythematosus, are initiated or aggravated by sunlight, and a long list of drugs given orally may give rise to photosensitivity (p. 320).

7. **Travel**. Ask about holidays, professional travel, and in the case of those born in other countries, about visits to or from relatives in their native country. Ask about details of recent air travel, including refuelling stops. Nowadays, many people, including medical students, travel long distances on holiday or to do

Table 4.2 Possible dermatological occupational and recreational problems

Nursing and hairdressing	Irritant hand dermatitis
Home decorating and repairs	Allergic contact dermatitis from epoxy resin glues
Violinist	Fiddler's neck—acne-like lesions
Sheep farming	Orf from infected animals
Photographic developing	Lichenoid dermatitis from colour developer
Jogging	Talon noir—small haemorrhages into the thick skin of the heels from ill-fitting shoes

elective periods of study. A history of a refuelling stop in the Middle East 6 weeks ago may help to explain a crusted sore on the wrist as a localized form of leishmaniasis (p. 161).

8. **Family and household contact history.** Many patients with skin disease are confused over infection and genetic transmission. Ask about first-degree relatives, as this can be a clue in conditions such as ichthyoses, and also ask about household contacts, as these are not always family members. Infections such as scabies may infect both relatives and others with whom the patient is in close contact. This can be a problem in, for example, a residential home for the elderly.

9. **The patient's thoughts on the cause of the problem.** Ask the patient what he or she thinks is wrong and what has caused it. The answer to this question may give you a clue to the diagnosis, and perhaps even more important, may also reveal unexpected theories and worries. Patients may tell you that they believe diet is the cause, and may have tried out unusual and sometimes very restricted diets for themselves or their children. Give the patient time to tell you about this towards the end of the history-taking, when he/she is relatively relaxed and you have gained his/her confidence.

These questions should be asked personally in a quiet and unhurried atmosphere, where the conversation cannot be overheard by other patients. A 'tick off' questionnaire to fill in while sitting in the waiting room is no substitute for a face-to-face discussion that will, for many patients, be the beginning of therapy.

Remember that almost all patients are embarrassed by skin disease and many are ashamed of their appearance. Treat them with understanding and sympathy, and they will remember their visits to you with gratitude, even if you cannot yet provide a cure.

Examination

In very few situations—for example, hand warts in children—it might just be acceptable to examine only the affected area of the body, but it is a very much better practice to ask all patients attending for the first time to put on a gown and to carry out a total skin examination. If this is done, both related and quite unrelated, but potentially serious problems will not be missed, and early curable skin cancers may be identified on body sites that are difficult to inspect personally, such as the back.

Key points

A total skin examination should be carried out to determine the full extent of the problem and possible unrelated conditions.

Examine the skin in a good light—daylight if possible—and look carefully at the pattern of involvement of the skin. Many skin diseases have a 'typical' or 'classic' distribution (Fig. 4.1). Drawing a sketch in your notes of the affected areas is useful.

Write down the **type** of skin lesions you see. Dermatologists define primary and secondary lesions, which are detailed in Table 4.3 together with references to where these lesions will be found illustrated in other parts of the book.

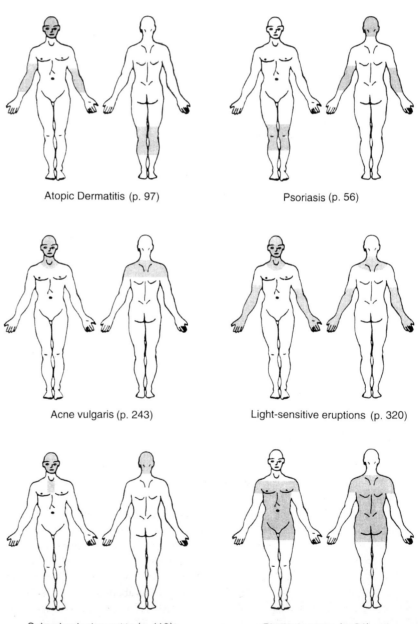

Atopic Dermatitis (p. 97)

Psoriasis (p. 56)

Acne vulgaris (p. 243)

Light-sensitive eruptions (p. 320)

Seborrhoeic dermatitis (p. 110)

Pityriasis rosea (p. 81)

Fig. 4.1 'Typical' distribution of lesions in common skin disorders.

Table 4.3 Primary and secondary lesions of the skin

Lesion	Description	Example—where to find it
Primary		
Macule	A flat, circumscribed area of altered skin colour	Vitiligo p. 227, pityriasis versi color, p. 161
		Peutz–Jegher lesions, p. 311
Papule	A small, circumscribed elevation of the skin	Molluscum contagiosum, p. 146
Nodule	A solid, circumscribed elevation whose greater part lies beneath the skin surface	Erythema nodosum, p. 213
Weal	A transient, slightly raised lesion, characteristically with a pale centre and a pink margin	Urticaria, p. 218
Vesicle (blister)	A small (less than 5 mm in diameter), circumscribed fluid-containing elevation	Dermatitis herpetiformis, p. 277
Bulla (blister)	Similar to a vesicle but larger	Bullous pemphigoid, p. 273
Pustule	A collection of pus	Acne, p. 243
Plaque	A flat-topped palpable lesion	Psoriasis, p. 56
Purpura	Visible collections of free red blood cells	Drug eruption, p. 289
Telangiectasia	Dilated capillaries visible on the skin surface	Topical steroid side-effect, p. 298
Secondary		
Scale	Thickened, loose, readily detached fragments of stratum corneum	Chronic disseminated lupus erythematosus (CDLE), p. 181
Crust	Dried exudate	Impetigo, p. 134
Excoriation	A shallow abrasion often caused by scratching	Atopic eczema, p. 97
Ulcer	An excavation due to loss of tissue including the epidermal surface	p. 209
Scar	A permanent lesion that results from the process of repair by replacement with connective tissue	CDLE, p. 181
Lichenification	Areas of increased epidermal thickness with accentuation of skin	Atopic eczema, p. 97

Is there any sign that the individual lesions have developed on a site of trauma or injury, such as a scratch or an operation scar? This is seen in a number of conditions, including psoriasis (p. 56), lichen planus (p. 78), and viral warts (p. 142). This is called the **Koebner phenomenon** and is a clue that the mechanisms involved in epidermal healing, possibly growth factors such as transforming growth factor, may be involved in the development of lesions in these diseases.

Remember that very few skin diseases are infectious and do not be afraid of touching the patient's skin. Patients with skin disease often develop a complex that they are 'untouchable' or 'unclean'. Ask the patient about such worries, and about whether or not there are problems with relatives and friends who are concerned about transmission of non-infectious problems, such as psoriasis and acne.

Investigations commonly used in dermatology

A number of investigations and lab tests are commonly used in dermatology. It is useful to know what samples are required and what to expect from the laboratory.

Identifying fungal infection

Superficial fungi that cause infections inhabit the outer layer of the skin—the stratum corneum—and skin scales or scrapings should be examined under the microscope. Take a scalpel blade and, with the affected area of skin stretched taut between two fingers, gently scrape the skin with a piece of paper, preferably black, held underneath. Scrape until a reasonable number of silvery scales are on the paper (Fig. 4.2). Try not to cause bleeding by scraping too deeply or too vigorously. This specimen can then be labelled and sent at normal temperature, through the post if necessary, to your local laboratory. Alternatively, this specimen can be examined directly, if a microscope is available, on a slide with a drop of 10% potassium hydroxide on it. A network of stick-like fungal hyphae may be seen (Fig. 4.3). Part of this sample should also be sent for culture, which may be positive, although no fungi were seen directly, and will allow exact identification of the type of fungus. The result of this test will not be available for 2–3 weeks.

If fungal infection of the hair is suspected, hair brushings, clippings, or scalp scrapings should be treated in the same way. In the case of possible fungal nail infection, take a clipping or scraping from the abnormal area of the nail.

Some fungi (for example, *Microsporum canis*) fluoresce brightly under ultraviolet light, and this fact can be used to make an instant diagnosis of scalp ringworm if a Wood's light—a UV source—is available. The fungi will fluoresce bright green.

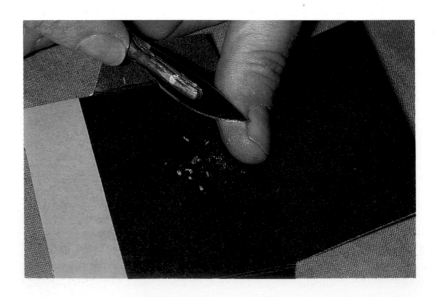

Fig. 4.2 The technique of taking scrapings for the identification of fungi in the epidermis. A piece of black paper makes it possible to see the scrapings accumulate as the epidermis is gently scraped with a scalpel blade. Do not cause bleeding.

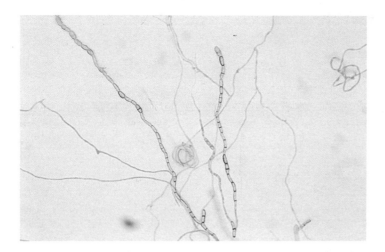

Fig. 4.3 Fungal hyphae. These will be easily seen down the microscope if the skin scrapings are mounted in 10% potassium hydroxide.

Skin biopsy

Many skin conditions require a biopsy to confirm the clinical diagnosis. This may involve taking a small ellipse of skin with a scalpel (Fig. 4.4) or using a sterile disposable skin biopsy punch with a diameter of 4–8 mm to take a small circle of skin (Fig. 4.5). The punch biopsy technique is extremely quick and, in the case of the smaller samples, may not require stitching.

Local anaesthetic (1–2% lignocaine preferably without adrenalin) should be infiltrated around the chosen lesion 5 minutes or so before biopsy. In the case of children, application of topical anaesthetic such as EMLA (lignocaine and prilocaine) under a dressing 1 hour before biopsy will help reduce discomfort. If in doubt, check with a senior colleague about which lesion to biopsy and from which body site. In general, a fresh lesion is preferred (present for less than 24 hours) and in the case of, for example, blistering diseases, this is essential. All biopsies will

> ### Key points
> Plan the site of your skin biopsy and the type of lesion biopsied with care.

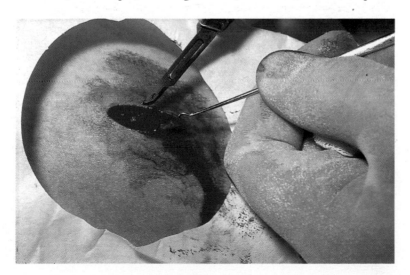

Fig. 4.4 The use of the scalpel and a skin hook in taking an elliptical skin biopsy. The hook should be inserted at one end of the ellipse and used instead of forceps, which will crush the tissue.

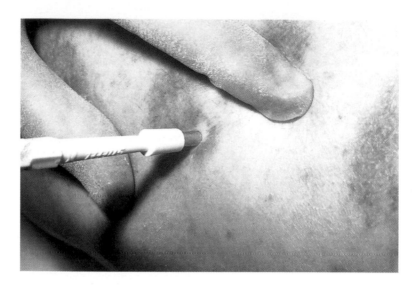

Fig. 4.5 The punch biopsy technique. This is quicker than a scalpel biopsy and requires less equipment. A disposable sterile punch, 4 mm in diameter, is applied with gentle rotating pressure to anaesthetized skin.

leave a small scar, so try to select a lesion on a site where this will not cause a cosmetic problem, such as the flank. Always try to avoid the shoulders and front of the chest, as the skin on these areas tends to form unsightly keloid scars. Figure 4.6 illustrates the skin tension or Lange's lines. If you orientate your biopsy scar along, rather than across these lines, it will in time be less visible.

What to do with the biopsy specimen

If in doubt, contact the laboratory **before** you begin to biopsy, rather than when you are holding the specimen in your hand. Does the pathologist want a fresh frozen sample, commonly required for blistering diseases, or do they also require

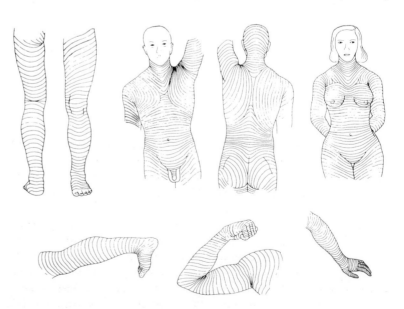

Fig. 4.6 Lange's lines. The long axis of a biopsy scar should be orientated along these lines.

material for electron microscopy, as well as light microscopy, which may be the case in rare dermatological disorders presenting in childhood? Label the biopsy pot or pots clearly and give the pathologist a brief, but relevant history. Always follow-up your biopsy clinics by reading the pathology report and if possible ask to see the slide yourself, either at a projection session or in the pathology department. Make sure that everyone who needs to know the result of the biopsy is informed. This is obviously particularly important if an unexpected result, such as a previously undiagnosed malignancy, is reported. An appropriate letter to the GP and, if necessary, an urgent return appointment for further treatment is a vital part of the biopsy process and will prevent possible future legal problems.

Confirming the diagnosis of scabies

The female scabies mite or *Acarus* can often be found in the superficial layers of the skin. A good place to look for the mite is the finger webs. A thread-like track may be seen that is the route along which the mite has burrowed into the skin. If the mite can be gently extracted from the skin with a needle and placed on a microscope slide, the patient can be invited to examine the cause of his/her itch. You are likely to have a patient who is quite horrified to see the evidence of the cause of his problem and who will therefore carry out the prescribed treatment with great attention to detail.

> **Key points**
>
> If at all possible, show your patient with scabies his tormentor. You will, in this way, ensure compliance with treatment.

Patch testing to confirm contact dermatitis

Allergic contact dermatitis (p. 118) is a relatively common problem in dermatology clinics. This is caused by a type 4 or lymphocyte mediated immunological reaction, and testing for it is done *in vivo*, usually using the patients back as the test area. It is important to accurately identify the allergen causing the problem so that the patient can be given instructions about avoidance of materials containing the allergen. If the responsible substance is handled at work, careful reduction of exposure to the material can make all the difference between a patient retaining his job or being forced to seek alternative employment. It is equally important to eliminate substances that the patient feels might be responsible for his problem by negative patch testing results.

Small quantities of a range of potential allergens, and also sometimes specially prepared and diluted samples of material the patient has supplied himself, are applied to inert metal chambers and large numbers of these—up to 50 is quite feasible—are applied simultaneously to the back (Fig. 4.7). After 48 hours, the patches are removed, and the skin examined for redness and/or swelling both immediately and after another 48 hours (Fig. 4.8). In practice, this means the patient being seen three times in one week, on day 1 for application of the patches and on days 3 and 5 for readings.

The exact materials to apply vary according to the patients' history and also in different parts of the world. In Europe, the normal practice is to routinely apply 20 substances in the 'European Standard Battery'—the substances found by collaborative research among all European dermatologists to be the most common causes of dermatitis (see p. 119). These are made up in little inert chambers on an adhesive backing. In addition to the Standard European Battery, specialist sets of mate-

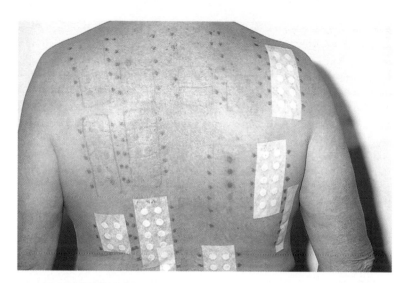

Fig. 4.7 The technique of patch testing. A large number of possible allergens have been applied to the back. Note the use of dye as a site marker.

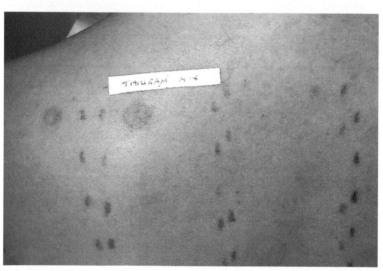

Fig. 4.8 A positive patch test showing erythema at 96 hours after application of the patches.

> ### *Key points*
>
> Patch testing may tell you the likely allergens. You have then to explain to the patient the relevance of your findings to his lifestyle

rials are available for certain body sites (e.g. footwear) or occupations (hairdressers, photographers), and are chosen according to the patient's history.

In North America, a slightly different set of allergens is used and monitored by the North American Contact Dermatitis Group.

'Allergy tests'

Many patients or parents of children with atopic dermatitis and urticaria in particular request allergy tests in the belief that it is possible to identify the allergen(s) involved in these conditions, and that, if these are then avoided, a cure will result. Unfortunately, this is not always feasible. Type 1 allergy tests or prick tests may identify clinically relevant allergens in respiratory atopy, but the patient with cutaneous problems will usually react on prick testing to many allergens, for example, house dust mite, pollens, cat and dog hair, and protein foodstuffs. The relevance of these reactions to the patient's eczema is often doubtful and, for this reason, these tests are usually only carried out in specialized allergy or contact dermatitis investigation units.

The quantitation of circulating serum IgE, measuring both total and specific IgE levels to inhaled and ingested allergens, using the radio allergosorbent or RAST test may be relevant, both in diagnosis and treatment. It is usually used or requested for children with severe atopic dermatitis. Parents, however, need to be warned that it may not be of practical value in that vigorous avoidance of all the allergens giving rise to a positive RAST may not improve the condition and, conversely, continued exposure to, for example, dog hair to which a positive RAST result has been obtained, may cause no problems. Careful clinical observation on the part of both doctor and patient or parent is more likely to produce clinically relevant information.

Photography

In dermatological records, one well-taken clinical photograph is frequently worth several paragraphs. They are very useful for ongoing monitoring of, for example, atypical naevi to try to prevent unnecessary excision of benign lesions, on the one hand, but also to identify at an early stage the lesions that are showing inappropriate change and should therefore be excised. Photographs are usually required if you are planning to present the case at a grand round, clinical meeting, or to write a case report for a journal.

Choose appropriate lighting and background, and place a centimetre scale next the area to be photographed. Often it is best to take a more distant orientation photo to show the body site involved, as well as a close up of the lesion. Always obtain the patients written permission for the photo and store this permission in the patient's records.

Special study module

Arrange an attachment both to the dermatology and the pathology departments in the hospital in which you are training.

Attend all the skin biopsy sessions and then personally follow all the samples through processing and reporting.

Keep a record of all the diagnoses made.

What have you learned about the correlation between clinical and pathological features of skin disease?

How often was the pathologist given appropriate information on the request form?

How has the surgical procedure affected management of this patient.

When was the patient informed of the result of the biopsy?

Did the patient understand the diagnosis and treatment plan?

Further reading

Lawrence, C.M. and Cox, N.H. (1993). *Physical signs in dermatology*. Wolfe London.

Myerscough, P.R. (1989) *Talking with patients*. Oxford University Press, Oxford.

Robinson, J. (1986) *Fundamentals of skin biopsy*. Chicago Year Book Publications, Chicago.

Zachary, C.B. (1991) *Basic cutaneous surgery*. Churchill Livingstone, New York.

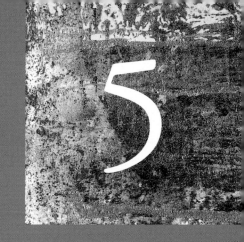

5

Psoriasis and other disorders of keratinization

- Problem cases
- Psoriasis
- Lichen planus
- Pityriasis rosea
- Pityriasis rubra pilaris
- Darier's disease
- The ichthyoses

Psoriasis and other disorders of keratinization

Problem cases

Read these case presentations, work your way through the information in this chapter, talk if possible to patients with similar problems, carry out an appropriate literature search if you have the facilities, and only then read the suggested management plans on p. 88.

Case 5.1

A 36-year-old, newly married accountant consults you about the management of her persistent widespread plaque psoriasis. She first developed psoriatic lesions when she was 14 and there is a strong family history. Although she attended the local dermatologist as a teenager 20 years ago, she found the rather messy tar preparations then prescribed unacceptable, and has not sought medical help for the last 15 years. She uses a little emollient to reduce scaling, and chooses clothes to cover her knees and elbows, which are particularly troublesome.

She wants to know if there are any new advances in psoriasis treatment that would help her, and in passing mentions that she hopes to start a family within the next year.

What will you tell her and suggest for her particular situation?

Case 5.2

A 73-year-old widower who lives alone has hypertension, chronic obstructive airways disease, and extensive widespread psoriasis, which is at times erythrodermic. In the past, a 10-day admission to the local hospital, once or twice annually, has kept his skin at least partly under control, but local bed reductions mean that this is no longer available. He finds applying topical therapy to his body regularly very difficult both because of his breathlessness and arthritis in his hands.

What treatment might be appropriate here? He is determined to continue to live in his own home.

Case 5.3

A 58-year-old woman comes to you with itchy papules on one wrist. They have been present for about 6 weeks. She thinks they may be insect bites. Her only medication is a diuretic that she has been on for 3 years for mild hypertension.

What conditions would you consider in the differential diagnosis and how would you establish a diagnosis?

Case 5.4

A 21-year-old male is brought to you by his girl friend. They have just returned from a sunny holiday on which he was badly sunburned. His back is covered with infected, crusted lesions and he feels generally unwell.

What conditions might this history suggest, and how would you arrive at a diagnosis?

Psoriasis

Psoriasis is one of the commonest of all skin diseases. All doctors need to be familiar with the many different types of clinical presentation, and to know the currently available range of treatments with their advantages and disadvantages for individual patients at different stages of their life.

Definition

A chronic relapsing and remitting scaling skin disease that may appear at any age and affect any part of the skin surface.

Prevalence

Among Caucasians, the prevalence of psoriasis is said to be 1–3%. This is probably a significant under-estimate, first, because patients with mild psoriasis may not seek medical help and, secondly, because incidence figures are often derived from hospital records so that those treated solely by family doctors or not seeking treatment at all will be excluded.

The sexes are affected equally and there appear to be two subgroups, one with onset most commonly in the second decade, and one with onset later in life in the fourth and fifth decades. These are often referred to as type 1 and type 2 psoriasis. Type 1 psoriasis patients, with the earlier age of onset, have a stronger family history.

Aetiology

It is clear that there are both inherited and environmental factors, which influence the development of psoriasis. Although a very wide range of biochemical and pathological abnormalities have been reported in psoriatic skin, the exact cause of psoriasis is not yet known.

Genetics of psoriasis

Psoriasis is a good example of a disease in which there appears to be multi-factorial inheritance. A number of genes may be abnormally expressed and this, in turn, predisposes to abnormal reactions to environmental agents, leading to clinical expression of psoriasis. Approximately one-third of patients have a positive family history and psoriasis is more likely to develop if both parents have a positive family history. Twin studies show concordance of around 75% for monozygotic twins and 25% for dizygotic twins. At present, many groups worldwide are actively searching for psoriasis susceptibility genes. To date at least seven genes, numbered psors 1–psors 7 have been identified, and it is likely that this list will increase over the next few years. Psors 1 is situated on chromosome 6p21.3 and is part of the major histocompatibility complex. This gene appears to be important in psoriasis in the UK and US, and confirms the previously known association of psoriasis with HLA-CW6 and HLA-B27. Other psoriasis susceptibility genes have been identified on chromosomes 1q, 10, 16q, and 17q. The gene on chromosome 16 is of particular interest as a mutation on chromosome 16q , nod 2, has recently been reported to be associated with Crohn's disease, which is clinically associated with psoriasis. Abnormal expression of this gene is associated with a very brisk response to infection, which does appear to be seen in at least some patients who develop psoriasis for the first time after a streptococcal infection.

Tumour necrosis factor

Tumour necrosis factor is a very potent pro-inflammatory cytokine and has, as one of its functions, the ability to increase migration of leucocytes into inflamed skin. Levels of tumour necrosis factor are elevated in the skin and joints of those with cutaneous psoriasis and psoriatic arthropathy. In addition, TNF receptors are up-regulated in the synovial fluid of patients with psoriatic arthritis. These observations, together with the promising results of anti-TNF therapy first in psoriatic arthropathy and, more recently, in cutaneous psoriasis suggest a major role for this cytokine in the clinical expression of psoriasis.

Immunological aspects of psoriasis

The lesions of psoriasis attract both neutrophils and lymphocytes at different stages of evolution of the psoriatic plaques. CD8 positive lymphocytes are seen mainly in the epidermis and CD 4 positive lymphocytes in the dermis. In addition to tumour necrosis factor discussed above, the cytokines interferon gamma, interleukin 2, and interleukin 12 are present in excess in psoriatic lesions. This is a Th1 or cytotoxic pattern, and its recognition has led to T cell targeted approaches to psoriasis therapy, including blocking of co-stimulatory molecule binding, the use of IL2 fusion toxins, and blockade of adhesion molecule formation. Drugs in current clinical trial include efaluzimab (Xanelin), which is directed against the CD11a component of LFA1 and alefacept (Amevive), a fusion protein of LFA3 and IgG1, which inhibits T cell activation by blocking LFA3 binding to CD2. The Th1 predominance in psoriasis is also currently being attacked with the use of IL10, which is a Th2 cytokine and is under investigation.

Epidermal keratinocyte proliferation in psoriasis

Psoriatic plaques have an increased epidermal cell proliferation rate. Radiolabelling techniques have been used to measure the transit time of epidermal cells maturing in their transit through the skin. In normal skin this is about 50–75 days, whereas in psoriatic skin it is only 8–10 days. With similar techniques, it has been shown that, while the germinative component of normal human epidermis is confined to the basal layer, in psoriatic skin it comprises the lower three layers of epidermal cells. It seems, therefore, that the rapid turnover of psoriatic cells is due both to an increase in the number of actively dividing cells, and to an acceleration in their rate of reproduction. As has been explained in Chapter 3 (p. 26) the two pairs of keratins found in the basal cells of normal epidermis are keratins 5 and 14, while keratins 1 and 10 predominate in the suprabasal layers. In psoriasis there is a persistence above the basal layer of keratins 5 and 1. In addition, keratins 6 and 16 are seen, which are associated with rapid cell division and tissue repair. Thus, psoriatic epidermis has some biological similarities to a healing wound of the epidermis.

The Koebner phenomenon

The Koebner phenomenon describes the tendency for psoriatic lesions to develop at sites of skin trauma, such as mechanical friction, sunburn, or lesions of child-

Key points

Tumour necrosis factor alpha appears to play a pivotal part in development of lesions of psoriasis.

hood illnesses, such as chickenpox. Possibly, the abnormal or unstable keratinocyte surface antigens or the abnormal keratin formed in those who are genetically predisposed are exposed by trauma to the immune system, which then reacts, triggering a hyperproliferative response in the epidermis.

Systemic drugs and psoriasis

Psoriasis may be both aggravated and precipitated for the first time by some systemic drugs. These include lithium, anti-malarials, non-steroidal anti-inflammatory agents, and beta blockers. Patients with psoriasis planning a tropical holiday must be aware that the anti-malarial chloroquine may cause their psoriasis to deteriorate. Alternatives, such paludrine and mefloquine, do not cause this problem.

Infection and psoriasis

Streptococcal infection, usually in the form of a sore throat, is a well-recognized precipitating event in patients with guttate psoriasis. It has been suggested that this may be due to the presence of super-antigens, and that there are shared antigens between the wall of the streptococcus and the keratinocyte. The development of guttate psoriasis is very strongly associated with the presence of the HLA-CW6 antigen.

Ultraviolet radiation and psoriasis

The majority of patients with psoriasis find that their lesions improve on exposure to natural sunlight, but about 15% find that UV exposure aggravates pre-existing lesions and may stimulate the development of new lesions. To date, no clear biochemical or immunological explanation has been proposed for these two subsets of psoriasis patients with opposing responses to UV.

Stress, smoking, and alcohol

In common with many skin conditions, psoriasis may develop for the first time during periods of stress or stress may aggravate pre-existing lesions. It is also established that stressed patients respond less well to standard anti-psoriatic treatment than more relaxed psoriatic patients. Both smoking and a high alcohol intake are associated with psoriasis, but to what extent this is a reaction on the part of the patient to the disease, rather than a cause of it in the first place is debated.

Pathology

The difference between normal epidermis and papillary dermis and that seen in active psoriatic lesions is shown diagrammatically in Fig. 5.1. The stratum corneum in psoriasis contains nuclei and is therefore parakeratotic. There is no granular layer and the prickle cell layer is expanded with bulbous, downward projections. Mitotic figures may be seen in supra-basal keratinocytes. In the papillary dermis, large dilated thin-walled blood vessels will be seen and above these vessels the epidermis is often relatively thin. This increased vascularization in psoriasis is another current target for therapeutic intervention and anti-angiogenic agents are currently in trial.

In both the dermis and epidermis there may be an infiltrate of leucocytes, and these may clump together in the stratum corneum to form so-called **Munro**

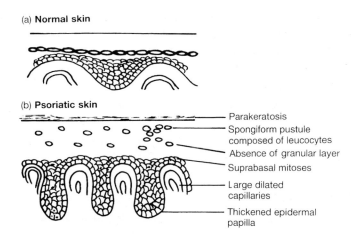

(a) **Normal skin**

(b) **Psoriatic skin**

— Parakeratosis
— Spongiform pustule composed of leucocytes
— Absence of granular layer
— Suprabasal mitoses
— Large dilated capillaries
— Thickened epidermal papilla

Fig. 5.1 Psoriatic and normal skin compared.

micro-abscesses or spongiform pustules. There is also a sparse lymphocytic infiltrate in early psoriasis lesions, both in the epidermis and the dermis. The epidermal lymphocytes are mainly CD8 positive cytotoxic T cells, while those in the dermis are CD4 T helper cells.

Clinical features

By far the commonest type of psoriasis is classic plaque psoriasis, but there are also several other less common clinical presentations listed below

- **classic plaque psoriasis**—much the commonest;
- **guttate-sudden onset of small lesions,** usually in a young person after strep infection;
- **seborrhoeic, flexural napkin,** or **inversus;**
- **erythrodermic;**
- **pustular**—generalized (von Zumbusch) or localized on the trunk and limbs or plamoplantar;
- **nail psoriasis.**

Plaque psoriasis

Classically, psoriasis vulgaris presents as red scaly plaques affecting the extensor aspects of the knees (Fig. 5.2) and elbows (Fig. 5.3), and the scalp (Fig. 5.4). Other common sites are the hands and the sacral area. The total area affected ranges from a few tiny plaques to almost all the body surface (Figs 5.5–5.7). Untreated, the individual lesions are raised, palpable, and topped by greyish-white silvery scale. Rubbing them after gently removing the scale reveals pinpoint bleeding from the dilated, superficial capillaries (Auspitz' sign). These dilated capillaries in the dermis can be seen on histological examination of a psoriatic plaque.

Guttate psoriasis

Guttate or 'raindrop' psoriasis is commoner in children than in adults, and presents as multiple small psoriatic lesions mainly on the trunk. This pattern is fre-

Key points

Find out what each individual patient with psoriasis hopes to achieve from treatment and develop a feasible treatment plan together.

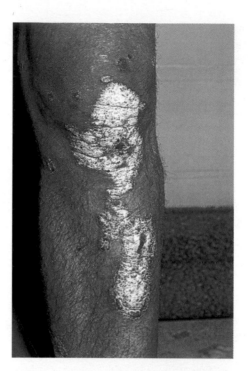

Fig. 5.2 Classic untreated lesions of psoriasis vulgaris. These lesions are commonly seen on the knees, elbows, and sacrum, and present as plaques topped by white or silvery scales.

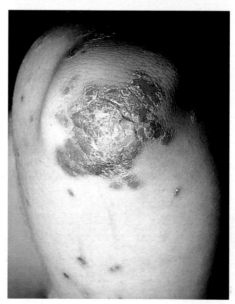

Fig. 5.3 Psoriasis of the elbows showing striking erythema and scaling.

quently preceded by a streptococcal throat infection (Fig. 5.8). It is quite common for a young patient to have only one episode of guttate psoriasis and thereafter no further problems. Virtually all affected patients carry the HLA-CW6 antigen.

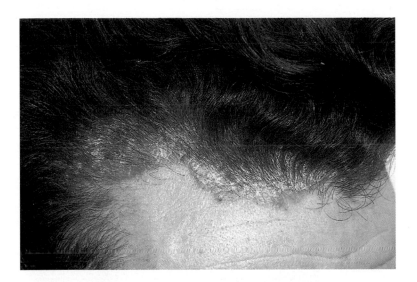

Fig. 5.4 Psoriasis of the scalp. This can be difficult to treat and can cause some hair thinning.

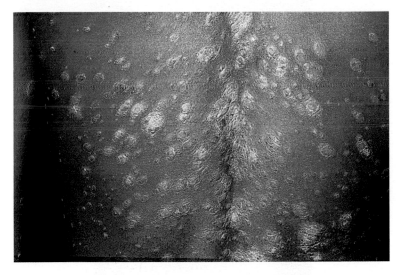

Fig. 5.5 Psoriatic plaques on the back of an individual with coloured skin.

Seborrhoeic psoriasis

Seborrhoeic psoriasis or **psoriasis inversus** describe psoriatic lesions in the body folds, especially the groins, axillae, and infra-mammary regions. Diagnosis may be difficult on both clinical and histological grounds, as the erythema and scaling can be very similar to that seen in seborrhoeic dermatitis. Similarly, napkin psoriasis in infants tends to involve the creases in the groin and is seen as red areas with associated fine scaling, rather than the classic more clearly demarcated psoriatic plaque. Psoriasis involving the body flexures can be difficult to treat as it is easily irritated by topical tars and dithranol, which are very effective in other sites.

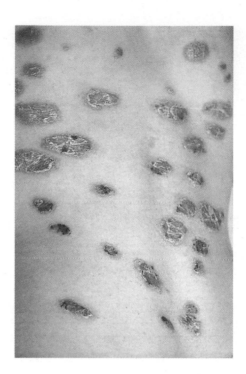

Fig. 5.6 Erythematus psoriatic plaques on a Caucasian back.

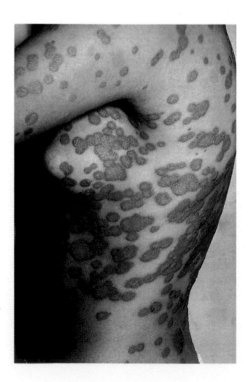

Fig. 5.7 Extensive psoriatic plaques developing on the trunk after chicken pox.

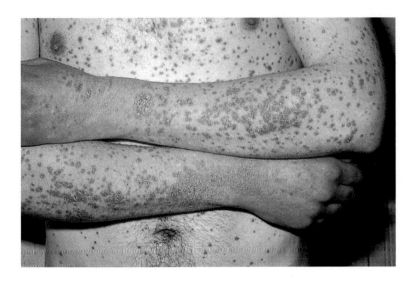

Fig. 5.8 Extensive guttate psoriasis.

Erythrodermic psoriasis

Erythrodermic psoriasis presents as an extensive erythema of the entire body surface with, at times, very few classical scaling psoriatic lesions (Fig. 5.9). Grossly increased blood flow through the skin may lead to loss of thermoregulation and to high output cardiac failure.

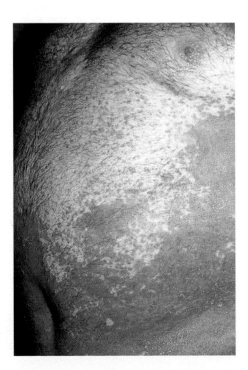

Fig. 5.9 Erythrodermic psoriasis involving mainly the lower part of the abdominal skin.

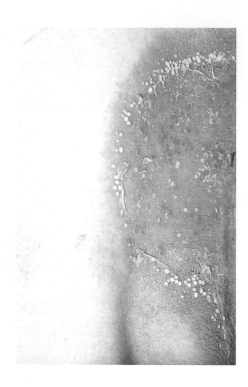

Fig. 5.10 Close-up of an expanding plaque of pustular psoriasis showing classic pustulation at the edge of the lesion.

Pustular psoriasis

Pustular psoriasis refers to varieties of psoriasis in which sterile pustules are present. Pustules tend to appear at the advancing edge of psoriatic lesions (Fig. 5.10). They may also be seen in erythrodermic psoriasis, and the combination of extensive erythroderma and sterile pustules is termed the **von Zumbusch** type of pustular psoriasis, a serious and, at times, life-threatening variety, due to associated fluid and electrolyte imbalance and high output cardiac failure.

Pustular psoriasis may also be seen as a non-life-threatening, but extremely chronic variant, on the palms and soles. These lesions respond poorly to currently available therapy (Fig. 5.11). There is a view and also genetic evidence to suggest that this condition, also called palmo plantar pustulosis, is distinct from psoriasis and should be considered separately. However, some anti psoriatic therapies are effective.

Scalp involvement

Psoriasis of the scalp is seen as thick, obvious scaling and redness, often most obvious at the hairline and behind the ears. Some patients with long-standing scalp psoriasis develop a degree of hair thinning, but it is not clear whether this is due to the psoriatic lesion or to treatment.

Nail involvement

A proportion of patients with long-standing psoriasis develop nail changes, including small pits on the nail plate and separation of part of the nail from the

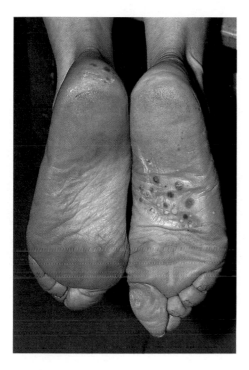

Fig. 5.11 Pustular psoriasis of the soles. The pustules are sterile.

nail bed (onycholysis) with sub-ungual hyperkeratosis. Discoloration of the nail resembling grease spots is also seen (Figs 5.12–5.14). These patients have a higher incidence of psoriatic arthropathy.

Psoriatic arthropathy

This is a distinctive seronegative arthropathy usually seen in patients with established cutaneous lesions of psoriasis. The sacro-iliac and distal inter-phalangeal joints are most commonly involved, but any joint may be affected by this mutilating variety of arthropathy. A higher incidence of arthropathy is seen in those with psoriatic nail changes. Occasionally, psoriatic arthropathy is diagnosed in the absence of overt skin lesions, but this is rare and other causes of arthropathy must first be carefully excluded. Many of the newer anti-cytokine and immunomodulating approaches to psoriasis treatment have initially been found to be effective in psoriatic arthropathy and subsequently used in trials of cutaneous lesions.

Many patients with actively developing psoriasis lesions complain of pruritus. Scratching may cause fresh lesions due to the Koebner phenomenon. After the first attack of psoriasis, relapses and remissions are frequent. A few fortunate individuals, after a single episode of guttate psoriasis, enter an almost complete and prolonged remission. More commonly, however, mild involvement of the scalp, knees, and elbows persists with, at varying intervals, episodes of more widespread involvement. Some psoriatics find their lesions improve over the years, whilst in others the process becomes more widespread and troublesome. Childhood psoriasis, although less prevalent than in adults, tends to be both persistent and difficult to treat.

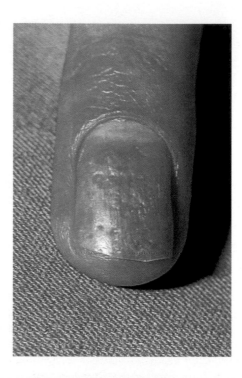

Fig. 5.12 Typical psoriatic nail changes. Note the separation of the distal part of the nail from the underlying nail plate (oncholysis) and the pitting of the nail.

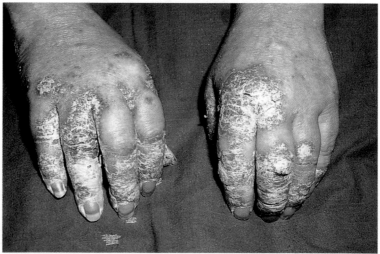

Fig. 5.13 Severe psoriasis of the hands with associated nail involvement.

Differential diagnosis

The differential diagnosis of psoriasis includes many scaling skin conditions, particularly those associated with underlying inflammation. Eczema (p. 97) is usually very pruritic and there is more inflammation than scaling. The distribution of the lesions is also usually a clue to the diagnosis, as eczema tends to affect the flexures. In most cases of ichthyoses, there is very little itch and a lot of scaling

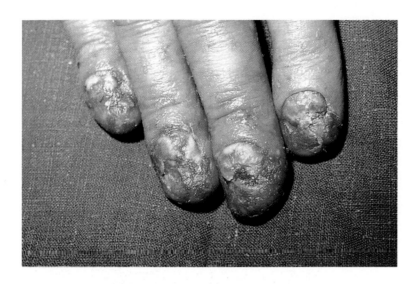

Fig. 5.14 Severe destructive psoriasis of the finger nails.

with little inflammation (p. 85). Reiter's disease (p. 170) can usually be excluded in the absence of genitourinary, rheumatological, or gastro-intestinal complaints. The histological features are diagnostic in lichenoid reactions including lichen planus (p. 78) so if in doubt a biopsy is justified. Biopsy and histological examination will usually differentiate seborrhoeic dermatitis, pityriasis rosea, and pityriasis rubra pilaris from psoriasis.

Be cautious about diagnosing an isolated plaque on the trunk of an elderly patient as psoriasis. Bowen's disease (p. 339) may look very similar. Once again, a biopsy will establish the correct diagnosis.

Investigations

Patients presenting with classic plaque psoriasis can easily be diagnosed on clinical grounds and a biopsy is not indicated unless there is clinical doubt. Occasionally, particularly when the presenting feature is a scaling lesion of the palm, taking scrapings for mycological examination to exclude a fungal infection is advisable.

In any patient with psoriasis and joint pain, radiological examination, and taking blood samples for rheumatoid factor and antinuclear antibody assessment will help differentiate rheumatoid arthritis from psoriatic arthritis. Patients with psoriatic arthritis have a seronegative arthropathy, and the small joints of the fingers are frequently involved.

Treatment

In considering appropriate treatment for a patient with psoriasis it is essential to consider:

- the patient's age and general health, including, if female, plans for pregnancy;
- the type of psoriasis;
- the body surface area involved and the areas worst affected;

Key points

Few patients nowadays will tolerate messy topical treatments for psoriasis in the long term.

- the previous treatments used and their success or failure;
- what the patient hopes for and needs to achieve for their life-style.

This last point is important and should be discussed with the patient at their first visit. An elderly patient with knee and elbow problems may only wish to spend time applying topical therapy for 2 or 3 weeks before an annual holiday, whereas a 20-year-old ballet dancer will need to keep her skin completely clear in order to pursue her career.

It is important at the time of the first consultation to explain to the patient the usually chronic nature of psoriasis and the fact that currently available treatments *control*, rather than cure the disease. The need for the patient's own active involvement, and possibly also that of a relative, in topical treatment should be explained.

Recently, there have been attempts to quantitate the degree of dermatological disability caused by a number of skin conditions. The psoriasis disability index is a well developed questionnaire on such items as time lost from work, interpersonal relationships, and other problems that were found on a much more detailed questionnaire to be the most common problems affecting the majority of psoriasis patients. This questionnaire administered before and after treatment can give some guide to the patient's view of the value of his treatment.

Many patients have unspoken fears that their psoriasis is infectious, or a form of cancer, or even both of these. The difference between an inherited susceptibility, which is present in psoriasis, and truly contagious infection, such as impetigo may require explanation and the truly non-malignant and non-premalignant nature of psoriasis should be emphasized.

Clear, useful patient information sheets are available on psoriasis. These are helpful and will reinforce the instructions given at the original consultation as much of this may be quickly forgotten.

Once the nature of the disease is fully understood, many patients with mild psoriasis may prefer to leave small plaques on knees and elbows untreated. There is no evidence that this will cause extension of psoriasis and it is an entirely acceptable option. A mild emollient, such as emulsifying ointment BP or white soft paraffin, will minimize scaling.

The majority of patients with psoriasis, however, will want a more active treatment programme. Methods of managing psoriasis have advanced considerably in the past few years, and the range of available topical and systemic therapies are itemized in Table 5.1 and examples of their use in Table 5.2.

For many patients topical therapy will be appropriate and relatively free of toxicity. Some initial help may well be needed to demonstrate exactly how to apply topical preparations, particularly those containing dithranol in their own homes, and it is very useful to arrange a practical hands on demonstration by a trained dermatological nurse of exactly how to use the creams and ointments prescribed, and what dressings to use. Initial application of topical preparations with advice in an out-patient treatment centre or psoriasis day-care centre will help compliance when the patient has to carry out treatment in their own home.

A small number of patients with very persistent large plaque psoriasis, or pustular psoriasis, or the erythrodermic variant will require in-patient care, but with

Key points

Newer systemic therapies for psoriasis are effective, but may have significant toxicity. Is this acceptable in a non-fatal disease?

Table 5.1 Topical and systemic preparations of value in the management of psoriasis

Therapy	Preparation	Advantages	Disadvantages
Topical	Dithranol-based	Long-term safety data reassuring	Some staining and irritation common. Difficult for out-patient use
	Tar	Long-term safety data reassuring	Messy and cosmetically relatively unacceptable. Recent concern about carcinogenicity
	Salicylic acid	Useful particularly for scalps, and hyperkeratotic palms and soles	Danger of salicylicism if high concentrations used on large areas of the body
	Topical steroids	Clean and cosmetically acceptable	Only moderate potency acceptable. Risk of topical side effects with more potent preparations
	Calcipotriol	Cosmetically acceptable	Very useful in primary care but of value only in mild to moderate psoriasis. Tends to improve, but not completely clear lesions
	Ultraviolet light	Cosmetically acceptable	Unknown future risk of malignancy.
	UVB-natural sunlight wavelengths		Improvement in psoriatic lesions tends to be associated with some erythema.
Systemic	Photochemotherapy (Psoralens + UVA = PUVA)	Cosmetically acceptable	Definite risk of malignancy (squamous cell carcinoma) in patients who have had more than 500 treatments
	Cytotoxic drugs (methotrexate, azathioprine, hydroxyurea)	Rapidly effective	Teratogenicity. Liver, marrow and renal toxicity
	Retinoid group of drugs acetretin (Neotigason)	Effective in 50% of chronic plaque psoriasis. Very effective in 80% of pustular psoriasis of palms and soles	Teratogenicity. Raised Cheilitis. Bony changes serum lipids.
	Cyclosporin (Neoral)	Effective	Rapid rebound on stopping treatment. Risk of permanent renal damage.
	Cytokine modulators	Useful in both skin and joint disease	Some current concern about side effects
	Immune modulating agents	Encouraging early results	Little data as yet on toxicity

Table 5.2 Examples of treatment for psoriasis of different types in different age ranges

Patient	Types of Psoriasis	Special considerations	Treatment	Comments
Boy aged 10	Guttate psoriasis	Usually self-healing type of psoriasis	0.1% dithranol in cream base or simple white soft paraffin	Check for recurrent sore throats and enlarged tonsils
Married woman aged 28	Chronic plaque	Wishes to add to family	Primary care trial of topical calcipotriol ointment. If ineffective, short contact dithranol up to 2%, 30 minutes daily	No currently available systemic treatment is appropriate for women who wish to become pregnant
Male aged 40	Severe pustular lesions	Hand lesions causing concern over losing job	Trial of topical dithranol. If not successful try topical steroids if these fail, consider for systemic acetretin therapy	
Female aged 56	Widespread plaques	Four recent hospital admissions. Post-menopausal. Relatively dithranol-resistant	Consider for PUVA therapy, or cyclosporin, or trials of new therapy	Appropriate only if patient lives reasonably close to PUVA centre. It is essential to keep an accurate record of the number of UVA exposures and the total dose of UVA
Male aged 72	Erythrodermic psoriasis	Severe chronic diseases obstructive airway makes home use of topical preparations very difficult	Consider methotrexate	Possible hepatic toxicity may be outweighed by improved quality of life.

newer more effective systemic anti-psoriatic agents, this number is dwindling steadily.

Topical therapy

This is the main form of treatment for the great majority of psoriasis patients. Appropriate preparations include:

- emollients;
- tar preparations;
- dithranol preparations;
- calciptriol and other vitamin D-based preparations;
- salicylic acid preparations;
- topical steroids;
- various combination of the above.

Emollients

Emollients are of great value in psoriasis in reducing scaling, and preventing the development of cracks and hacks, particularly on the palms and soles. Patients should be given a pack of small samples of several emollients to try and choose the most effective for their skin. Usually, a lighter preparation is preferred for the trunk and limbs, and a heavier one for the hands and feet. This will reduce scaling, but will not affect erythema or prevent new plaques developing. Evidence-based studies are lacking, but emollients are worth recommending on the grounds that they have virtually no side effects and are likely to produce at least cosmetic improvement.

Tar preparations

These have been used to treat psoriasis for over 100 years and appear to have anti-mitotic activity. They are relatively cosmetically unacceptable and their use is therefore declining. They are available as creams, pastes, and ointments, and need to be covered with stockinet dressings. Evidence-based dermatology and recent comparative clinical trials suggest that the maximum benefit from topical tar will be achieved by concentrations no higher than 5%, and that there is no logical reason to use higher concentrations, which are messy, and stain both clothing and bedding. A few patients develop a sterile folliculitis when tar is applied to hair-bearing areas. This is self-limiting.

The traditional Goeckermann regime includes the use of both tar and ultraviolet light (UVB), and there is some evidence to suggest that the combination of UVB and tar will clear psoriatic plaques more quickly than either alone.

There are a number of cleaner proprietary tar preparations available. These are slightly less effective than crude coal tar preparations, but for out-patient use this is more than compensated for by their cosmetic acceptability. These include 5% tar and 2% allantoin in a 'vanishing cream' base (Alphosyl), Clinitar, Pragmatar; 10% tar in a water miscible base (Carbodome), and Zetar (USA).

Dithranol (anthralin)

Preparations containing dithranol act in psoriasis by inhibiting mitosis and thus slowing down the accelerated rate of keratinocyte division in psoriasis. They are widely used and are useful for most types of psoriasis. The concentration of dithranol used may vary from 0.1 to 3% or higher in an appropriate base. This is commonly Lassar's paste (zinc paste with 15% salicylic acid added). Traditionally, this paste has been applied to psoriatic plaques night and morning under a stockinet gauze dressing after protecting the surrounding normal skin with white soft paraffin, a very important point in patient education, as normal non-psoriatic skin is easily irritated by dithranol.

The Ingram regime combines topical dithranol applications with tar baths and ultraviolet light therapy (UVB). This treatment is safe and effective, with psoriatic plaques clearing in 2–3 weeks. As the psoriatic lesions clear, the skin may temporarily become stained a grey-brown colour. This staining wears off 7–10 days after stopping treatment.

Ready-prepared dithranol preparations in the UK include a range of concentrations of dithranol in Dithrocream, Micanol, and Psorin. In the USA, an equivalent proprietary preparation is Drithocream.

Dithranol—short contact treatment

A patient-acceptable and effective method of applying dithranol is by the 'short contact' technique, which is based on the observation that dithranol applied to plaques of psoriasis remains on the psoriatic epidermis in small quantities even after washing. Evidence-based studies suggest no significant therapeutic benefit of short contact over conventional dithranol application, but the greater convenience of the short contact approach is in its favour.

In the short contact regime, the patient applies the appropriate concentration of dithranol (usually between 0.25 and 1%) to his skin for 10–30 minutes daily, and after this time bathes or showers to remove all visible dithranol. This can be done in the early morning or late evening, and is a very convenient approach, avoiding the need for dressings or staining of clothing.

Comparative studies have shown that this approach will result in a slightly longer time taken to clear the lesions than traditional 24-hour contact with bandaging, but the greater convenience of short contact therapy compensates for this for most patients.

Salicylic acid-containing preparations

These are most commonly used on the scalp, and on very thick hyperkeratotic areas on the palms and soles. Salicylic acid is a keratolytic and can be used on the scalp in concentrations up to 10–20% in aqueous cream or emulsifying ointment, and in lower concentrations for the palms and soles. Cocois, Ionil T, and psorin all contain salicylic acid.

Topical steroids

Topical steroids are very useful in the management of psoriasis in certain body sites. Strong topical steroids should not, however, be the mainstay of treatment of chronic plaque psoriasis. Although the plaques will initially respond, many patients will subsequently develop 'unstable' or erythrodermic psoriasis. Other problems of inappropriate long-term steroid use are described on p. 298.

Moderate potency topical steroids are useful for the management of flexural psoriasis provided the duration of use and quantities prescribed are controlled. Pustular psoriasis of the palms and soles may respond to stronger topical steroids—for example, beclomethasone dipropionate (Propaderm) or fluocinolone acetonide (Synalar)—and here also the quantity of steroid used and the duration of treatment should be carefully monitored.

Combinations of topical steroids and other anti-psoriatic preparations described above can be useful. The combination of a topical steroid and salicylic acid (Diprosalic) is useful as a lotion for stubborn scalp psoriasis.

Other steroid-containing gels and lotions (for example, Betnovate scalp application, Synalar gel) are clean and easy to use, but quantities prescribed should be reviewed regularly and, in the case of chronic persistent lesions, alternatives such as Cocois (12% coal tar solution, 2% salicylic acid, 4% precipitated sulphur in coconut oil and wax) considered.

Vitamin D derivatives (calcipotriol, calcipotriene, tacalcitol, calcitriol)

A number of vitamin D analogues are now available for topical use. They appear to have very little effect in mobilizing the body's calcium stores and, therefore, hypercalcaemia has only been observed to date in patients who have used very large quantities for long periods of time. They act by promoting normal epidermal differentiation, and a large systematic review suggests that they are at least as effective as topical steroids tars and dithranol, and much more cosmetically acceptable. Patients using topical vitamin D analogues notice a rapid reduction in scaling of their psoriatic plaques and a slower reduction in underlying erythema, which does not always clear completely. They have the advantage of being clean and odour free, and are therefore justifiably popular for out-patient use. The current recommendation is that no more than 100 g weekly should be used to avoid any risk of hypercalcaemia.

A popular and patient-acceptable current combination is to alternate a topical vitamin D derivative with a topical steroid, to reduce the irritant affect of the vitamin D preparation, and to minimize the undesirable atrophogenic effect of topical steroid. Current available preparations include tacalcitol (Curatoderm), calcitriol (Silkis), and calcipotriol (Dovonex).

Topical retinoids (e.g. tazarotene)

Topical retinoids may help promote differentiation of psoriatic skin and randomized controlled trials have shown short-term benefit, but with some irritation of the normal skin around the psoriatic plaque, particularly in very fair skinned individuals. Tazarotene (Zorac) is currently available. Because of concern about possible percutaneous absorption, this should not be prescribed for pregnant or potentially pregnant young women, as there is a risk of foetal malformation.

Ultraviolet light (UVB)

The action of both tar and dithranol is enhanced by exposure to ultraviolet light in the UVB range (280–315 nm). These are the predominant wavelengths found in natural sunlight, and are usually administered in carefully measured doses from appropriate light sources in the Goeckermann regime with tar or the Ingram regime with dithranol. Well-controlled studies suggest a definite advantage for dithranol and UVB in the Ingram regime compared with dithranol alone.

Narrow band UVB, using tubes emitting ultraviolet radiation only in the 310–312-nm range, is even more effective in rapidly clearing psoriatic plaques than broad band UVB, and is currently the UVB regime of choice either singly or in combination.

Shampoos

While it is traditional to prescribe tar-based and salicylic acid containing shampoos for mild psoriasis, there is little proof of their efficacy by comparison with regular use of a standard shampoo. Some patients find them soothing, but to be effective they must be left in contact with the scalp for several minutes. In many countries tar-containing shampoos are only available on prescription because of the theoretical risk of carcinogenesis.

Systemic therapy

- PUVA photochemotherapy
- Oral retinoids
- Methotrexate
- Cyclosporin
- Hydroxyurea
- Systemic steroids
- Mycophenolate mofetil
- Anti cytokine experimental drugs
- Experimental drugs which inhibit T cell activation

While topical therapy, properly applied, will control the great majority of psoriatic lesions, a small proportion of patients will require systemic therapy. These will usually be patients who are under the regular supervision of a dermatologist either as an out-patient or for short periods as an in-patient.

The choices here lie between photochemotherapy (PUVA), the retinoid group of drugs (currently only available in the UK on hospital prescription), cytotoxic drugs (including methotrexate and hydroxyurea), and the immunosuppressive drugs cyclosporin or mycophenolate mofetil. These treatments should not be considered until a very adequate trial of topical treatment has failed. None are safe for women in the child-bearing years without adequate (usually oral) contraception. Systemic steroids should only very rarely be used to control psoriasis. Although initially effective, the dosage needed to maintain control rises steadily and patients end up suffering more from the side effects of systemic steroid therapy than they ever would from psoriasis.

At present a large number of experimental immunomodulating drugs are in trial for patients with psoriatic arthropathy or severe cutaneous psoriasis. These can be broadly divided into those that reduce the number of pathogenic T cells, those which inhibit T cell activation and migration, those which redirect the immune system and those with anti-cytokine activity. Some of these show impressive short-term benefit, but longer-term efficacy and side effect profiles are not yet fully established.

Photochemotherapy (PUVA)

This treatment involves the use of an oral photosensitizing agent, a psoralen, and subsequent total body exposure 2 hours later to ultraviolet light in the UVA range (320–365 nm; psoralen + UVA = PUVA) in a specially designed cabinet (Fig. 5.15). This form of therapy should only be used for clearing psoriasis—induction therapy. Growing evidence of the increased risk of both melanoma and non-melanoma skin cancer associated with high dose long-term PUVA means that maintenance PUVA therapy cannot be recommended, and that an upper lifetime limit of 1000 J/m^2 prescribed UVA is regarded as the maximum safe total lifetime dose.

The combination of both oral retinoids and PUVA—RePUVA—is for some patients an effective method of psoriasis control, which allows lower doses of both UV and retinoids to be given. The normal pattern is to start oral retinoid treatment 10–14 days before introducing PUVA.

Psoralen is deposited in the lens of the eye, and PUVA-treated patients must therefore wear dark glasses during treatment and for 24 hours thereafter.

Current reviews of psoriasis therapies in regular use show a sharp decline in the number of patients with psoriasis receiving PUVA therapy, probably due to the now well-established carcinogenicity risk

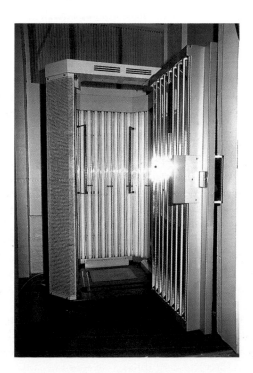

Fig. 5.15 A typical photochemotherapy (PUVA) cabinet.

Key points

Oral retinoids are not suitable antipsoriatic therapy for women of child bearing age.

Retinoids

Retinoids are synthetic vitamin A-like derivatives. The retinoid currently commercially available and most effective for disorders of keratinization is acetretin (Neotigason, Neotegason). The exact mode of action is not understood, but it is well recognized that vitamin A is necessary for normal keratinization. The usual starting dose is 25–30 mg orally daily for 2–4 weeks. Some heavier patients will require a slightly higher dose. Neotigason can be used relatively long-term to control psoriasis, provided patients are carefully monitored. Minor side effects include drying of the lips and nasal mucosa, and are easily dealt with by the liberal use of emollients. Retinoids may be associated with elevation of serum cholesterol and triglycerides, and assessment of fasting lipids pre-treatment and thereafter at 3–6-month intervals is therefore wise.

The most important point is that retinoids are teratogenic, and that young female patients must use a totally reliable form of contraception, both during retinoid therapy and for 2 years after cessation of therapy, as retinoids can be stored for long periods in the body fat. This means that oral retinoids are not appropriate psoriasis therapy for a younger female who has not yet completed her family.

As indicated under PUVA, the combination of an oral retinoid and PUVA can be effective, and reduce total dose requirements of either preparation.

Methotrexate

Methotrexate is a very useful cytotoxic drug for control of severe psoriasis. Control can usually be obtained with relatively small doses given at weekly intervals. Its particular advantage is its speed of action, as improvement of psoriasis may be seen within 48 hours of administration of methotrexate. It also has the advantage of having been in use for over 30 years, so side effects are well established.

Methotrexate can be given orally, intramuscularly, or intravenously. The usual dose required varies from 5 to 20 mg orally once weekly. Careful monitoring of haematological and hepatic function is essential. The most likely side-effects are marrow depression and hepatic fibrosis. Marrow depression is rare at the usual doses, provided there are no adverse drug interactions, and liver damage is related to the cumulative total dose and to any past hepatic problems, such as alcohol excess. Patients starting methotrexate should be counselled about avoiding or minimizing alcoholic intake, while on methotrexate.

If long-term methotrexate use is envisaged, a pre-therapy liver biopsy should be considered, as at present there are no non-invasive tests that give the equivalent information. This, however, has to be balanced against the fact that liver biopsy itself has a recognized morbidity and even mortality rate. Any patient who develops abnormal liver function tests while on methotrexate should have methotrexate discontinued and the need for liver biopsy again be considered. Patients who are on long-term methotrexate should also be considered for liver biopsy when they reach a cumulative total dose of 1.5 g.

Drug interactions are particularly important in patients on methotrexate. Non-steroidal anti-inflammatories, trimethoprim/sulphonamides, and systemic steroids are the main problems, and concomitant therapy with these should be avoided in patients on methotrexate. Patients on methotrexate should carry a patient information sheet and drug interaction warning card.

Cyclosporin

Systemic cyclosporin is an effective method of controlling severe psoriasis. It is given orally at a dose of 2–4 mg/kg/day, which can be reduced to a maintenance dose of 0.5–1 mg/kg/day as lesions clear. Initially, psoriatic plaques will clear rapidly, often within a week of starting treatment. However, psoriasis may return just as rapidly, when cyclosporin is withdrawn. Cyclosporin is thought to act on psoriasis by inhibition of calcineurin phosphatase. It is used mainly to achieve short-term control of severe unstable psoriasis, as long-term use is very often associated with toxicity.

The main toxicity associated with cyclosporin is renal damage and full renal function studies should be carried out prior to commencing a patient on cyclosporin. Blood pressure, serum creatinine, and urea should be measured and two creatinine clearance tests should be carried out. While on cyclosporin, blood pressure serum creatinine and urea should be measured monthly, and creatinine clearance repeated 3 6 monthly. The dose of cyclosporin should be reduced or withdrawn if creatinine climbs more than 25% above base line values and/or the diastolic blood pressure exceeds 95 mmHg. Known drug interactions in the case of cyclosporin include aminoglycosides, trimethoprim, ketoconazole, phenytoin, rifampicin, isoniazid, and non-steroidal anti-inflammatories. Again, patients should carry a patient information sheet and drug interaction warning.

Hydroxyurea

This drug is rarely used in the management of psoriasis, and would not normally be considered unless retinoids, cyclosporin, and methotrexate were inappropriate or treatment with these had failed. A 60% improvement in 60% of patients is reported. The dose is 1 g/day, and the main toxicities are bone marrow depression and teratogenicity. Patients on hydroxyurea, therefore, need regular haematological assessment and females must avoid pregnancy for 6 months after stopping the drug.

Mycophenolate mofetil

This drug has been used for several years in transplantation clinics to prevent organ rejection. The success of cyclosporin in controlling psoriasis led to trials of mycophenolate mofetil in psoriasis. The dose of mycophenolate mofetil (Cellcept) is up to 2 g orally daily, but many patients with psoriasis respond to much lower doses. It is generally effective, but takes 2–3 weeks to show benefit. Some patients cannot tolerate mycophenolate mofetil due to severe nausea.

Immune modulators that reduce the number of pathogenic T cells: Alefacept and denileukin diftitox

These drugs are fusion proteins Alefacept combines the binding site of lymphocyte function associated antigen 3 with the Fc portion of human IgG and denileukin diftitox combines IL2 with a subunit of diphtheria toxin. Current trials show good responses with a reassuring safety profile.

Drugs that inhibit T cell migration and activation: Efalizumab

This is a humanized anti-CD 11a monoclonal antibody, which affects T cell adhesion and subsequent migration. Results to date are promising.

Key points

Watch for drug interactions in patients on long term methotrexate

Drugs that divert the immune system Recombinant IL 10.

IL 10 down-regulates the excessive TH^1 response characteristic of psoriasis. Trials show an improvement in PASI scores with no toxicity

Cytokine modulating agents Etanercept and infliximab

There is current interest and enthusiasm for the experimental use of tumour necrosis factor alpha inhibitors in severe psoriasis. These preparations have shown considerable benefit in patients with psoriatic arthropathy and their use has now been extended to those with severe cutaneous psoriasis. Two currently available preparations are etanercept (Enbrel) given by subcutaneous injection and infliximab (Remicade) given by intravenous infusion. Both show dramatic improvements in lesions of psoriatic arthropathy and severe cutaneous psoriasis. However, the side effect profile of these preparations is not yet fully established, and there is concern about serious infection, sepsis, and reactivation of tuberculosis. Careful post-marketing surveillance should establish the true risk/benefit ratio of these exciting new approaches to psoriasis control.

Management of psoriasis of the nails

Severe nail involvement in psoriasis is probably impossible to treat in isolation. However, many systemic therapies used for psoriasis produce at least short-term improvement in nail problems.

Management of psoriatic arthropathy

Psoriatic arthropathy may respond, at least in part, to systemic methotrexate or to cyclosporin, Patients with severe problems of both cutaneous and psoriatic arthropathy should be managed jointly by a dermatologist and rheumatologist. It is obviously very important to avoid severe drug interactions with systemic therapy used for cutaneous psoriasis and non-steroidal anti-inflammatories prescribed for joint problems The anti-cytokine and immune modulating agents discussed above are likely to be used for these patients.

The Psoriasis Association has branches in many countries and publishes useful literature for patients. Many psoriatics find membership of this Association of value (e-mail: mail@psoriasis.demon.co.uk).

Lichen planus

Definition

This is a cutaneous disorder with itchy, flat-topped papules most commonly seen on the inner surfaces of the wrists and the lower legs. The mucous membranes are usually affected. Spontaneous resolution usually takes place in a period of 3 months to 2 years.

Prevalence

This disease accounts for 0.2–0.8% of dermatological out-patient consultations in Britain and North America.

Aetiology

The cause of lichen planus is unknown. A drug eruption virtually indistinguishable from so-called idiopathic lichen planus can be precipitated by a wide variety of drugs and the lesions of acute graft-versus-host disease are also very similar. This suggests that the problem has an underlying immunological basis. Lichen planus lesions can also be precipitated by trauma—the so-called Koebner phenomenon. There appears to be an association between lichen planus and primary biliary cirrhosis in some series, but the mechanism for this association if any is not understood

Clinical features

Classically, the onset is acute with intensely itchy, red or violet, shiny, flat-topped papules. The flexor surfaces of wrists, the forearms and legs are the usual sites (Fig. 5.16). The oral mucous membrane is often affected with white, spongy, slightly raised lesions, sometimes with a trabecular or lacy appearance, on the inner surfaces of the cheeks (Fig. 5.17). These lesions are commonly asymptomatic and, unless specifically looked for, they may well be missed. They are, however, an important point in establishing the diagnosis. Similar lesions may be seen on the genitalia.

The cutaneous lesions may persist for many months and characteristically develop a fine white network on their surface—a pattern called Wickham's striae. Pruritus generally tends to diminish in time. Rarer variants of lichen planus include:

- an annular or linear pattern;

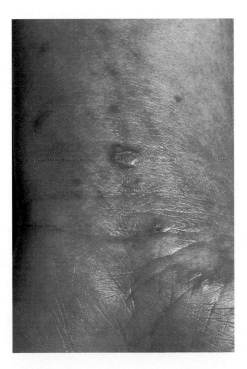

Fig. 5.16 Lichen planus seen on the classic site of the inner wrist area. Note the bluish-red, flat-topped papule with an overlying white network. This pattern is referred to as Wickham's striae.

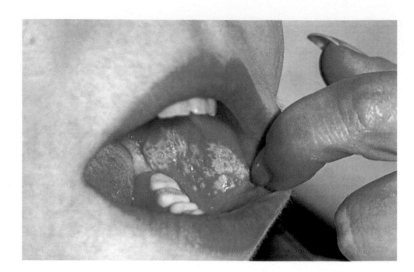

Fig. 5.17 Lichen planus of the oral mucous membranes. Note the white, web-line pattern on the inner surface of the cheek.

- atrophic;
- ulcerative;
- hypertrophic forms.

All of these tend to be more persistent and resistant to therapy than the classical type.

Involvement of the nails is seen in about 10% of patients, usually those with the more chronic skin lesions. Fine ridging or grooving, severe dystrophy, and even complete destruction of the nail bed may occur.

Pathology

The pathology of lichen planus is that of the lichenoid tissue reaction, a pattern that is seen in a number of skin conditions, such as lichenoid drug eruptions. 'Liquefaction degeneration' or selective destruction of the basal layer of the epidermis gives the dermo-epidermal junction a ragged, 'saw-toothed' outline. A mixed cell infiltrate is seen in the papillary dermis. This infiltrate varies in density, but tends to be found in close contact with the overlying epidermis and to contain some free melanin. Discrete round deposits of amorphous pink material may also be observed in the papillary dermis. These so-called 'colloid bodies' are thought to consist of disintegrating basal cells. There is a prominent, sometimes wedge-shaped, granular layer, and the epidermis is thinned in the atrophic and thickened in the hypertrophic form of the disease.

Immunofluorescence studies show large quantities of immunoglobulin on the colloid body surface. This is usually IgM and, although the resulting 'bunch of grapes' immunofluorescent pattern is striking, it is not diagnostic, as colloid bodies can be seen in a variety of states associated with basal cell degeneration.

Differential diagnosis

Lichen planus is normally fairly easily diagnosed on clinical grounds and histological confirmation is not always required. It is essential to take a good history to exclude the possibility of a lichenoid eruption due either to drugs (thiazides, anti-malarials, and gold) or to external contact with photographic colour developers. Occasionally, when the clinical picture resembles psoriasis, biopsy will be required. Persistent ulcerative or hypertrophic lesions should also be biopsied to confirm the diagnosis.

Therapy

The most important aspect of treatment of lichen planus for the patient is control of itch. Moderately potent topical steroids are the most useful preparation and, for persistent itch, systemic sedating antihistamines may help. Stubborn lesions associated with severe and persistent itch may respond to intra-lesional steroid injections.

Some dermatologists advocate a short course of systemic steroids for early severe cases, but the evidence that this is effective is lacking.

Synthetic retinoids given systemically have been reported to be of benefit in some studies of treatment of severe cutaneous or oral lichen planus and systemic cyclosporin A has also been reported of benefit in a few cases. These drugs should not be used in mildly itchy cases involving only a small surface area, as the condition is usually self-limiting in 3–4 months.

Pityriasis rosea

Definition

A self-limiting disorder characterized by the development of asymptomatic erythematous scaling macules on the trunk.

Incidence and aetiology

Pityriasis rosea is most commonly seen in children and young adults. An increased incidence in spring and autumn, and outbreaks in institutions suggest that an infective agent, possibly viral, may be the aetiological agent. Recent studies of involvement of the human herpes viruses 6 and 7 have produced equivocal results.

Clinical features

The first clinical lesion in pityriasis rosea is the herald patch, an isolated pink or red patch with a peripheral collarette of scale. This is usually seen on the trunk, up to a week before the main eruption appears and is followed by the development of oval macules, also with peripheral scaling, on the trunk, thighs, and upper arms. The trunk lesions tend to have their long axes parallel to the ribs, giving a so-called 'Christmas tree' distribution of the lesions (Fig. 5.18). Involvement of the hands, feet, or scalp is rare, and lesions are usually asymptomatic although there may be mild pruritus.

Pityriasis rosea generally remits spontaneously in 4–8 weeks, but atypical or severe forms may last longer.

Pathology

This is non-diagnostic, and an accurate history and careful clinical examination are more reliable aids to diagnosis. If a biopsy is performed a moderately dense,

> ### *Key points*
> Pityriasis rosea is self-limiting, usually affects the young, and causes asymptomatic, oval macules on the trunk, upper arms, and thighs.

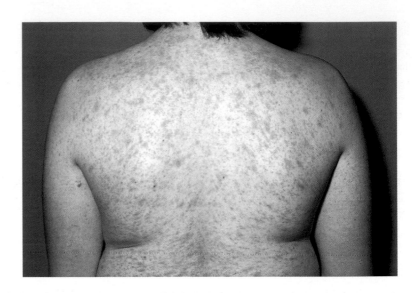

Fig. 5.18 Pityriasis rosea with typical involvement of the trunk. Secondary syphilis is an important differential diagnosis to consider.

mainly lymphocytic dermal infiltrate, papillary oedema, and a few extravasated red blood cells may be seen. Spongiosis may be seen in the epidermis at the edge of a developing lesion. This histological picture is very similar to that of secondary syphilis. Serological tests will differentiate between the two conditions.

Differential diagnosis

Secondary syphilis, drug eruptions, pityriasis versicolor, and occasionally guttate psoriasis may all cause confusion. Serological studies will exclude syphilis and negative mycological examination will exclude pityriasis versicolor. A good history will eliminate a drug eruption and, occasionally, a biopsy may be required to rule out psoriasis.

Therapy

Itch can be relieved by a moderate potency topical steroid until the lesions clear spontaneously.

Pityriasis rubra pilaris

Definition

A rare red scaly skin condition with characteristic papules concentrated around the hair follicles.

Incidence and aetiology

Pityriasis rubra pilaris (PRP) is uncommon. There are several clinical variants including a familial type with autosomal dominant inheritance. The cause is not yet known. It can easily be confused clinically with psoriasis.

Clinical features

In typical cases there is, on the trunk, extensive erythema in which occasional islands of normal skin can be seen. Follicular papules, said to look like a nutmeg grater, appear on the backs of the fingers, and a striking yellow-coloured hyperkeratosis develops on the palms and soles (Fig. 5.19). There are no symptoms and the patient is well.

The condition usually clears spontaneously in 6 months to 2 years.

Pathology

There is hyperkeratosis and parakeratosis around hair follicle openings, a mild inflammatory infiltrate in the papillary dermis, and apparent enlargement of the arrector pili muscles.

This is a non-specific picture and diagnosis should be based on clinical, rather than on histological appearances.

Differential diagnosis

Occasionally, a biopsy will be needed to differentiate between PRP, and either psoriasis or seborrhoeic dermatitis.

Therapy

This is difficult and unsatisfactory. A proportion of patients do well on acetretin (neotigason) 20–30 mg/day for 4 months or less if the condition resolves. Low doses of oral methotrexate 5–15 mg weekly may also be helpful. Topical treatment with a keratolytic containing 2% salicylic acid may be useful to help reduce hyperkeratosis of the palms and soles, and moderate potency topical steroid may reduce itch. PRP does not respond well to oral steroids.

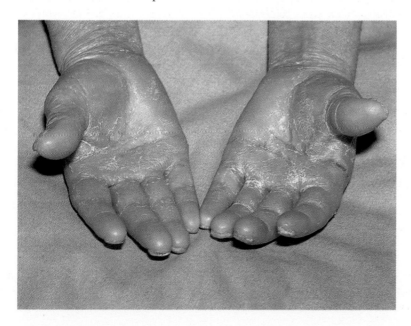

Fig. 5.19 Palms in pityriasis rubra pilaris, showing typical thickened yellow appearance of the epidermis.

Darier's disease

Definition

A genetically determined disease characterized by abnormal keratinization based mainly on the hair follicles and causing a greasy, reddish-brown papular eruption.

Aetiology and incidence

The gene for Darier's disease is situated on the long arm of chromosome 12 and is the ATP2A2 gene that codes for the sarcoplasmic/endoplasmic reticulum calcium ATPase, SERCA A2. The disease is transmitted by autosomal dominant inheritance, but as many patients have a negative family history, new mutations appear to be common. The reported prevalence varies from 1/30,000 to 1/100,000.

Clinical features

Darier's disease is usually first seen in young adults as greasy brown papules on the chest and scapular area. It may be aggravated by sunlight and may have an acute onset after sunburn (Fig. 5.20). Small pits on the skin of the palm of the hand and irregular nicks at the distal end of the nails are also present (Fig. 5.21). Cutaneous infections with herpes simplex may give rise to very severe widespread infection—so-called Kaposi's varicelliform eruption in patients with Darier's disease, suggesting that they have a localized immune defect.

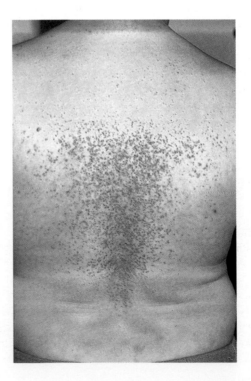

Fig. 5.20 Darier's disease. The greasy papules on this young man's back appeared for the first time as a severe episode of sunburn was fading from the mid-zone of his trunk.

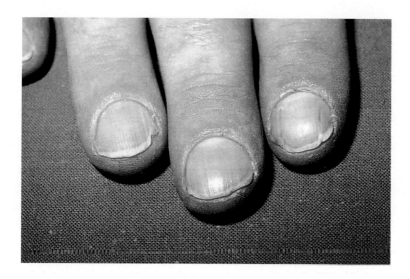

Fig. 5.21 Nails in Darier's disease showing striking nicking at the free margin.

Pathology

Abnormalities of keratinocytes are seen in the lower layers of the epidermis. Prematurely keratinized cells (corps ronds) and distorted keratinocyte nuclei ('grains') are seen causing parakeratosis.

Treatment

Some patients with very mild Darier's disease may require no specific treatment. For others, with the more severe forms of the disease, acetretin (Neotigason) 20 mg/day is very effective. As with the treatment of severe psoriasis with retinoids, caution must be taken to ensure that the drug is not given to pregnant women, and that contraception is maintained for a minimum of 2 years after stopping the drug because of teratogenicity and a long half-life of acetretin. Cheilitis is a common minor side effect and temporary elevation of triglycerides may occur, particularly if the patient is obese.

Moderate potency topical steroids for itch and salicylic acid preparations to reduce scaling have largely been superseded by the retinoids.

The Ichthyoses

Definition

Disorders of keratinization, usually genetically determined, characterized by excessively dry and visibly scaly skin. There may also be associated erythema and in the neonate some of these conditions may present as a blistering problem.

Currently, two groups of relatively rare skin problems, the ichthyoses and the inherited group of blistering disorders, epidermolysis bullosa, are attracting considerable attention from geneticists and molecular biologists. Mutations associated with subtypes of these two groups of skin diseases are being reported with increasing frequency. These developments clearly increase our academic knowledge of these diseases and it will be important to see if this increased knowledge at the molecular level can be translated to therapy.

- autosomal dominant ichthyosis vulgaris;
- autosomal recessive or lamellar ichthyosis;
- X-linked recessive ichthyosis;
- bullous ichthyosiform erythroderma (epidermolytic hyperkeratosis).

The majority of patients with ichthyosis present in infancy and childhood. The remainder first show clinical signs of the condition in adolescence or adult life. It has been reported in some series that a proportion of patients with adult-onset ichthyosis may have an underlying neoplasm, usually of haematological origin.

Autosomal dominant ichthyosis vulgaris

In the UK, autosomal dominant ichthyosis is common, having a prevalence of 1:250 to 1:300. There is an underlying disorder of keratinization seen on light microscopy as an absent epidermal granular layer.

Clinical features

Affected children present in early childhood with a rough, dry skin, most marked on the extensor surfaces of the arms and worst in winter. The scales are fine and white. Many children have rough, horny papules, seen best on the extensor surfaces of the upper arms, thought to be due to faulty keratinization around hair follicle openings (Fig. 5.22). The skin of patients with atopic dermatitis is dry, but the relationship of this xerosis (dry skin) to true ichthyosis is uncertain. Dominant

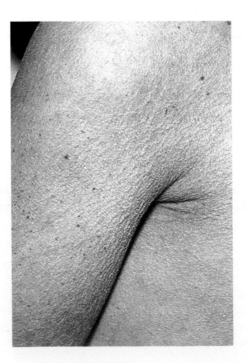

Fig. 5.22 Autosomal dominant ichthyosis. Fine, white scales are most profuse on the upper arms.

ichthyosis vulgaris tends to improve slowly during childhood and puberty, but may also persist into adult life.

Treatment

This depends on the use of lubricants and emulsifying preparations. Excessive use of soap should be discouraged and emulsifying ointments substituted. Water-soluble oils should be added to bath water or used after bathing. Preparations containing urea in a water-miscible base may help to maintain adequate hydration of the stratum corneum, (for example, Calmurid), but some patients complain of intense stinging for a few minutes after their application. Topical steroids should not be used routinely to lubricate dry skin.

Autosomal recessive or lamellar ichthyosis

A serious scaling condition in which the infant may present at birth in a transparent membrane. This infant is referred to as a collodion baby. There may be serious associated ocular problems due to ectropion. The infant then develops extensive thick scales on an underlying erythematous base. Alopecia and nail dystrophy are also common.

Some of these children have mutations in the gene coding for glutaminase on chromosome 14q11, while other associated mutations have been reported on chromosomes 2q, 3p, 17p, and 19p.

Treatment is symptomatic with copious use of emollients and avoidance of over-heating.

Sex-linked recessive ichthyosis (ichthyosis nigricans)

Prevalence and aetiology

This is very much rarer than the autosomal dominant variety and, although the fully developed disease is seen in males only, female heterozygotes may have mild degrees of the condition, mainly on the lower legs. An associated abnormality is a deficiency of the enzyme steroid sulphatase seen in both affected children and carrier mothers. This enzyme deficiency can be detected in the placenta, but does not appear to be associated with any increased incidence of perinatal problems, although affected mothers may give a history of excessively long labours. The gene appears to be in the Xp22.32 locus

Clinical features

There are large, greasy, polygonal, yellow, or brown scales mainly on the trunk (Fig. 5.23) and limbs with some sparing of the flexures. There may be associated ocular problems with corneal opacities.

Pathology

There is a striking increase in the granular layer with a thickened overlying stratum corneum.

There is little tendency for the condition to improve with time. Removing the scales with abrasion and copious emollients are the usual methods of controlling the disease. Use of systemic retinoids has produced conflicting reports, but gene transfer is a possible future approach.

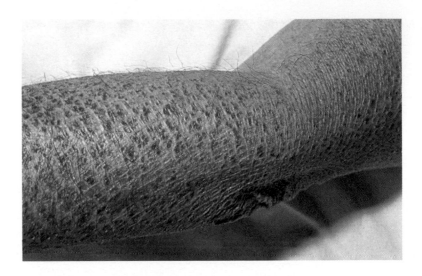

Fig. 5.23 Ichthyosis nigricans (sex-linked ichthyosis vulgaris). The scales are large, greasy, and yellowish in colour.

Bullous ichthyosiform erythroderma

A rare disorder in which patients have both erythrodermatous skin and blisters in varying combinations. This condition is inherited by autosomal dominant transmission, and is caused by mutations in the genes for keratins 1 and 10 on chromosomes 12q and 17q.

Biopsy of affected skin shows very characteristic blister formation within the epidermis, even if the area chosen for biopsy is not clinically bullous. Affected babies usually have extensive blistering and desquamation at birth, sometimes giving rise to fluid balance problems. In later life, scaling on an erythematous base predominates.

Treatment

Liberal use of emollients is the best approach. Oral retinoids have again not been uniformly successful.

Other very rare ichthyotic conditions include those with systemic associations such as Refsum's syndrome, due to a specific defect in phytanic acid metabolism, and characterized by ichthyosis, retinitis pigmentosa, and neurological defects.

Discussion of problem cases (see p. 55)

Case 5.1

The important points in this woman's history are, first, that she wishes for a cosmetically acceptable method of controlling her psoriasis and, secondly, that this remedy must not be teratogenic in view of her wish to conceive. At her age, time is not on her side.

In general, in younger adults, it is preferable to try to control psoriasis with topical treatment as all systemic approaches to psoriasis management have some toxicity. PUVA can give rise to cutaneous malignancies, methotrexate is toxic to the liver

Discussion of problem cases continued

and cyclosporin can cause renal toxicity. All of these complications are related to the cumulative total dose, so starting systemic treatment of any type as late in life as possible makes sense in the case of a chronic relapsing and remitting disease. None of the above systemic agents are safe for use in young women of child-bearing potential who are not taking full contraceptive precautions, usually the oral contraceptive.

Oral retinoids are less toxic to the patient him or herself long term, but are absolutely ruled out in this woman's case as they are potent teratogens. In addition, they are stored in the body fat for as long as 2 years after discontinuation of oral administration, so if a 36-year-old were given a retinoid she could not even attempt to conceive until she was 38, whether or not this successfully cleared her psoriasis.

We, therefore, come to the choices of topical therapy in various combinations with or without added UVB therapy. Topical tar is effective, but messy to apply and the cleaner proprietary tars tend to be less effective. Topical dithranol is effective, but may irritate the surrounding normal skin and must therefore be used with care. Calcipotriol or calcipotriene is moderately effective, but rarely removes all traces of psoriasis.

Any of these three preparations can be used in association with UVB radiation therapy. Current evidence suggests that the use of narrow band UVB therapy in the 310–312 nm range is more effective than broader band UV and has less risk of long-term side effects, particularly carcinogenesis, as lower cumulative total doses are needed.

Our patient wanted a full discussion of the possible treatment options including a full explanation as to why none of the 'psoriasis pills' were appropriate for her. She opted for a weak concentration of proprietary dithranol (0.25% with gradually increasing concentrations to 1.0% dithocream). This was applied as short-contact dithranol with the patient using it for 20–30 minutes each morning before showering and dressing for work. In addition, she had a 6-week course of narrow band UVB therapy, attending three times a week after work at the local out-patient treatment centre. On this regime her psoriasis cleared well and remained clear for the next 4 months, during which she had a 2-week Mediterranean holiday that was almost certainly of additional value in maintaining her clearance.

Six months later she returned with mild psoriasis and 8 weeks pregnant. Her psoriasis remained virtually clear throughout pregnancy, quite a common observation, but flared again 6 weeks after delivery. A further course of UVB at the local out-patient treatment centre cleared the lesions and did not interfere with breast feeding.

She asks you about the chances that her son will develop psoriasis. How will you reply?

Case 5.2

This elderly gentleman lives alone and the nearest dermatology out-patient treatment centre is 20 miles away. His psoriasis is seriously affecting his ability to continue to live independently and his arthritis makes it very difficult for him to use topical treatments. Possible approaches here would include:

1. Regular (daily or 3–4 times a week) topical applications with help from the local district nurse or practice nurse.

Discussion of problem cases continued

2. Systemic treatment with retinoids, methotrexate, or cyclosporin A.

Initially, a trial of district nurse management was conducted. She came in three times a week to help in applying first weak tar and then calcipotriol. However, on both of these routines, his psoriasis flared and became irritable. Topical, moderate potency steroids were also tried but also with little benefit. After some discussion, the patient was then given a 6-week trial of oral methotrexate, 10 mg weekly, once it had been established that his liver function was normal and his creatinine clearance adequate for his age. He was counselled to avoid all alcohol, while he was taking methotrexate. His psoriasis cleared within 3 weeks on this regime with no elevation of liver function tests or serum creatinine, or fall in white cell count. His arthropathy also improved to the extent that he planned his first holiday in 6 years. He continues to take his oral methotrexate 10 mg orally weekly under district nurse supervision, attends the general practitioner monthly for liver function tests and white cell counts, and sees his local consultant dermatologist quarterly.

1. What advice **must** this patient be given about drug interactions and methotrexate?

2. What specific investigation should be considered as a base line in patients in whom you are contemplating methotrexate therapy long term?

3. What are the risks and benefits of carrying out this particular investigation?

4. If this patient responds poorly to methotrexate, would you discuss cytokine inhibitors, e.g. TNF alpa inhibitors with him?

Case 5.3

While the description of the lesions might suggest insect bites, they do not usually last as long as 6 weeks. Again, the timing and duration of therapy do not suggest that a drug eruption is a likely diagnosis. The site of the lesions and the itch both suggest lichen planus as a possible diagnosis. On examination, the patient had white patches in her mouth. A small punch biopsy was taken from the wrist and showed a lichenoid tissue reaction, compatible with a diagnosis of lichen planus. The lesions cleared slowly over the next 5 months during which moderate potency topical steroids were prescribed.

Case 5.4

The history here suggests the possibility of impetigo complicating severe sunburn or possibly secondary viral infection on pre-existing eczema. However, there is no past personal or family history of eczema.

Swabs were taken for bacteriological and viral culture, and the young man started on topical and systemic anti-staphylococcal antibiotics. Two days later the virologists reported a heavy growth of herpes simplex type 1 and he was started on full doses of systemic acyclovir. The infection cleared rapidly, leaving raised papules on his back. A biopsy of one of these showed disruption of the epidermis with grains and corps ronds. This pattern is diagnostic of Darier's disease. Darier's disease appears frequently for the first time after sun damage, and is a condition associated with severe secondary h. simplex infection or Kaposi's varicelliform eruption. What other signs might this young man have?

Special study module projects

1. Ask as many patients as you can approach with psoriasis who you see in general practice, in the out-patient department treatment centre, or in the dermatology ward for 5 minutes of their time. Prepare a brief 2-page questionnaire asking how they feel about their psoriasis and how this has affected their lives. Include questions on family problems, difficult situations at work, on holidays, on relationships with the opposite sex, and possible problems relating to the hairdresser and buying clothes. Ask them if there was a complete cure for psoriasis how much they would be willing to pay for it. Relate the sum they quote to their lifestyle and apparent income.

   What are the common features, and what has this study told you about psoriasis and disability?

   Could any of the points brought up by these patients you have spoken to be relevant to any other dermatological conditions?

2. Make a list of the systemic drugs used in the management of patients with psoriasis. Draw up an appropriate information and drug interaction warning card for patients who are on each of these systemic therapies to carry. Think carefully about any necessary regular investigations and how often these should be done. If you were the general practitioner of patients on these drugs, what specific points would you look for in the letter from the local dermatologist.

Further reading

British Association of Dermatologists (1995) *Guidelines for the management of patients with psoriasis*. BAD, London.

Camisa, C. (1994) *Psoriasis.* Blackwell Scientific, Oxford.

Roenigk, H.H. and Maibach, H.I. (eds) (1990) *Psoriasis*, 2nd edn. Marcel Dekker, New York.

Van der Kerkhof, P. (ed.) (1999) *Textbook of psoriasis*. Blackwells, Oxford.

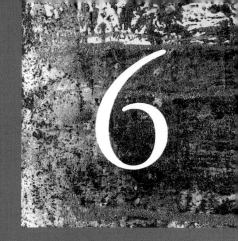

6

Dermatitis and eczema

- Problem cases

- The terms dermatitis and eczema

- Mechanisms of cutaneous inflammation

- Acute, subacute, and chronic dermatitis

- Atopic dermatitis

- Nummular or discoid dermatitis

- Asteatotic eczema (eczema craquelé)

- Seborrhoeic dermatitis

- Contact dermatitis

- Dishydrotic eczema

- Neurodermatitis

- Prurigo nodularis

- Stasis dermatitis

- Patient association

- Discussion of problem cases

- Special study module

Dermatitis and eczema

Problem cases

Case 6.1

A young couple come to see you together to ask for your help in treating their first child, a boy now aged 9 months, who has had red apparently itchy skin since the age of 3 months. He is very irritable, sleeps badly, and scratches continually. His parents say they are desperate. What is the likely diagnosis, are any investigations required, and how would you manage the child?

Case 6.2

A 28-year-old postdoctoral scientist in your local University consults you about persistent dandruff, sticky eyes, a rash in the nasolabial fold, and a vague generalized itch. He is very concerned about scabies. What diagnosis does this presentation suggest and what is your management plan?

Case 6.3

An 18-year-old hairdresser consults you about dry, scaly patches on the dorsum of her hands, which have developed over the past year. She started hairdressing 2 years ago and has a past history of asthma as a child. She herself blames the perm lotion, which comes into contact with her skin even though she wears rubber gloves most of the time. What is the likely diagnosis and what investigations and treatment are indicated?

Case 6.4

A 69-year-old, obese, retired teacher consults you about dermatitis around her right ankle with obvious underlying varicose veins. The skin is red, irritable, and inflamed. She has been applying a cream to it given to her by her sister, but thinks that this may have made the problem worse. What investigations and treatment might be appropriate here?

Suggested diagnoses and treatment plans will be found on p. 127–8.

The varieties of eczema and dermatitis that will be discussed in this chapter are:
- atopic dermatitis;
- nummular dermatitis (discoid dermatitis);
- asteatotic eczema (eczema craquelé);
- seborrhoeic dermatitis;
- contact dermatitis: direct irritant, including napkin dermatitis and allergic contact dermatitis;
- dishydrotic eczema (pompholyx);
- neurodermatitis (circumscribed lichen simplex);
- prurigo nodularis;
- stasis dematitis.

The terms dermatitis and eczema

The term dermatitis simply means inflammation of the skin and can be qualified according to the likely cause, but eczema has no clear universally agreed definition. In the past, there has been a suggestion that one could think of this group of disorders as either exogenous—due to an obvious external cause—or endogenous—no obvious external cause and assumed to be due to genetic susceptibility. This led to the idea that the term eczema should be used to describe endogenous problems and dermatitis for exogenous problems. This distinction has become artificial as we understand better, for example, the interaction between environmental and genetic factors in atopic dermatitis. For these reasons, most dermatologists prefer the term dermatitis, rather than eczema to describe this group of disorders, qualified by the type of dermatitis, as it is simply and clearly defined as inflammation of the skin, and the pathological appearance is also well established.

Mechanisms of cutaneous inflammation

Cell marker studies have established that the T lymphocyte is preferentially recruited into the dermis and epidermis in the great majority of cutaneous inflammatory processes, and in most situations the CD4$^+$ helper T lymphocyte is found in much larger numbers than the CD8$^+$ T cytotoxic or suppressor subset. In patients with atopic dermatitis, the majority of these T helper lymphocytes are of the TH2 subset.

If timed sequential biopsies are carried out of skin on which inflammation has been deliberately induced, polymorphonuclear leukocytes will be found about 4–6 hours after applying the inflammatory stimulus. By 24 hours, virtually all the cells present are lymphocytes. Both lymphocyte function associated antigen (LFA) and gamma interferon are also expressed in the epidermis, and on cells in the papillary dermis early in the dermatitis reaction. The role of tumour necrosis factor alpha in these interactions is also currently under investigation.

The role of the Langerhans cell in the inflammatory reaction in the skin and particularly in the induction of allergic contact dermatitis, is now partly understood. Langerhans cells can function as antigen-presenting cells, although they are not as efficient as macrophages. Potentially antigenic materials absorbed through the skin become bound to the surface of Langerhans cells, which can then traffic in the lymphatic system to the local draining lymph nodes, where the development of a specifically sensitized clone of lymphocytes takes place. What is not understood is the reason why any one contact with, for example, nickel, results in sensitization and subsequent contact dermatitis, while many other apparently identical events, both in other individuals and in the patient himself prior to his developing dermatitis, do not.

Acute, subacute, and chronic dermatitis

Dermatitis of any of the clinical varieties discussed below may be acute, subacute, or chronic. Each of these three stages has distinct clinical and pathological appearances. It is necessary to be able to identify these three phases or stages in the dermatitis reaction as they all require different approaches to treatment. At any time, one lesion on a patient may be acute, while a second lesion on another part of the body may be subacute or even chronic. This is particularly true of atopic dermatitis.

Table 6.1 Clinical and pathological features of the acute, subacute, and chronic phases of the dermatitis reaction

	Acute	Subacute	Chronic
Clinical	Redness, swelling, oozing,	Redness, swelling, crusting	Scaling, thickening of the skin and increase in
	Formation of small blisters,	Scaling, secondary infection	skin markings—lichenification. Itch
	Pain, heat, tenderness	Itch—may be severe	Scaling, parakeratosis
Pathological	Dermal and epidermal oedema (spongiosis)	Crusting and parakeratosis	Marked acanthosis (epidermal thickening)
	Dilated and congested dermal capillaries	Early acanthosis Oedema	Coarsening of papillary dermal collagen
	Dermal infiltrate very early leucocytes, later lymphocytes	Perivascular lymphocytic dermal infiltrate Few lymphocytes also in dermis	

Acute dermatitis is painfully inflamed oedematous oozing epidermis, which is seen on biopsy as an area of gross oedema within the epidermis, pushing individual keratinocytes apart, and thus causing the development of vesicles or small blisters.

Subacute dermatitis is the presence of visible scale and crust associated with inflamed skin, and on biopsy one sees the scaling and crusting, and also the epidermal disruption with a lymphocytic infiltrate among the keratinocytes.

Chronic dermatitis is seen as a thickened, often purple or violaceous, elevated plaque, and this on biopsy is seen as epidermal acanthosis or thickening of the keratinocyte layer with a lymphocytic infiltrate in the papillary dermis.

Atopic dermatitis

Definition

A chronic extremely itchy form of dermatitis with a strong genetic aetiological component, usually beginning in infancy, and frequently associated with asthma and rhinitis.

Prevalence and aetiology

Atopic dermatitis currently affects up to 20% of children in the UK, and similar or higher prevalence figures are reported from the US, Scandinavia and Australia. It is a skin disease that must be recognized and understood by all those working in dermatology, in paediatrics, and in primary care worldwide. In adults the incidence is lower, but the severity of the disease and the disability it causes tend to be greater. Children with atopic dermatitis are a very high proportion of those attending paediatric dermatology clinics and the disease is an important cause of childhood morbidity with significant loss of time from education for those most severely affected. It is also an expensive disease, both for families and for the health care systems worldwide. In certain ethnic groups, such as the Chinese, it seems to be rarer, but more severe and persistent than in Caucasians.

Table 6.2 lists some complications of atopic dermatitis.

Table 6.2 **Problems associated with atopic dermatitis**

Dermatological
Severe infection with herpes simplex type 1—eczema herpeticum
Increased colonization of the epidermis by *Staphylococcus aureus*
Dry skin—either xerosis of atopy or autosomal dominant ichthyosis
Dry and prominent hair follicles, particularly on upper arms—keratosis pilaris
Juvenile plantar dermatosis; shiny, tender soles of feet with tendency to fissure formation
In female adults, nipple dermatitis
Increased incidence of persistent and stubborn warts and *Molluscum contagiosum*
Ocular
Cataract and keratoconus
Gastrointestinal
Food intolerance and food allergy

Environmental triggers to development of atopic dermatitis

Cohort studies of children born in the UK over the last 20 years show that the incidence and prevalence of all types of atopic disease are rising, and appear to be rising faster in higher income small families. This has led to a hypothesis that increased levels of hygiene and decreased natural exposure to micro-organisms in infancy delay or prevent maturation of the immune system, and thus lead to atopic dermatitis. This 'hygiene hypothesis' is, however, not in keeping with the observation that exposure to high levels of house dust mite in infancy are associated with development of atopic dermatitis.

Genetics of atopic dermatitis

Most patients with atopic dermatitis have a positive family history of the atopic triad—dermatitis, asthma, and allergic rhinitis. The concordance for atopic dermatitis is high in monozygotic twins at 85% and much lower at around 20% in dizygotic twins, clearly indicating a large genetic susceptibility element, which interacts with the environment in leading to development of atopic dermatitis. Many past studies of the genetics of atopy have concentrated on respiratory atopy, but recent genetic work looking specifically at atopic dermatitis has revealed a major susceptibility locus at chromosome 3q21 with other possible susceptibility loci at 1q21, 17q25 and 20p. Some of these loci are very close to those identified as possible psoriasis susceptibility sites (see p. 56), suggesting that they may be loci associated with genes important in cutaneous reactivity and inflammation in general.

Maternal and infant diet and atopic dermatitis *

This area has been researched in great detail over the past decade with conflicting results. A small proportion of children and adults with severe atopic dermatitis have clinical allergies to eggs, cows milk, other dairy products, and peanuts, and a higher proportion of these patients have elevated levels of specific IgE to these foodstuffs, but no clinical evidence of adverse allergic reactions to these substances. This has led to trials of elimination diets both in affected children and adults, and also in pregnant mothers with a strong family history of atopic dermatitis. Results suggest that in a small proportion of severely affected patients, specific exclusion diets may be beneficial. There have been many studies carried out to establish a relationship between breast-feeding and a reduction in the incidence of atopic dermatitis, but the most recent reports do not suggest that breast-feeding, short term or prolonged, prevents development of atopic dermatitis, despite the many other advantages of breast-feeding.

Immunological aspects of atopic dermatitis

Serum levels of immunoglobulin E are elevated in 80% of atopic dermatitis patients, but within the normal range in the remaining 20%. Conversely, about 5% of the normal population have elevated IgE levels, but are clinically normal. Thus, an elevated IgE level is neither necessary nor sufficient for a diagnosis of atopic dermatitis.

The results of radioallergosorbent testing (RAST) to determine the specific antigens against which IgE is synthesized, differ in infants and older children. In infants, high RAST levels will be found against foods—usually eggs, dairy products, and fish. At around 1 year of age the pattern changes and the bulk of the elevated IgE is directed against inhaled allergens, such as the house dust mite (*D. pteronissinus*), animal hair, and pollens.

Our current understanding of the complex immunological abnormalities observed in patients with atopic dermatitis suggests the there is a disorder of immune regulation involving an imbalance in number and function of T cell subsets. In atopic dermatitis there is over activity of the TH2 lymphocyte subset. These lymphocytes produce interleukin 4 and interleukin 5, which in turn stimulate IgE production by B lymphocytes. In contrast, the numbers and activity of TH1 lymphocytes is low. TH1 lymphocytes stimulate production of gamma interferon and the fact that the cord blood levels of gamma interferon are low in babies born to atopic mothers and who subsequently develop atopic dermatitis themselves, suggests that this could be a primary, rather than a secondary immunological event in the development of atopic dermatitis. These low levels of gamma interferon may be due to increased activity of cyclic AMP phosphodiesterase, which cause increased synthesis of prostaglandin E2 that, in turn, inhibits gamma interferon production, thus perpetuating a cycle of over-activity.

Atopic dermatitis, and bacterial or viral infections

Patients with atopic dermatitis frequently have skin that is colonized by staphylococci. There is not always obvious secondary bacterial infection visible, but these patients do tend to improve if an anti-staphylococcal antibiotic is added to their treatment regime. It is thought that the reason for this is that staphylococci secrete super-antigens, which even in minute quantities stimulate T cells and thus cause release of pro-inflammatory cytokines.

Sufferers from atopic dermatitis also tend to have a very severe reaction to exposure to the herpes simplex type 1 virus, and may develop eczema herpeticum (see p. 102). This over-brisk reaction to the virus may also be triggered by super-antigen activity.

Both viral warts and molluscum contagiosum (p. 142) appear to be commoner and more persistent in children with atopic dermatitis.

> ### *Key points*
> Atopic dermatitis sufferers are prone to severe superimposed herpes simplex infection.

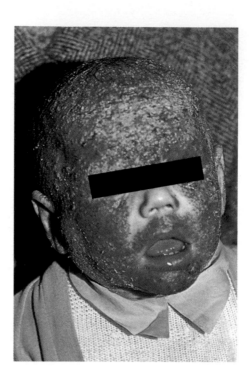

Fig. 6.1 Atopic dermatitis in infancy. The face and scalp are often affected in young children, and relative sparing of the perioral and nasal region is common as seen here.

In atopic dermatitis there are also vascular abnormalities as the cutaneous vasculature responds abnormally to stimulation. Instead of a normal 'weal and flare' response, firm rubbing of the skin elicits **white dermographism** as a simple white linear streak along the site of pressure with no erythema.

Clinical features

Sixty per cent of those who have atopic dermatitis first develop it in infancy. It may appear as early as 6 weeks, with apparently itchy scaly lesions on the scalp, face, and trunk. The infant will be irritable and wakeful, and tries to rub the affected areas. In babies the cheeks, wrists, and hands are usually red, scaling, and scratched, but even in severe disease there may be sparing of the central panel of the face (Fig. 6.1). Most children and adults with atopic dermatitis have a very dry skin and, in some cases, they have autosomal dominant ichthyosis.

In toddlers and older children, the common sites of involvement are the elbow, knee, and buttock flexures, the ankles, the dorsa of the feet under straps of shoes, the retroauricular fold, and the antecubital fossae (Fig. 6.2). In severe cases there may be extensive involvement of all four limbs with gross excoriation and secondary infection. Some children with atopic dermatitis develop shiny hacked skin on the soles of the feet. This is called juvenile plantar dermatosis and may also be seen in non-atopics. Despite the suggestive appearance, these children do not have a footwear allergy.

In a high proportion of affected children atopic dermatitis clears spontaneously between the ages of 2 and 5 years, but if it continues into adolescence and adult life it develops into the more chronic type, with striking lichenification in the

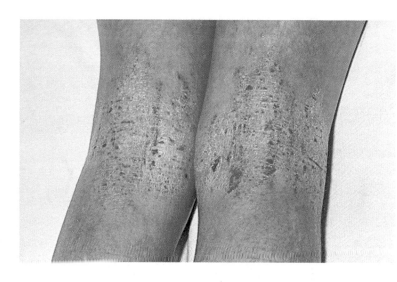

Fig. 6.2 Atopic dermatitis involving the knee flexures in a 10 year-old child. Note both lichenification and recent excoriations.

popliteal and antecubital fossae, and on the nape of the neck (Fig. 6.3). Prominent infra-orbital creases are also seen, giving the child or adult a weary and prematurely aged expression. Thinning of the lateral half of the eyebrows (Hertoghe's sign) is frequently present, due to continual rubbing. Shiny fingernails result from buffing rather than scratching the lesions.

Adults with atopic dermatitis tend to have a generalized dry skin associated with diffuse, itchy plaques involving large areas of the trunk and face. Some women with atopic dermatitis develop difficult and painful lesions around the nipples.

Some patients with atopic dermatitis also have autosomal dominant ichthyosis vulgaris and 'keratosis pilaris' may also be present. This consists of horny papules at the orifices of the hair follicles, and is most easily seen and felt on the outer surface of the upper arm.

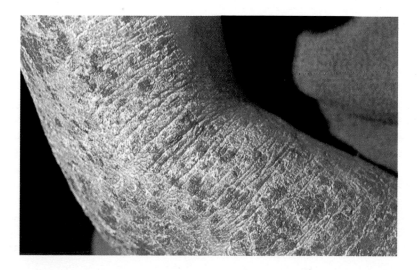

Fig. 6.3 Severe atopic dermatitis in an adult. Note gross lichenification and superimposed excoriations.

Many patients with atopic dermatitis also have asthma, which may either be very active at the same time as the skin or flare independently.

Atopic dermatitis and contact dermatitis

Large epidemiological studies suggest that patients with atopic dermatitis have a lower incidence of allergic contact dermatitis, but are more susceptible than non-atopics to irritant contact dermatitis. It is most important, therefore, to offer atopic adolescents guidance about careers and to indicate those occupations that are inadvisable. Many atopic girls are interested in a nursing career because of their knowledge of hospital life, but this may be difficult as continual exposure to soap disinfectants and water is likely to cause the skin to flare. Many student nurse training courses will not take individuals with a past history of atopic dermatitis for this reason.

Investigations

Internationally agreed criteria for the diagnosis of atopic dermatitis have been established, based on clinical features of the disease. The UK modification of these criteria is that to make the diagnosis of atopic dermatitis the presence of itch for the preceding 12 months is required plus two or more of flexural dermatitis, onset before the age of 2 years, a personal history of asthma or hay fever, and dry skin. Specific investigations are, therefore, rarely required to confirm the diagnosis in patients with atopic dermatitis and the diagnosis should be made on clinical grounds.

As stated above, not all patients with atopic dermatitis have a raised IgE so a normal level will not exclude the diagnosis. Blood should not be taken routinely from infants with suspected atopic dermatitis as IgE levels are usually within the normal range until after 6 months, even if the infant has severe dermatitis.

Prick tests to a wide range of allergens can be carried out on older children and adults, but they tend to give a wide range of positive results, which are not all of any clinical relevance. They are not recommended as a therapeutically useful routine investigation and can be very distressing to young children.

Bacteriological swabs taken from affected areas of skin will usually show a heavy growth of *Staphylococcus aureus*, but again this is non-specific and it may be difficult to decide if this is simple secondary bacterial colonization, which will clear with routine treatment, or if specific anti-staphylococcal therapy is needed.

A test that may be of therapeutic relevance in patients with vesicles and suspected atopic dermatitis, or with an unexplained flare of pre-existing atopic dermatitis, is to swab the skin for herpes simplex virus. Atopic patients are prone to severe herpes simplex type 1 infections as discussed above (p. 99) and require systemic anti-viral therapy.

Kaposi's varicelliform eruption (eczema herpeticum)

The most important complication of atopic dermatitis is the development of eczema herpeticum or Kaposi's varicelliform eruption after exposure to herpes simplex type 1 virus. This is seen as the presence of small blisters in areas of dermatitis and general malaise with fever. This can cause severe systemic upset,

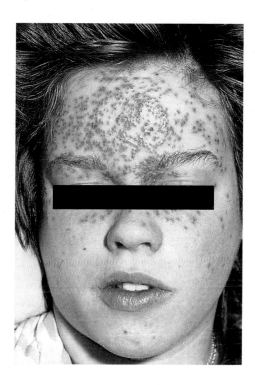

Fig. 6.4 Patient with atopic dermatitis and Kaposi's varicelliform eruption. Note striking eruption on forehead.

which prior to the availability of effective systemic anti-viral therapy could be fatal. It is, therefore, very important that parents of children with atopic dermatitis know that their child should not come into contact with individuals who have simple cold sores, as atopic children are at risk of a much more extensive and serious herpes simplex infection (Figs 6.4, 6.5, and 6.6).

Treatment

Many organizations such as the American Academy of Dermatologists and the British Association of Dermatologists publish guidelines on the management of atopic dermatitis. It may be useful to consult the appropriate website for the current version of such guidelines.

The start of management of the atopic patient or the parent of an atopic child is to explain the nature of the disease and that control, rather than cure is the aim. It is reasonable, however, to be optimistic concerning spontaneous regression, particularly in the case of young children. There are now useful quality of life questionnaires available even for young children with atopic dermatitis. These will give some indication of the degree of distress the child is suffering and can be used to monitor response to treatment.

Prescriptions for topical treatment should be accompanied by a practical hands on demonstration from a trained dermatological nurse of how to apply emollients, creams and ointments, and also how to use bandaging for maximum comfort and to prevent damaging scratching. This can be done in an out-patient centre, health centre or, best of all, in the patients own home with the help of a community liaison nurse who will be able to adapt the treatment regime to the home circumstances.

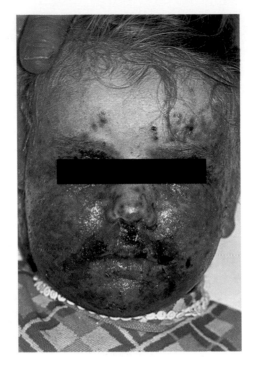

Fig. 6.5 Kaposi's varicelliform eruption in a 3-year-old child with mild atopic dermatitis. Herpes simplex virus was isolated from the lesions.

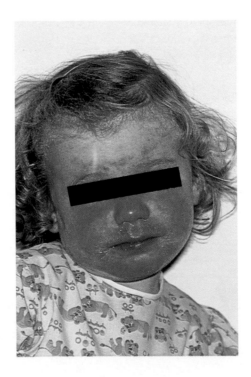

Fig. 6.6 Same child as in Fig. 6.5, 3 months later. Note complete healing and absence of scarring.

The following treatments are useful for patients with mild and moderate dermatitis:

- emollients;
- topical steroids;
- sedating antihistamines;
- antibiotics;
- wet wrap dressings;
- ichthyol impregnated bandages;
- ultraviolet light (UVB);
- environmental change, e.g. trying to reduce house dust mite exposure.

For more severe cases the following treatments may be required:

- photochemotherapy (Narrow band UVB usually, rarely PUVA)
- cyclosporin orally for short periods
- azathioprine
- mycophenolate mofetil
- topical tacrolimus ointment (FK 506)
- topical ascomycin SDZ ASM 981 picrolimus
- acyclovir for superimposed herpes simplex infections
- dietary restrictions
- alternative medicine approaches—Chinese herbs and hypnotherapy

Emollients

Most patients with atopic dermatitis have dry skin. Use of emollients can greatly reduce discomfort and itch. They can also reduce the quantity and potency of topical steroids needed. Preparations such as emulsifying ointment BP, Epaderm or 50% liquid paraffin in white soft paraffin should be used in place of soap to prevent further drying. Emollients can be prescribed for use both in and after the bath or shower. A wide range is available and it is useful to initially prescribe small quantities of several preparations with different textures so that patients can find what suits them best. Bath additives include Diprobath, Hydromol, and Oilatum; after bath preparations include Doublebase Ultrabase, Unguentum M, and Dermol, which contains an antimicrobial. The addition of urea to emollients in preparations such as aquadrate and calmurid may increase their efficacy, but some children and adults find they cause quite severe stinging.

Topical steroids

Weak and moderately potent topical steroids are of great value in the regular management of atopic dermatitis. It is, however, important not to prescribe them for long periods of time without regular clinical review to see if the steroid potency can be reduced. Patients should be taught that while red skin needs some topical steroid, dry skin needs only an emollient. Care should be taken not to use steroids

Key points

If a child with atopic dermatitis is responding poorly to topical steroid prescription, check with the parent that this is being applied. Many parents are nervous of topical steroid side effects.

more potent than 1% hydrocortisone on the face for longer than 1–2 weeks without review, as it is usually the thin skin of the face that is first to show the atrophy and telangiectasia associated with topical steroid overuse. It is also important to avoid over prescription of topical steroids in children to avoid both topical and systemic side effects, which can occur as a result of absorption of topical steroids through inflamed skin.

Many parents are very well aware of topical steroid side effects and may underuse topical steroids because of concern about these. This is a relatively common current cause of apparent non-response to prescribed treatment

Antibiotics

The combination of a topical steroid and anti-staphylococcal antibiotic is often useful as staphylococcal infection can aggravate atopic dermatitis and treating the staphylococcal colonization is frequently associated with clinical improvement. The antibiotic can be used either as a topical steroid antibiotic combination (for example, fucidin hydrocortisone), or a single topical agent [for example, mupirocin (Bactroban)], or given orally as a 5-day course of flucloxacillin or other appropriate antibiotic based on bacteriological sensitivity. There is ongoing concern about the emergence of methicillin resistant staphylococci so, as with topical steroids, patients should be reviewed regularly.

Antihistamines

Sedating antihistamines will help control the itch of atopic dermatitis and prevent night time scratching, but the more modern non-sedating antihistamines are of less benefit. Promethazine and hydroxyzine hydrochloride are both useful and should be used alternately as patients tend to become used to one preparation after 3–4 weeks with loss of sedating effect.

Wet wraps

This is a specialized bandaging technique and the term describes the use of a damp stockinet bodysuit held in place by a dry suit with either a weak antiseptic, such as Burrows solution (aluminium acetate), or a diluted topical steroid in contact with the skin. This is easiest to use at night and the beneficial effect is probably a combination of good hydration, the therapeutic affect of the chosen application, and the fact that two layers of stockinet make scratching very difficult. The technique is mainly used for short periods of time for small children and infants, and care must be taken to avoid hypothermia. Trained nurses should give families a demonstration of how to apply these wraps for home use

Occlusive bandaging

Ichthyol impregnated bandages (ichthopaste) over a topical steroid are also useful in preventing scratching and keeping the steroid in contact with the skin for the maximum amount of time. They can be left in place for 48 hours or longer. This technique is particularly useful for stubborn lesions on the limbs. An alternative, but similar approach is to use 1% ichthyol in zinc ointment over a thin layer of topical steroid held in place with conventional bandaging.

Environmental change

It is sensible to try to reduce allergen exposure as far as is compatible with leading a fairly normal life. The house dust mite collects in carpets curtains and bedding, so a wooden floor, blinds in place of curtains, and a non-permeable cover for the mattress and quilt may all help, as will keeping the environment at a relatively low level of temperature and humidity. Hair-bearing pets should be discouraged and clothing should be of cotton, rather than wool, which can be very irritant.

The management of severe atopic dermatitis

The treatments suggested below should only be considered when the more established methods suggested above have failed. Remember that, although atopic dermatitis is distressing, it is benign. Many of the treatments discussed below have potentially serious side effects and should not be used without thoughtfully balancing the risk/benefit ratio, particularly in young children.

Photochemotherapy: narrow band UVB or PUVA

Patients with severe atopic dermatitis may benefit from a 4–6-week course of ultraviolet light treatment to clear stubborn atopic dermatitis. It is very important to keep a careful note of the cumulative total dose of UV. Current evidence suggests that narrow band UVB is as effective at clearing or improving atopic dermatitis as photochemotherapy at lower total UV doses and without the need for systemic photosensitizing agents. PUVA should therefore only be used very rarely for atopic dermatitis.

Cyclosporin

The immunosuppressive drug cyclosporin (Neoral or Sandimmun) is extremely effective in controlling severe atopic dermatitis. However, high doses usually in the 2–5 mg/kg/day range are needed and these may cause renal toxicity. If a patient has atopic dermatitis of a severity requiring consideration for cyclosporin treatment, two creatinine clearance studies should be carried out, and blood pressure, serum urea, and creatinine monitored regularly, while on treatment. A 6–8-week course of treatment that can be repeated is recommended. Elevation of creatinine levels 25% or more above baseline levels should be an indication for withdrawal of cyclosporin. Low dose maintenance treatment has been suggested, but results are not always satisfactory. Oral cyclosporin should only be used in exceptional cases in childhood dermatitis and then only for short periods

Azathioprine

The cytotoxic drug azathioprine or imuran will also control atopic dermatitis. Doses of 50–100 mg/day are usually effective, but patients must be monitored carefully for marrow depression and hepatic damage.

Mycophenolate mofetil (cellcept)

This drug has been used for some years by nephrologists to prevent rejection of transplanted kidneys and therefore has a well-established safety profile. It has been used in adult patients with severe atopic dermatitis with benefit. Nausea is the main recorded side effect.

Tacrolimus (Protopic 0.03–0.1% tacrolimus ointment)

Tacrolimus is a topical ointment developed from the immunosuppressive agent FK 506. Extensive trials have shown efficacy and safety in both adults and children with atopic dermatitis. Some patients complain of irritation and a burning sensation during the first week of therapy, but this generally settles. At present in the UK it is licensed for use in children over the age of 2 years and in adults.

Pimecrolimus (Elidel 1% pimecrolemus cream)

Topical ascomycin (Pimecrolimus), previously known as ASM 981 has been developed as Elidel cream for resistant atopic dermatitis. Clinical trials show efficacy with a low toxicity profile. It has the added advantage of having been used in trials in infants as young as 3 months of age.

Management of eczema herpeticum (topical herpes simplex infection superimposed on atopic eczema)

Always consider the diagnosis of eczema herpeticum in any atopic dermatitis patient who develops vesicles or who shows rapid deterioration, particularly if the patient is feverish and generally unwell. Swabs and blister fluid should be taken to identify herpes simplex virus and the patient should then be commenced on systemic acyclovir without waiting for laboratory results. If the patient is febrile, acyclovir should be given intravenously for the first 28–72 hours at a dose of 5 mg/kg/day for adults. Topical steroids should not be applied to the infected skin. Once there is obvious evidence of herpes virus infection, topical acyclovir is unlikely to be effective

Dietary restriction

Many parents and some patients have the impression that their atopic dermatitis is exacerbated or caused by certain foods. These are usually dairy products, eggs, fish, and nuts. Dietary exclusion may be effective in a small subset of patients with severe atopic dermatitis, but is demanding on the patient who must be enthusiastic and able to co-operate. In this situation, a time limited trial of elimination of certain foods may be worthwhile. The assistance of a qualified dietitian is essential, particularly in the case of children, to ensure that the remaining diet is adequate, particularly in calcium intake. The best trial of dietary treatment is total compliance and rigorous exclusion of specific foods in rotation for 4–6 weeks. The diet should be stopped if there is no benefit.

Alternative or complementary medicine: Chinese herbal therapy and hypnotherapy

Many parents will enquire about herbal and other less conventional approaches to treatment for their children with atopic dermatitis in the belief that such treatments are safer than conventional topical or oral medicines. A randomized double blind study has shown benefit in patients with diffuse widespread atopic dermatitis when given a decoction of a particular blend of Chinese herbs. The active ingredients have not been identified. Patients who wish to use Chinese herbs should have liver function checked regularly as hepatotoxocity has been reported.

Conclusion

This long list of possible approaches to atopic dermatitis control clearly indicates that at present there is no reliable, proven, effective, and safe method of permanently suppressing symptoms. Fortunately, in the great majority of patients, the condition is self-limiting and clears spontaneously by the age of 5 years. For older patients the prognosis must be more guarded.

Patient support group

The National Eczema Society provides support and information for patients with all types of dermatitis and eczema, but is particularly helpful to families with a child with atopic dermatitis. They provide useful information sheets, local meetings and networks, a regular magazine and useful information on where to purchase pure cotton clothing, etc. (website: www.eczema.org).

Nummular or discoid dermatitis

Definition

A chronic, recurrent pattern of dermatitis with discrete coin-shaped lesions tending to involve the limbs.

Incidence and aetiology

This variety of dermatitis usually affects adults, many of whom will have a past history of atopic dermatitis. The aetiology is unknown. Although secondary infection is common, a primary infective cause has not been proven.

Clinical features

The lesions are usually circular or oval, ranging from 4 to 10 cm or more in diameter, and are often distributed symmetrically on the legs (Fig. 6.7). The dermatitis reaction on these sites is usually subacute with erythema, mild oedema, and in some cases, vesiculation. The surface may be moist and appear infected. Pruritus is variable and can be absent.

Diagnosis

Classic nummular dermatitis is generally easy to diagnose, but atypical cases may resemble a primary infective problem, psoriasis, or allergic contact dermatitis. The distribution of the lesions, generally sparing the knees, elbows, and scalp, is unlike psoriasis. Patch testing will identify most patients with allergic contact dermatitis, a few of whom, particularly women with nickel dermatitis and hand lesions, have a nummular pattern of dermatitis.

Treatment

Topical corticosteroids are the most effective means of controlling this condition. As secondary infection is common, the use of a steroid–antibiotic combination [for example, betamethasone valerate + chinoform (Betnovate C)] is logical and may

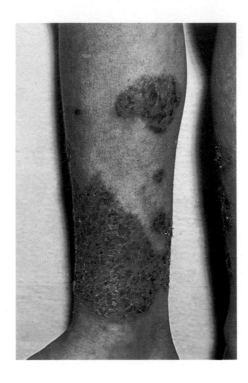

Fig. 6.7 Nummular dermatitis.

clear the lesions. In more persistent cases, the application of 0.5–2% tar or ichthyol in zinc paste will be beneficial. Systemic anti-pruritics are rarely required.

Asteatotic eczema (eczema craquelé)

This term is used to describe the dry irritable skin seen mainly on the limbs of elderly patients. The skin is dry and has large scales with a 'crazy-paving' appearance (Fig. 6.8, see opposite page). It appears to be the result of loss of epidermal lubrication together, in many cases, with inadequately removed soap after washing. The problem is extremely common in communities of elderly people.

Treatment

This consists of replacing the missing lubrication. Soap should be withdrawn and Epaderm, emulsifying ointment BP, Unguentum M, or a similar preparation used. Adequate lubrication may require very regular application of emollients and a reduction in bathing. Topical steroids should be avoided as the underlying skin is already thin and fragile.

Seborrhoeic dermatitis

Definition

Seborrhoeic dermatitis is seen in two distinct subsets of patients, small infants and young adults. The infantile form is characterized by large yellowish scales mainly on the scalp, face, and napkin area, and is usually self-limiting. The adult form

Key points

It is very easy to aggravate seborrhoeic dermatitis by over treatment.

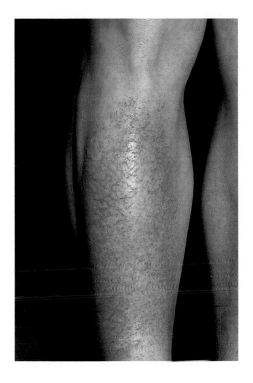

Fig. 6.8 Eczema craquele. Note redness and scaling on shin area.

affects the face, scalp, and anterior chest, and is associated with itch and irritability of the skin, which seems out of proportion to the relatively mild degree of scaling and erythema seen.

Prevalence and aetiology

Infantile seborrhoeic dermatitis is a relatively common condition in young babies and may cause confusion with infantile atopic dermatitis. The aetiology is unknown. There does not appear to be any link between the infantile and adult forms of seborrhoeic dermatitis, and there is no evidence that children who have seborrhoeic dermatitis as infants are at greater risk of adult dermatitis in their later lives.

Adult seborrhoeic dermatitis is less common, but much more persistent. It appears to be most often seen in young adult males and is often associated on the trunk with involvement of the hair follicles, seborrhoeic folliculitis. In spite of the name, neither qualitative nor quantitative changes in sebaceous secretion have been found in either the infantile or the adult form. The micro-organism *Pityrosporum ovale* has been found in greater numbers than on normal skin in patients with seborrhoeic dermatitis and a proportion of patients respond to topical anti-fungal therapy. This suggests that *P. ovale* is an aetiological agent, although it is not yet established whether this is in a primary or a secondary role.

Clinical features

In infants, the child usually presents in early infancy with large yellow scales on the scalp extending down onto the forehead (Fig. 6.9). The child usually also has involve-

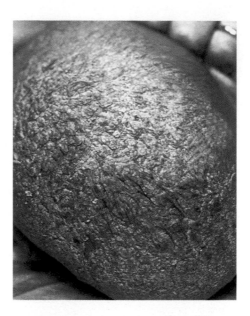

Fig. 6.9 Infantile seborrhoeic dermatitis. Severe scalp involvement with large yellow adherent scales.

ment on the trunk (Fig. 6.10), napkin area, and the axillae. There does not appear to be any pruritus, as the child is usually eating and sleeping well. This is a valuable diagnostic point in favour of seborrhoeic dermatitis and against atopic dermatitis.

In adults, the eruption consists of discrete, asymptomatic, or mildly pruritic, red to yellow, glazed-looking lesions, mainly on the trunk. The pre-sternal area, the axillae, submammary folds, groins, and external ear are common sites. Facial lesions are commoner in men and may be very persistent (Fig. 6.11), particularly in the nasolabial fold. Mild erythema and fine scaling are the usual clinical fea-

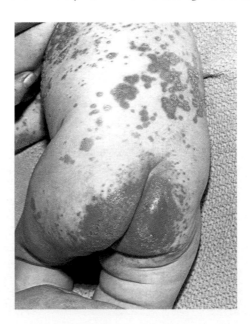

Fig. 6.10 Infantile seborrhoeic dermatitis. Erythema and scaling are present, but there is no apparent pruritus.

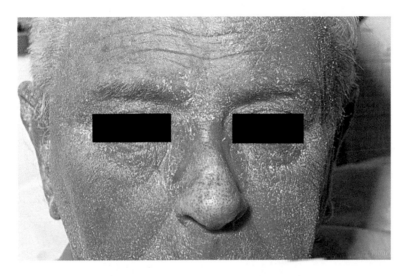

Fig. 6.11 Seborrhoeic dermatitis. Note erythema and scaling.

tures. Lesions on the trunk (Fig. 6.12) may be circular, pale pink, and at times difficult to see despite symptoms.

The scalp is frequently involved, and the presenting complaint may be of severe and persistent dandruff (pityriasis capitis, seen as scaling and erythema on the scalp). Eyebrow and eyelid involvement is common with early morning stickiness of the eyelids. This blepharitis can be very unresponsive to therapy.

Overall, seborrhoeic dermatitis tends to be chronic with seasonal variations peculiar to the individual. Severe and persistent seborrhoeic dermatitis is seen in a high proportion of patients who are HIV positive (see p. 171).

Diagnosis

Confusion may arise with allergic contact dermatitis, psoriasis, and pityriasis versicolor. Patch testing will generally exclude a true contact allergy, and the greasy

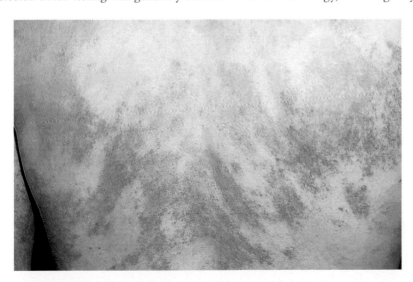

Fig. 6.12 Seborrhoeic dermatitis involving the trunk of an adult patient.

Fig. 6.13 Seborrhoeic folliculitis. The lesions are often minimal relative to the degree of discomfort.

yellow appearance of the lesions and their distribution are pointers against psoriasis, but this may easily be confused, particularly when there are only scalp lesions present. In psoriasis, however, the lesions are easily palpable and well delineated with large coarse silvery scales, whereas in seborrhoeic dermatitis they are more diffuse with finer smaller scales. Mycological examination of scrapings from individual lesions will exclude pityriasis versicolor and may show the presence of large numbers of the yeast, *P. ovale*.

Seborrhoeic folliculitis is often associated with seborrhoeic dermatitis of the trunk. This consists of multiple small papules based on the follicles, and is thought to be due to excessive colonization of the follicles by *P. versicolor* (Fig. 6.13). It can be very resistant to treatment.

Treatment

Seborrhoeic dermatitis is a chronic problem that tends to recur whatever treatment is used. These include a topical imidazole anti-fungal, such as ketoconazole cream and shampoo (Nizoral, UK and USA), sulconazole (Exelderm, UK), miconazole (Daktarin, UK), clotrimazole (Lotrimin, USA, and Lotriderm, UK), econazole (Spectazole, USA). Oral imidazoles are effective, but should only be considered if topical measure fail and should not be used continuously on a long-term basis.

The associated problem of seborrhoeic folliculitis is particularly difficult to treat and may only respond to systemic imidazoles.

Weak potency topical steroids are also of value (for example, 1% hydrocortisone cream to face and flexures), but as with imidazoles, the condition tends to recur.

Contact dermatitis

Contact dermatitis comprises two quite distinct problems. These are:

* caused by a **direct irritant action** of a substance on the skin;

Key points

Contact dermatitis may be caused by a direct irritant or by allergic contact.

- **allergic contact dermatitis**, which occurs only in patients whose skin has previously been sensitized by a contact with an allergen. Fresh contact with the antigen elicits a dermatitis reaction mediated by specifically sensitized T lymphocytes. The role of the epidermal Langerhans cells in presenting the allergen and in making subsequent contact with T lymphocytes, either in the skin or local lymph nodes an important area of dermato-immunological research.

Some of the differences between direct irritant contact dermatitis and allergic contact dermatitis are shown in Table 6.3. Current figures show that in the UK direct irritant dermatitis is a much commoner problem than the allergic contact variety.

Table 6.3 Differences between direct irritant and allergic contact dermatitis

	Direct irritant	Allergic contact
Prevalence	Very common	Much less common
Prior exposure to substance	Not required	Essential
Affected sites	Sites of direct contact with little extension	Sites of contact and distant sites
Susceptibility	Everyone susceptible	Only some patients susceptible
Other associated skin diseases	Atopy predisposes	Prolonged use of topical medicaments for chronic skin disease (e.g. leg ulcers) predisposes
Timing	Rapid onset 4–12 hours after contact	Onset generally 24 hours or longer after exposure
	Lesions develop at first exposure	No lesions on first exposure

Direct irritant contact dermatitis

Definition

Dermatitis caused by exposure to a substance, which has a damaging effect on the normal barrier function of the epidermis.

Incidence and aetiology

Irritant contact dermatitis is very common and may be:

- **acute** due to a single exposure to an irritant substance;
- **subacute** due to repeated exposures of a small area as in napkin dermatitis;
- **chronic** 'wear and tear' due to repeated exposures to materials that deplete the normal protective film of lipid in and on the epidermis.

Acute irritant dermatitis is seen after one single, usually accidental, exposure to a strong skin irritant, such as acid, alkali, phenol, halide, or quaternary ammonium compounds. The onset is rapid and lesions appear exactly at the sites of contact.

Subacute irritant dermatitis is seen as ongoing irritation as in infantile napkin dermatitis.

Chronic irritant dermatitis   A classic example of **cumulative exposure** to a mild cutaneous irritant is 'barmaid's hands' due to continual contact with detergents and/or alkalis, which degrease the skin and remove the protective lipid film.

Mild examples of cumulative insult irritant dermatitis are extremely common among persons regularly exposed to detergents and degreasing agents, either at work or at home, and patients with atopic dermatitis are particularly susceptible. Many sufferers are convinced that they have an allergy and may find it difficult to accept that this is not the cause of their problem.

Clinical features

After exposure to a strong irritant, the affected skin becomes reddish-brown and vesicles develop. The lesions appear rapidly, usually within 6–12 hours of contact, are very well localized to the site of contact, and are painful and itchy. If there is no further contact with the irritant, recovery is rapid and it is unusual for lesions to develop at distant body sites. Identification of the aetiological agent depends on a careful history and, as the site and timing of the lesions are clear-cut, the patient himself will usually identify the substance in question.

In subacute dermatitis, repeated exposure to the irritant confuses the clinical and pathological picture. There is erythema with crusting and sometimes blistering. There may also be early acanthosis and skin thickening. In infantile irritant napkin dermatitis (Fig. 6.14) the child has extensive erythema, sometimes with erosions and blistering on the napkin area, with striking sparing of the skin folds, which have been relatively protected from the direct irritant effect of urine and faeces. This is in contrast to napkin candidosis in which the occlusive environment of the skin folds encourages candida overgrowth.

Chronic irritant dermatitis tends, initially, to present as dry, hacked, or fissured areas of skin, which are susceptible to secondary infection. This is seen typically in young mothers and others such as domestic workers whose hands are repeated-

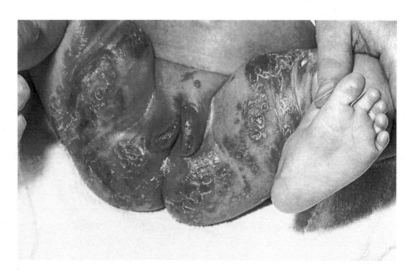

Fig. 6.14 Napkin dermatitis. Severe involvement with relative sparing of skin flexures.

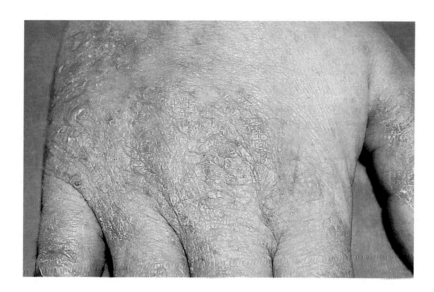

Fig. 6.15 Chronic wear and tear dermatitis on the backs of the hands.

ly exposed to soap, detergents, and water (Fig. 6.15). These substances tend to accumulate under rings and, with the added effect of local trauma, may provoke severe reactions, which are clinically very similar to those seen as a result of allergic contact sensitivity to metals.

Treatment

Identification of the irritant and its subsequent avoidance is the cornerstone of successful therapy. The cause is identified on the patient's history. Patch testing to standard allergens may be needed to rule out allergic contact dermatitis.

For the active phase, removal of soap for cleansing, and substitution of emollients, such as Epaderm with, in addition, a topical steroid cream or ointment are usually effective. If the lesions are acute with vesicles and weeping, wet dressings applied as soaks or lotions may be needed until the subacute phase is reached, when topical steroids can be substituted. Suitable wet dressings and lotions include aluminium acetate lotion 5% in sterile water and calamine lotion BP (15% calamine, 5% zinc oxide, and 5% glycerine). Prior soaking of the area in a weak solution of 0.01–0.1% potassium permanganate in water for 5 minutes may be soothing and help to prevent secondary infection. The choice of topical steroid for the subacute phase is wide and, as the surface area involved may be small and the condition of short duration, the use of a relatively strong steroid is justified. Suitable examples are 0.1% betamethasone 17-valerate with 3% clioquinol in a water miscible base (Betnovate C), fluocinolone acetonide (Synalar), or beclomethasone dipropionate 0.025% (Propaderm). As acute reactions seldom become chronic, keratolytics are rarely indicated.

Children with napkin or diaper dermatitis should have all napkins removed and be nursed in a warm dry environment with the skin exposed. Lesions will rapidly resolve if this is done and improvement will be accelerated by the use of a mild steroid anti-fungal combination, such as miconazole/hydrocortisone (Daktacort). The mother should, however, be warned that this should not become the child's regular napkin cream and topical steroids should be withdrawn when the skin returns to normal.

The management of chronic cumulative irritant contact dermatitis involves protection of the area involved, most commonly the hands, from exposure to the cause and the liberal use of emollients to replace the lipid barrier. Patients should be warned that up to 6 months daily application of emollients and continuing avoidance of soap for cleansing may be needed before the skin regains its barrier function and can be considered normal.

Prevention of irritant dermatitis is theoretically simple. All individual workers at risk should be issued with appropriate advice, barrier creams, and protective clothing. Chronic detergent contact with hands should be prevented by using occlusive vinyl (not rubber) gloves and underneath these a thin pair of cotton gloves to absorb perspiration. This is much more effective than flock or cotton-lined rubber or vinyl gloves. Thorough rinsing of the hands after essential soap and water exposure is important as is the regular use of emollient preparations to hydrate the skin (for example Epaderm, Doublebase, emulsifying ointment BP, Unguentum M). Routine use of topical steroids for this purpose is not recommended.

Allergic contact dermatitis

Definition

Dermatitis caused by prior exposure to an allergen leading to specific cell-mediated sensitization.

Prevalence and aetiology

Allergic contact dermatitis affects 1–2% of the population in most parts of the world. Certain groups are at greater risk. For example, patients with chronic skin conditions, such as leg ulcers, tend to develop allergies to medicaments and workers exposed to common sensitizers, such as chromates in the building industry, or dyes and tanning agents in leather manufacture, have a higher incidence than the population at large.

The commonest sensitizing agents in Europe and North America have been identified, and they can be used as a standard or routine battery of around 20 patch tests for investigating patients with this type of dermatitis. Substances in this battery are changed as appropriate according to observed changes in clinical problems, but include nickel and chromates, rubber breakdown products, preservatives, topical antibiotics, and topical steroid molecules. The current European battery is listed in Table 6.4. In addition, smaller groups of relevant allergens are used when investigating specific problems, for example, a 'footwear battery' for chronic foot dermatitis, a medicament battery for leg ulcers, and a cosmetic battery for facial problems.

In theory, once the offending allergen has been identified by patch testing and thereafter avoided, rapid clearance of the skin lesions should occur, but in practice this is not always the case. Certain common allergens are very difficult to avoid in the course of everyday life and nickel is a good example. It is found in cutlery, coins, cooking implements, gardening and motoring equipment, jewellery, house-

Table 6.4 Materials currently used in the European Standard Battery for patch testing

0.5% Potassium dichromate	20% Neomycin
1% Thiuram mix	PPD mix
5% Cobalt chloride	1% Quaternium 15
1% Formaldehyde	20% Colophony
Carba mix	25% Balsam of Peru
1.0% PPD	30% Wool alcohols
2% Mercapto mix	1% Epoxy resin
16% Parabens	1% Ethylene diamine
Clioquinol 6%	0.1% Thiomersal
1% PTBP formaldehyde resin	5% Nickel sulphate
2% Mercapto mix	8% Fragrance mix
1% Tixocortol pivalate	0.01% Primin
0.1% Budesonide	Caine mix

hold furniture, and many other items, and it can be extremely difficult, even for an intelligent and motivated patient, to avoid nickel contact. Even trace amounts of nickel in the diet from foodstuffs or cooking implements may play a part in perpetuating the skin lesions.

The medico-legal consequences of allergic contact dermatitis acquired through exposure to allergens at work are complex. Contact dermatitis is classified as an industrial injury in the UK and some patients are entitled to financial compensation. Prevention by removing the sufferer from the allergen-containing environment or by removing the allergen from the process for which the patient is responsible is theoretically possible, but clearly requires collaboration between the work force, occupational health physicians and others.

Clinical features

Allergic contact dermatitis usually presents with acute or subacute dermatitis lesions at sites where the allergen is or has been in direct contact with the skin and also with milder involvement of more distant areas where there has been no obvious direct contact. As sensitization may develop after many years of trouble-free daily contact with the allergen, the patient may be unaware that he is reacting to this particular substance. Even after positive patch testing, it may be very hard to convince him that a material handled regularly for many years is now to be avoided.

Common sites of involvement are the ear lobes and nape of neck (nickel in jewellery, Fig. 6.16 and 6.17), the wrist (metal or leather watch straps or bracelets), and the feet (tanning agents used in curing leather, adhesives used for fixing insoles, dyes used for leather or socks, glue used in assembling shoes, Fig. 6.18). Topical steroids themselves may elicit an allergic contact dermatitis. This should always be considered when a patient has dermatitis, which appears to deteriorate while on steroid therapy.

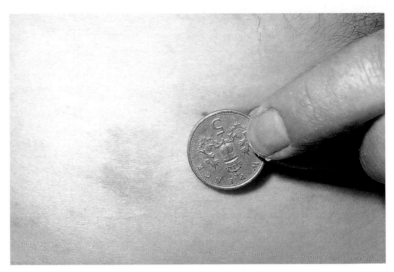

Fig. 6.16 Nickel dermatitis showing striking reaction to nickel coin.

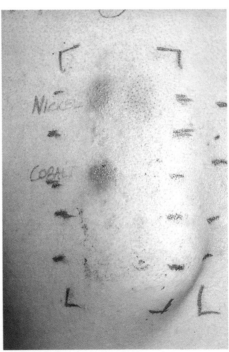

Fig. 6.17 Same patient showing striking reaction on conventional patch testing to both nickel and cobalt.

In the early stages the affected area is inflamed and itchy, with papules and vesicles. Continued exposure to the allergen will lead to dryness, scaling, and fissuring. This picture may be complicated when renewed exposure causes an acute or subacute exacerbation to develop on the background of a long-standing chronic dermatitis. The lesions frequently spread well beyond the area of contact with the allergen and also even to distant body sites, which have not been in contact with the allergen. The main site of involvement may give a useful clue to the

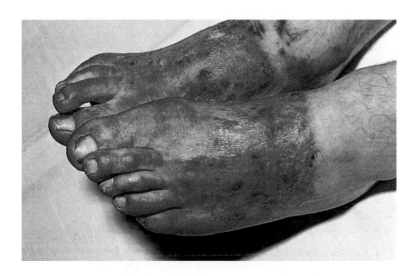

Fig. 6.18 Shoe dermatitis. After topical treatment patch tests were performed and a positive result obtained to potassium dichromate.

Table 6.5 Principal sites of allergic contact dermatitis and likely causes

Site	Likely cause
Face	Cosmetics, perfume in toilet soap, nickel, plastic spectacle frames, medicaments (e.g. antibiotics in eye or ear drops) (Fig. 6.19)
Scalp	Hair dyes (paraphenylenediamine—PPD), lotions and tonics containing Balsam of Peru
Mouth	Denture materials
Neck and ear lobes	Nickel containing jewellery
Wrists	Nickel, PPD, chromates–jewellery and leather watch straps
Hands	Plants (e.g. primulas), nickel (begins under rings), material handled in occupation or recreation, lanolin (hand creams, medicaments)
Body	Nickel jean studs or rubber material in underwear, clothing dyes
Feet	Dyes used in socks and shoes glues, chromates, etc., in shoes

Key points

In chronic persistent hand dermatitis, arrange for patch tests to identify unexpected allergens. Eighty per cent of all contact dermatitis involves the hands and forearms.

cause and Table 6.5 lists such common sites and likely agents. Exposure to sensitizing plants, particularly to primula, tends to cause a blistering eruption relatively rapidly on the sites of actual contact and also a general facial erythema due to airborne allergen. The compositae family of plants are another common source of problems at the present time. These include chrysanthemums and even the common dandelion.

Hand dermatitis tends to be a common and persistent problem in individuals sensitive to nickel. In all cases of persistent hand dermatitis, it is good practice both to patch test to exclude an allergen, such as nickel and to examine scrapings for fungi to exclude a fungal infection.

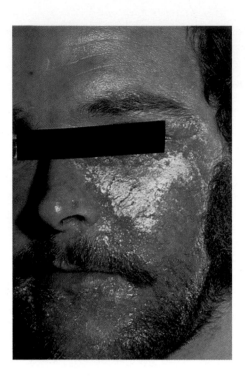

Fig. 6.19 Medicament dermatitis. This patient had recently received an eye ointment containing neomycin.

Treatment

The management of allergic contact dermatitis is divided logically into four stages.

1. **Detection of the likely sensitizing agent** by taking a careful occupational, recreational, and medicament history. Knowledge of the common sensitizers and the sites they may affect is obviously necessary at this stage.

2. **Preparation for valid patch testing** to identify the allergen. Ideally, the patient should avoid all materials thought to be possibly responsible for the eruption, while applying a topical steroid preparation to clear the dermatitis. The presence of active lesions even at distant body sites while patch testing is carried out will result in both false positive and false negative results, and all lesions should therefore be cleared *before* patch tests are performed.

   Topical steroid preparations are helpful. The strength of steroid used should be chosen according to the site involved—facial lesions should receive a mild preparation (for example, clobetasone butyrate, Eumovate), while the thicker skin of the hands and feet require a stronger preparation (for example fluocinolone acetonide, Synalar). Most centres prefer to avoid patch testing until the skin has been relatively free of inflammation for 4–6 weeks and the area to which the patches are to be applied has free of topical steroids for 1–2 weeks, but this is not always possible. Pregnancy has an effect on the immune system and thus on the results of patch testing, so if possible it is best to delay patch testing until after delivery to obtain a relevant result. Recent sun exposure particularly if the patient has developed erythema will also confuse results of patch testing. It is therefore wise to plan patch testing for a time before not immediately after a sunny holiday.

3. **Patch testing to the suspected substances** (for the technique, see p. 49). In practice it is common to test patients with all substances in the European standard battery plus any other likely allergens, for example, small pieces cut from the inner aspects of shoes in foot dermatitis. This can be done using chemicals stored in syringes and applied to inert metal chambers or by using prepared strips of patches (Trutest). The patches are left in position for 48 hours, removed, and the area examined for redness and swelling at that time and also 48 hours later, i.e. at 48 and 96 hours post-application. Patch test results can be surprisingly difficult to interpret, as some allergens are also irritants and irritant reactions can, to the non-expert, look very like a true positive result. In general, the 96-hour reading is regarded by most experts as the most likely to be reliable

4. **Counselling on avoidance of responsible allergens** following patch test results. This is not always straightforward. For example, although it may be easy to avoid the plant in primula dermatitis, it is much more difficult to obtain appropriate allergen-free footwear in shoe dermatitis. There are difficulties in industry when a skilled worker finds it hard to avoid exposure to an allergen encountered in his daily work, and factory or industrial medical officers may be of great assistance in such cases.

It is essential that these four stages of treatment and investigation be followed. A delay in response to treatment prior to patch testing (stage 2) may be due to continuing exposure to the aetiological agent. This is particularly common in medicament-induced contact dermatitis, and in such cases topical preparations containing lanolin or preservatives (for example, parabens) should be avoided. The possibility of topical corticosteroid sensitivity should also be considered.

Latex allergy
Clinical features

Throughout the 1990s there has been a very steep rise in the number of reported cases of latex allergy giving rise to severe and at times life threatening type 1 allergic reactions. This has been attributed to the steep rise in the use of inexpensive rubber gloves because of concern over transmission of infection including HIV and hepatitis. Patients with latex allergy develop itching burning or swelling at the site of latex contact within an hour. Those at particular risk of latex sensitization include patients with atopic dermatitis, those with spina bifida, others who require regular general anaesthesia, dentists, and other health care workers. All of these groups come into latex contact more frequently than the rest of the population. Everyday objects that may trigger an alarming anaphylactic reaction include dummies or pacifiers for infants, balloons, condoms, and anaesthetic intubation tubes. There may also be confusing cross-reactions with foodstuffs that include bananas, kiwi fruit, melons, tomatoes, carrots, celery, and even potatoes.

Diagnosis

This may be based first on clinical suspicion, with the patient, for example, giving a history of swollen lips after inflating balloons. The suspicion can be confirmed by a RAST test looking for anti-latex IgE antibodies, or by conventional patch tests, or by immediate prick testing. None of these are infallible, and it is wise to err on the side of caution and work on the assumption that an individual with a suggestive clinical history is indeed latex sensitive even in the absence of positive laboratory evidence.

Treatment

Patients should avoid all rubber contact and use vinyl products instead. They should carry a card with this information for their dentist, doctor, anaesthetist, midwife, etc. If there is concern about a very severe anaphylactic reaction, the patient may be supplied with a self-injectable source of adrenaline for emergencies (epipen).

Dishydrotic eczema (pompholyx)

This term is used to describe a very characteristic pattern of intensely itchy vesicles of the skin of the hands—cheiropompholyx—and, occasionally, also the feet—cheiropodopompholyx. The sides of the finger are frequently involved and clinically the individual lesions have a 'sago grain' or 'frog spawn' appearance due to translucent deeply-set papules (Fig. 6.20). These are often easier to feel than to see.

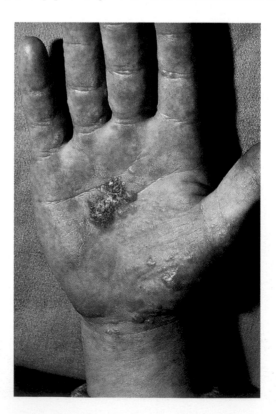

Fig. 6.20 Cheiropompholyx involving the palms and side of the fingers.

The cause of this pattern of dermatitis is not understood. In some cases, patients have allergic contact dermatitis, especially to nickel. In other cases, no specific allergen is found, but the problem appears to be aggravated by stress.

Treatment

Systemic antihistamines will help control the need to scratch and thus prevent secondary infection. The intense, but usually short-lived, itch is best treated for a short time with potent topical steroids. If the lesions are very moist, wet soaks, using calamine lotion may be helpful.

Neurodermatitis (circumscribed lichen simplex)

Definition

A well-demarcated area of chronic lichenified dermatitis, which is not due to either external irritants or identified allergens.

Aetiology

In predisposed persons, the lesions are induced by continual scratching or rubbing of a localized area of itchy skin. The initial pruritic stimulus, which seems to be related to stress or emotional disturbance, generates an itch-scratch-itch cycle. This, in turn, stimulates a reactive epidermal hyperplasia recognized clinically as lichenification (Fig. 6.21).

Neurodermatitis is relatively uncommon and the diagnosis should be made after excluding commoner causes of dermatitis, for example, irritant or allergic contact dermatitis. It is commoner in women than in men.

Clinical features

Usually the isolated, well-circumscribed, lichenified, slightly elevated plaques are seen on the nape of the neck, the forearms, or the legs. They have a characteristic

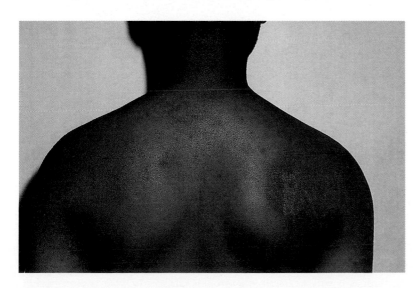

Fig. 6.21 Neurodermatitis showing dark thickened area over skin of right scapula.

mauve colour and accentuation of normal skin markings. Affected patients are often tense and obsessive, and there appears to be an association with atopy.

Diagnosis and treatment

A biopsy may occasionally be necessary to confirm the diagnosis when individual lesions resemble psoriasis or even lichen planus. An atypical fungal infection could also cause confusion. Mycological examination will exclude this possibility.

Treatment should be aimed at breaking the itch-scratch-itch cycle and consists of antihistamines by mouth to reduce pruritus, topical corticosteroids to suppress inflammation, and tar or ichthyol-containing preparations for their anti-pruritic and keratolytic effects. Occlusive dressings prevent scratching and are the most effective treatment. For lesions on a limb, a tar or ichthyol impregnated bandage (for example, Coltapaste, Ichthopaste) applied for a week may totally clear the lesion. Unfortunately, however, recurrence after removal of occlusion is frequent. In some cases intra-lesional injections of a steroid preparation, such as triamcinolone may be beneficial.

Prurigo nodularis

This problem can be regarded as a variant of neurodermatitis. As a result of itch and subsequent scratching, lichenified nodules develop. They may be as large as 1–5 cm in diameter and the clinical differential diagnosis may include skin tumours. The history of chronic severe itch is helpful, but a biopsy may be necessary to establish the diagnosis. Potent topical steroids under occlusive dressings are the most useful form of treatment.

Stasis dermatitis

Definition

An area of dermatitis on the lower legs, commonly seen in association with venous insufficiency or frank ulceration.

Incidence and aetiology

A large number of obese, usually female, patients have a degree of venous insufficiency or frank varicose veins of the lower limbs. Prior to the development of frank stasis ulcers (p. 209) a mild dermatitis reaction associated with epidermal atrophy, purpura, and pigmentation due to haemosiderin may develop. These changes are related to extravasation of blood into the tissues and poor oxygenation.

Clinical features

The inner aspects of both lower legs above and around the medial malleolus are chiefly involved. The skin is shiney, atrophic, and usually has large numbers of small blood vessels clearly visible (Fig. 6.22).

Treatment

Treatment of underlying varicose veins is the most important form of therapy. The use of topical steroids, although symptomatically valuable, is not recommended long-term as it will accelerate the atrophic changes in what is already thin epi-

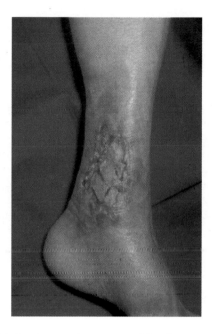

Fig. 6.22 Varicose eczema showing atrophy and tissue breakdown around the malleolus.

dermis. Protective ichthyol or tar-impregnated bandages are useful both in preventing scratching, and in protecting from other forms of minor trauma.

Patient association

The National Eczema Society is a patient support group with branches in many countries, which offer support and practical advice to sufferers from all types of dermatitis and eczema, although a high proportion of members have atopic dermatitis. The Society produces a number of well-researched and medically approved information packs (website www.eczema.org).

Discussion of problem cases (see p. 95)

Case 6.1

The history is strongly suggestive of atopic dermatitis. The mother gives a history of seasonal rhinitis, so the child has an atopic background. No laboratory tests are necessary to confirm the diagnosis. The parents needed time and a careful explanation of the nature of atopic dermatitis, including the fact that it is usually self-limiting. Printed leaflets will help enforce verbal explanations. The child was carefully examined to exclude the possibility of secondary problems, particularly eczema herpeticum. Emollients and a soap substitute were prescribed and the mother asked to avoid woollen clothing next the baby's skin, substituting cotton. One per cent hydrocortisone ointment was prescribed as the initial steroid and oral promethazine for night time sedation. A dermatology nurse spent time with the parents showing them how to apply dressings. The parents were given the address of the National Eczema Society.

The mother returned 2 weeks later with the child who was much improved, but still scratching and rubbing his legs. A moderate potency steroid was prescribed for

Discussion of problem cases continued

this area and 1 month later his skin was itchy, but looked relatively normal. He continued to require prescriptions for hydrocortisone and night sedation for the next 9 months, and his skin flared with episodes of teething, and minor coughs and colds. By the age of 2 years his skin was dry, but non-inflamed and apparently non-pruritic.

The parents ask you about the likelihood of any further children being affected. How would you reply?

Case 6.2

This presentation tends to be a bit of a heart sink case for a dermatologist. The history and presentation strongly suggest seborrhoeic dermatitis and associated seborrhoeic folliculitis. Both are very difficult to clear completely. The pattern of involvement on the face and scalp with sparing of the fingers does not suggest scabies.

The patient was given topical imidazole (ketoconazole) cream and shampoo, and this improved the problems on his face and scalp, but did not affect the itch on his trunk. At his request and, after discussion, he was given a 4-week course of oral imidazole (fluconazole), again with little benefit. This was stopped and he had a 6-week course of UVB therapy, but was concerned about future skin cancer risks, so this also was stopped and he was given simple 2% menthol in calamine cream with a little symptomatic relief. At the next visit, he tells you he is emigrating to the US.

Are there any other treatment options to consider here?

Case 6.3

Young individuals embarking on a hairdressing career often have hand dermatitis problems, particularly in the first year when they are working as juniors and spend a lot of time shampooing—thus in contact with water and detergent. Most salons will not let them wear latex or rubber gloves, so the cumulative drying effect to the skin is considerable.

This is the most likely explanation in this case. Patch testing was carried out to exclude an allergic cause and as expected the results were negative, although difficult to interpret because of some irritant reactions.

She was advised to use copious amounts of emollients and to wear cotton under rubber gloves as much as possible. Her skin slowly improved on this routine and she was able to continue to train as a hairdresser.

Case 6.4

The patient has visible varicose veins and the history suggests associated stasis dermatitis. Once the dermatitis has been treated she should be referred for consideration for surgical treatment of her varicose veins. The preparation she was using on her leg was a lanolin-containing steroid cream, not a recommended therapy for stasis dermatitis because of the skin thinning effect of topical steroids. However, in the short-term they should not actually aggravate pre-existing dermatitis.

Because of this history, the patient was patch tested and was found to be sensitive to lanolin. Her leg was treated with ichthopaste bandages and, when the dermatitis had settled, her varicose veins were surgically treated. Three months later the skin around her ankles was relatively normal.

What advice do you give her about her lanolin allergy?

Special study module

Attach yourself to the local contact dermatitis investigation service or patch test service

Follow 20 patients through patch testing gaining experience of taking a relevant history, applying appropriate patch tests, and interpreting results. What are the patients told and what do they understand?

If possible go with the consultant dermatologist on one or two workplace visits to see the relationship between the patch test service and the working environment.

How would you audit the service?

How could you improve the service?

Further reading

Bieber, T. and Leung, D.Y.M. (2002) *Atopic dermatitis*. Marcel Dekker Inc., New York.

Fisher, A.A. (2001) *Contact dermatitis*, 5th edn. Lippincott, Williams and Wilkins, Philadelphia.

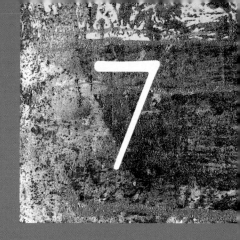

7

Cutaneous infections and infestations

- Problem cases
- Bacterial infections
- Mycobacterial infections
- Viral infections
- Spirochaetal infections
- Fungal infections
- Protozoal infections
- Cutaneous infestations
- Sexually transmitted disease
- Dermatological complications of infection with the human immunodeficiency virus infection (HIV 1)
- Discussion of problem cases
- Special study module project

Cutaneous infections and infestations

Problem cases

Case 7.1

A 7-year-old boy is brought to you by his mother. He has a history of atopic dermatitis, which still troubles him in the winter months, mainly on his face and in the popliteal fossae. In the past 3 days he has developed widespread, but superficial crusting on his cheeks. He is otherwise well.

What is the differential diagnosis here, what investigations might be useful, and what therapy would you prescribe?

Case 7.2

A young mother comes to your surgery 2 weeks after Easter. The family spent Easter in a farm cottage and helped with young lambs. She has had a painful ulcerated lesion on her hand for 4 days and her young son now has a similar lesion, also on his hand. She is febrile and has enlarged lymph glands, and is very worried that she is spreading a serious disease to her family. What might be the problem here and how will you manage it?

Case 7.3

A young Asian couple bring their 2-year-old daughter to see you because of loss of normal pigmentation on her right forearm. The child is otherwise well, but the parents are clearly very concerned. The child was born in Pakistan and only came to the UK 3 months ago.

What are the causes of painless loss of normal pigmentation and how would you establish a diagnosis?

Case 7.4

You are consulted by the mother of an 18-year-old girl, who is on dialysis and awaiting a kidney transplant, about an unrelated matter. In passing, she mentions that her daughter has both hand and genital warts. The mother wants to know if she should be treated now or wait until after the transplant when she will feel fitter.

What is the best approach in this case?

Case 7.5

A 38-year-old college lecturer consults you about a red, painful right calf. He has just returned from a weekend walking in the New Forest area of the UK and wonders if he has an allergy to his new walking boots.

Discuss the possible differential diagnosis, the appropriate investigations, and the suggested treatment.

Problem cases continued

> ### Case 7.6
>
> You are asked to visit a retirement home. Five elderly ladies all have scaling and itch involving most of the trunk and limbs, and you are told that a nurse who has just gone on holiday has the same problem. Before you have seen the patients topical hydrocortisone has been applied to the affected areas with very little benefit. The senior nurse in charge is concerned about a change in the detergent used for laundry.
>
> What are the possible causes of this outbreak, what investigations might be helpful, and what treatments would be appropriate?

In Britain, Europe, and North America the numbers of patients with bacterial cutaneous infection has fallen over the past two decades. It is still important, however, to be able to recognize and treat these conditions promptly. Unfortunately, there has been no such decline in the incidence of viral or fungal cutaneous infections, but recent advances in therapy has made it possible to treat previously intractable problems.

Bacterial infections

Impetigo

Definition

A superficial cutaneous infection caused by either staphylococci or streptococci.

Incidence and aetiology

Impetigo is easily spread in situations such as day nurseries, where there is frequent contact between children.

The organisms commonly identified in impetigo are *Staphylococcus aureus* and group A streptococci. The disease is much commoner in children and can present as a very thin-roofed, quickly ruptured blister, especially when caused by staphylococci.

Clinical features

The hallmark of impetigo is a superficial lesion covered with a heavy honey-coloured crust, usually on the face and hands. Impetigo can develop very rapidly and may complicate a pre-existing skin condition such as atopic dermatitis or acne (Fig. 7.1).

Management

Removal of crusts with warm saline or olive oil soaks, and the application of a topical antibiotic, such as aureomycin, fucidin, or mupirocin (Bactroban), are the essential points in management. The infection in impetigo is extremely superficial and, therefore, most cases will respond quickly and heal with no scarring.

While the use of systemic antibiotics in impetigo is only essential if streptococci have been shown to be present, as the aim is to prevent post-streptococcal

> ### Key points
>
> Impetigo (a superficial infection by staphylococci or streptococci) usually responds quickly to topical antibiotic, but systemic antibiotics are required to prevent post-streptococcal glomerulonephritis.

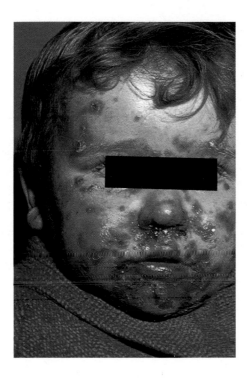

Fig. 7.1 Staphylococcal impetigo superimposed on mild atopic dermatitis. Note gross honey-coloured crusting.

glomerulonephritis, it is common practice in the majority of severe cases also to prescribe full doses of oral penicillin or erythromycin for 5–7 days.

Erysipelas

Definition

A cutaneous streptococcal infection characterized by sharply demarcated unilateral lesions, commonly on the face.

Clinical features

Erysipelas presents as a bright red, brawny, oedematous area. The face is most frequently affected. The organism gains entry through a minor abrasion and infects the superficial lymphatic vessels. The lesions are unilateral, and associated with leucocytosis and fever (Fig. 7.2).

Diagnosis and treatment

Prompt response to full doses of oral penicillin is the most useful diagnostic test for erysipelas. Although swabs should be taken routinely for bacteriological confirmation, the results should not be awaited before starting therapy. Topical therapy is unnecessary, but many dermatologists routinely prescribe a topical antibiotic. Topical steroids should be withheld, as they will delay response to systemic antibiotic therapy.

In a proportion of cases recurrent erysipelas develops on the same site, leading in time to chronic lymphoedema. Management of this complication is difficult and, although long-term antibiotic therapy is used, results are not always satisfactory.

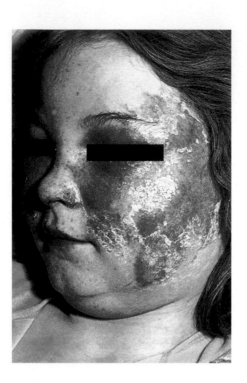

Fig. 7.2 Erysipelas. Note well-demarcated edge to the lesion. Response to oral penicillin within 24 hours is normal.

Cellulitis

Definition

A cutaneous infection, usually due to streptococci, but with deeper involvement of the subcutis than in erysipelas.

Clinical features

Cellulitis presents as a raised, hot, tender, erythematous area of skin (Fig. 7.3). The organism enters through a cut or abrasion, or a pre-existing dermatological disorder such as a leg ulcer. The affected area is larger and more diffuse than in erysipelas and the edges are not so well demarcated. Fever and leucocytosis are common. The draining lymph nodes are usually palpable and tender.

Diagnosis and treatment

Diagnosis is usually straightforward and therapy should be commenced immediately with full doses of a systemic antibiotic. Bacteriological swabs should be taken to identify the causative organism and to test for its antibiotic sensitivity. When these results are available the antibiotic can, if necessary, be changed. The initial choice of antibiotic will depend on the patient and his environment. In an otherwise healthy young person seen outside hospital, streptococcus is likely to be the cause and full doses of penicillin V are appropriate. On the other hand, in the elderly or in patients who have impaired immunity, a variety of organisms may be responsible and a broad-spectrum antibiotic (for example, flucloxacillin) should be used. Blood cultures should be taken before starting therapy in this situation.

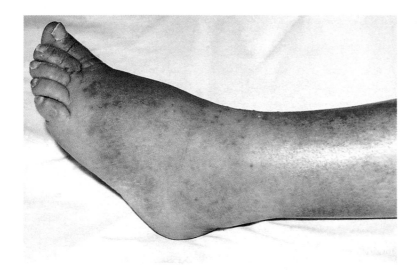

Fig. 7.3 Cellulitis involving the skin of the lower leg and ankle. Note intense swelling and erythema.

Erythrasma
Definition

A cutaneous infection caused by *Corynebacterium minutissimum*.

Clinical features

Erythrasma causes an asymptomatic, reddish-brown area of skin, commonly in body flexures, particularly the groin. It does not appear to be contagious and, if untreated, it spreads slowly with a well-demarcated advancing edge.

Diagnosis and treatment

Erythrasma can be diagnosed both by bacteriological identification of *Corynebacterium minutissimum* and by the coral-red fluorescence seen under Wood's light. Clinical confusion with a superficial fungal infection is resolved by these procedures.

Topical imidazoles such as clotrimazole or miconazole, or topical erythromycin are all effective. Full doses of erythromycin by mouth (250 mg four times per day for 7 days) are also curative, but rarely needed.

Mycobacterial infection
Tuberculosis

Although 'classical' tuberculosis is now uncommon in Britain, it must still be remembered and promptly treated in the elderly, the immunosuppressed, and immigrant populations with less natural resistance to *Mycobacterium tuberculosis*. In many parts of the world there is, at present, an upsurge of tuberculosis infection in immunosuppressed individuals and, in many cases, there appears to be resistance to classic anti-tuberculous drugs. In this section of the population, tuberculosis can appear in atypical forms, and it is important always to consider tuberculosis in any stubborn and atypical skin problem in immunocompromised individuals.

> ### *Key points*
> Classic tuberculosis is uncommon in Britain, but may be present in some populations (the elderly, the immunosuppressed, and some immigrants), where its appearance may be atypical.

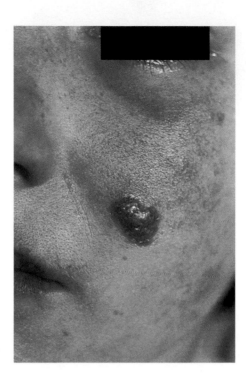

Fig. 7.4 Lupus vulgaris. Note yellow-brown translucent tinge to lesion.

Lupus vulgaris
Definition

The commonest form of cutaneous tuberculosis occurring after primary infection in individuals with good natural resistance to *M. tuberculosis*.

Incidence and aetiology

Lupus vulgaris (LV) is most common in northern Europe and affects females more often than males. Children are more frequently affected and in the elderly it may present with reactivation of old lesions following inadequate treatment in the past.

Clinical features

Lupus vulgaris most commonly affects the face and neck and is seen initially as firm, translucent, brown nodules (Fig. 7.4). These are called 'apple jelly nodules' because of their appearance on diascopy. This is gentle pressure on the lesion with a transparent glass slide or coverslip to impede local blood flow.

Untreated, the lesions will slowly spread laterally, giving rise to disfiguring scarring and contractions (Fig. 7.5). Malignant change has been reported in these scars, even in patients who have not received therapeutic X-rays or large doses of UV light in the past.

Pathology

Discrete, well-formed, tuberculoid granulomata are seen in the mid-dermis. Caseation is rare and the mycobacteria will only exceptionally be identified in Gram-stained sections, or by culture or guinea-pig inoculation.

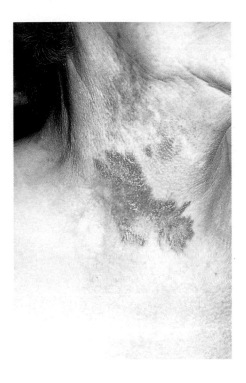

Fig. 7.5 Lupus vulgaris showing striking scarring and continuing activity on skin on right side of the neck.

Diagnosis and treatment

Biopsy and culture should be performed to confirm the diagnosis and then the patient should receive full anti-tuberculous therapy for at least 1 year. Current practice is to give three anti-tuberculous drugs. The current drugs of choice are rifampicin, isonicotinic acid hydrazide (INAH), and pyrazinamide. Ethambutol is used if resistance is suspected and rifabutin is useful as prophylaxis in those with low CD4 counts.

Scrofuloderma

Definition

Cutaneous tuberculosis due to spread of the organisms via sinuses from underlying caseous lymph nodes.

Clinical features: an ulcerated area is seen usually on the neck, overlying palpable lymph nodes (Fig. 7.6). Recognition is easy as *M. tuberculosis* can be identified both in the nodes and in the material draining onto the skin surface.

Treatment

Full anti-tuberculous therapy is required. The recommended drugs are as for lupus vulgaris.

Leprosy (Hansen's disease)

Air travel and the presence of a large immigrant population in parts of many countries make it important for both family doctors and dermatologists to recog-

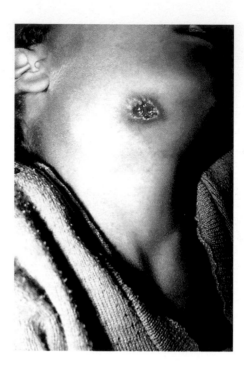

Fig. 7.6 Scrofuloderma. Here, *M. tuberculosis* can be cultured from the ulcerated area that is in direct contact with an infected lymph node underlying the ulcer.

Key points

Do not forget leprosy as a cause of pigment loss in dark skinned individuals.

nize or at least suspect the commoner presentations of leprosy. Although the condition is rare in Europe and North America, undiagnosed cases of leprosy can spread infection amongst a wide range of contacts, particularly the young and the elderly.

The polar varieties of *Mycobacterium leprae* infection are tuberculoid and lepromatous, but in current practice, most patients have borderline or mixed infection. The tuberculoid form is associated with low infectivity and a high degree of natural resistance to the organism, whereas the lepromatous type is associated with large numbers of easily identified micro-organisms, a high degree of infectivity, and little natural resistance to the mycobacteria. In between these two extremes lies a range of presentations combining features of both polar forms. Borderline or dimorphous leprosy, and indeterminate leprosy are terms used to describe these clinical problems.

Clinical features

In tuberculoid leprosy the infection is mainly in the peripheral nerves and the cutaneous manifestation is likely to be an anaesthetic macule or plaque with pigmentary changes. On white skin this may show as an erythematous or brown discoloration, but on coloured skin depigmentation is commonly seen. Palpable peripheral nerves may be felt near the area of discoloration. As skin appendages are damaged by the process, sweating and hair growth are diminished or absent. The lesions tend to develop adjacent to scars and vaccination sites, and they are sparse in the pure tuberculoid type (Fig. 7.7). These depigmented areas may clinically resemble vitiligo, which is much commoner than leprosy in the UK. Remember that dark skinned families from countries where leprosy is commoner

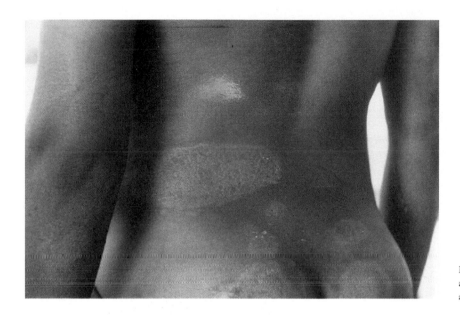

Fig.7.7 Tuberculoid leprosy. Note obvious areas of depigmentation that were also anaesthetic.

may be very concerned that a relatively innocuous patch of vitiligo (p. 227) is, in fact, leprosy and may need vigorous reassurance.

In borderline cases the lesions are similar, but more numerous.

In lepromatous leprosy macules, papules, nodules, and ulceration develop at sites where tissue temperature is low, such as the nostrils, which are frequently involved, leading to septal perforation, collapse of the nasal bones, and a characteristic deformity. Hair growth and sweating over the lesions is not impaired, and normal sensation is preserved. A generalized thickening of the involved facial tissues gives rise to a leonine facies, and severe and intractable leg ulcers may develop.

Pathology

In tuberculoid leprosy well-formed granulomata invade the dermis from within the nerve trunks, which are the primary site of infection. Cutaneous nerves may have been destroyed by this process and *M. leprae* will rarely be seen despite careful microscopy.

In lepromatous leprosy the granulomata generally lie deeper in the dermis and contain a large proportion of foamy histiocytes (macrophages). *M. leprae* are presented in large numbers in these cells and can be easily identified with special stains (for example, Ziehl–Nielsen).

Diagnosis and treatment

The diagnosis should be confirmed and treatment started at a centre that has some experience of leprosy. A full-thickness skin biopsy, skin snips, a peripheral nerve biopsy, and the lepromin test are all diagnostic aids. The choice of which of these to use in individual cases depends on the clinical presentation.

Treatment is based on systemic sulphones, rifampicin, and clofazimine, although resistance is becoming a problem and in the initial stages it can be complicated by reactions, particularly in lepromatous leprosy. In the UK, there is a leprosy panel organized by the Department of Health, who will give advice on best current therapy (Tel. no. 0207 972 1522). The duration of treatment varies. The tuberculoid variety should be treated for 1–2 years after disease activity has ceased, but in the lepromatous variety treatment should continue for life. Children who are household contacts should be followed up as they can harbour the organism for many years and develop the disease in adult life. Adult contacts rarely become infected.

Viral infections

Warts

Definition

Common benign cutaneous tumours caused by the human papilloma virus (HPV).

Warts are usually self-limiting cutaneous tumours caused by a range of DNA viruses, the human papilloma viruses (HPV). They vary significantly in their clinical presentation and different types of wart virus may be associated with specific clinical presentation (for example, genital warts). The wart virus is transmitted by direct contact. A small number of the over 90 varieties of human papilloma virus currently recognized have oncogenic potential. This is of particular importance in immunosuppressed individuals such as organ transplant recipients.

There are a number of different types of wart:

- **Common wart (Verruca vulgaris):** These easily identified lesions are usually multiple, raised, hyperkeratotic, and are commonly found on the hands. They are particularly common in children aged 5–10 years and may be painful, especially when periungual. Common warts demonstrate the *Koebner phenomenon* (p. 45), and develop on sites of trauma. All types of warts are more persistent in those whose cell-mediated immunity is suppressed. Renal transplant recipients, for example, tend to have large numbers of warts that stubbornly resist treatment (Fig. 7.8).

- **Plane warts:** These occur most frequently on the face and the backs of hands. Each is a slightly raised circular or oval plaque. Despite their relatively banal appearance, they are surprisingly resistant to therapy (Fig. 7.9).

- **Plantar warts (Verruca plantaris):** Constant pressure and friction on the soles prevents the normal outward expansion of warts in this site and instead they grow inwards towards the dermis (Fig. 7.10). Pressure on nerves can cause considerable pain. Children, sportsmen, athletes, and others who use communal showering facilities are particularly at risk.

Human papilloma viruses types 1 and 3 are the commonest types associated with cutaneous warts described above. They are not considered oncogenic varieties of HPV.

- **Genital warts:** These warts tend to develop in large clusters. They affect the penile and vulvar skin, mucous membrane, and also the peri-anal area (Fig.

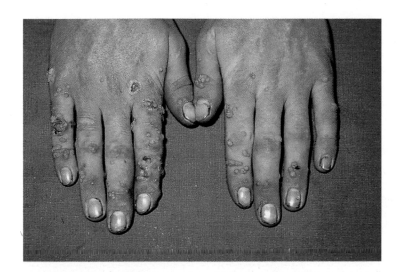

Fig. 7.8 Multiple hand warts. Note extensive lesion on the dorsal of all fingers.

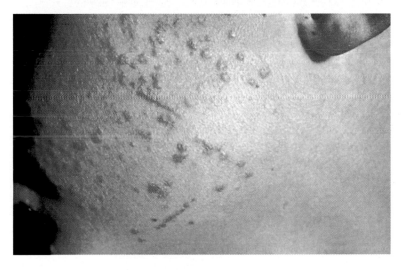

Fig. 7.9 Plane warts. Note the Koebner phenomenon caused by scratching.

7.11). Sexual partners should attend for examination and treatment, as otherwise re-infection is very common. All patients with peri-anal warts should have a proctoscopic examination to exclude rectal involvement. In children with genital warts the possibility of sexual abuse must be considered. HPVs types 16 and 18 are commonly found in genital warts, and there is current controversy about their oncogenic potential.

Pathology

Biopsy is rarely required to confirm the clinical diagnosis. The histopathology is, however, characteristic. Hyperkeratosis and acanthosis are accompanied by large numbers of keratohyalin granules in the Malpighian layer. Some epidermal cells are vacuolated and may also contain basophilic inclusions. The wart virus can be clearly seen and identified by electron microscopy.

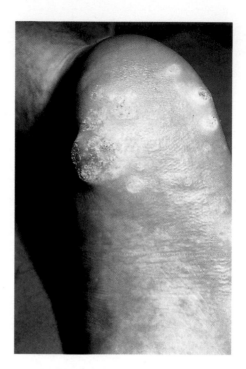

Fig. 7.10 Multiple plantar warts. These can be both painful and difficult to treat.

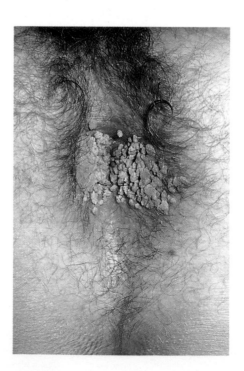

Fig. 7.11 Extensive perivulvar warts. In this situation full gynaecological examination is essential to rule out continuing infection.

Diagnosis

Diagnosis of warts is usually made by the patient. Occasionally, the periungual fibromata of tuberous sclerosis are misdiagnosed as periungual warts, but close examination and a search for other signs of this condition (p. 316) should clarify the situation. Plantar warts may be confused with either corns or, if haemorrhage into the lesion has occurred causing discoloration, with invasive malignant tumours such as malignant melanoma.

Paring down the lesion with a sharp scalpel blade can be of diagnostic help as in plantar warts punctate bleeding points will be seen. In corns, one sees only a thickened epidermis, while in a malignant tumour, such as melanoma, dark friable vascular tissue will be revealed. If a malignant tumour is suspected the patient should be referred without delay for a diagnostic excision biopsy. It is preferable to excise unnecessarily the occasional plantar wart than to treat a malignant melanoma inappropriately.

Genital warts may be confused with condylomata lata of syphilis and, as both conditions are transmitted by sexual contact, they may co-exist. Full serological screening for venereal diseases should therefore be performed routinely on all cases of genital warts.

Treatment

A large proportion of **common warts** will involute spontaneously and, therefore, either no treatment or placebo treatment for the first 3–4 months after presentation is quite acceptable, particularly in the case of small children. If therapy is considered necessary, a salicylic acid paint (for example 12% salicylic acid, 10% acetone, and collodion to 100%—Salactol, Duofilm) is recommended. Paints containing glutaraldehyde (Glutarol) are also useful. For lesions persisting despite a 3–4 month trial of such paints, cryotherapy with liquid nitrogen, or a slush of carbon dioxide snow and acetone can be used. Warts should be frozen for sufficient time to cause the surrounding skin to develop a white halo. Some discomfort is inevitable, and blistering may develop 24–48 hours after treatment. The procedure should be repeated at 3-weekly intervals until the warts are gone. Curettage, or electrocautery, or diathermy under local anaesthesia are standard methods for dealing with more persistent warts. Radiotherapy has been used in the past, but nowadays is not to be recommended even for persistent lesions.

With all forms of therapy the recurrence rate is relatively high.

Plane warts, particularly on the face, should be treated by bland, non-scarring preparations. Salicylic acid paints may accelerate spontaneous clearance.

For **plantar warts** slightly different methods are more likely to be successful. The first step is to pare away as much of the overlying hard skin as possible, and then apply salicylic acid or gluteraldehyde-containing paint (Salactol, Glutarol), and covering with occlusive plaster. In some countries 25–50% podophyllin in liquid paraffin or white soft paraffin (posalfilin)is used. This causes tissue necrosis if an occlusive bandage is kept in place for 10–14 days. The remaining wart virus-infected tissue can be curetted away after this period.

Formalin soaks are also of value. The patient applies a protective layer of Vaseline to the surrounding normal skin, then immerses the wart for 10–20 minutes in a saucer containing 3–6% formalin in an aqueous solution. This is repeated daily, and after 2–3 weeks warts become smaller and desiccated, and can be curetted out with ease and little pain.

Genital warts can be persistent and difficult to treat. Full vaginal and/or rectal examination should be performed to establish the extent of the problem before starting to treat the visible lesions. Cryotherapy can then be commenced, and used weekly or twice weekly for as long as is necessary. This is at present the best method of out-patient management, causing relatively little discomfort. Alternatively, daily applications for 3–4 days of podophyllin 25–50% in soft paraffin is effective, but it leads to considerable maceration and discomfort. It is difficult to use on an out-patient basis.

Situations in which warts must be regarded as a more serious problem are pregnancy and immunosuppression. Young pregnant women with a few mild genital warts tend rapidly to develop large, fungating, cauliflower-like masses of lesions. The use of podophyllin in pregnant women is *not* recommended because of sporadic case reports of foetal damage. Early and efficient treatment of small lesions with cryotherapy is the treatment of choice.

In the immunosuppressed patient warts can grow with alarming speed and give rise to major problems. Children on long-term chemotherapy for leukaemia and other malignancies tend to develop large and very persistent lesions. Such patients should be treated promptly and effectively as spontaneous resolution is most unlikely to occur. It is also good practice to examine such children for warts prior to commencing chemotherapy and treat any lesions before further chemotherapy-induced immunosuppression develops. Transplant recipients tend to be very difficult to treat once they develop warts and it is good practice to vigorously treat all warts prior to transplantation to prevent future problems. Very persistent warts in transplant patients may require specialist measures, such as intra-lesional bleomycin or systemic interferon.

Molluscum contagiosum

Definition

An infectious cutaneous lesion caused by a pox virus.

> **Key points**
>
> Molluscum contagiosum and orf are caused by a pox virus.

This benign, but troublesome condition is a common cause for dermatological out-patient referral in the under-fives, and occasionally in older children and adults. Multiple lesions are common in young children, but in adults isolated lesions, sometimes of considerable size, are more common.

Clinical features

The lesions are most commonly seen on the face and neck, although the trunk may also be involved. The lesions are elevated, smooth, reddish papules, and all have a small central punctum, which is an important diagnostic point to be sought (Figs 7.12 and 7.13). Troublesome lesions may develop around the eyelids and at the vermilion border of the lip. In adults, isolated lesions may develop on any body site and in recent years crops of mollusca on genital skin have been seen more commonly.

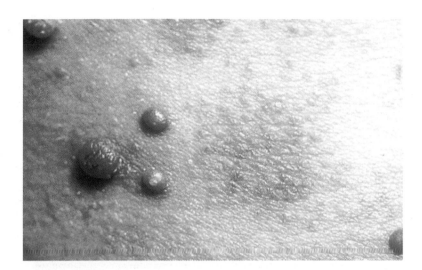

Fig. 7.12 Molluscum contagiosum. Note central punctum, seen best on the largest lesion.

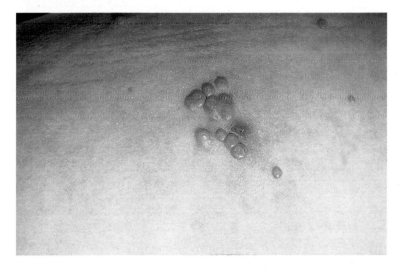

Fig. 7.13 Molluscum contagiosum. Note cluster of pearly lesions with central umbilication.

Pathology

Biopsy is rarely required and is usually performed on a large isolated lesion to exclude other more serious conditions. The histological changes are confined to the epidermis and consist of acanthosis, hyperkeratosis, and an increase in the numbers of keratohyalin granules. As epidermal cells in the centre of the lesion are destroyed they are replaced by large, amorphous, eosinophilic structures, the molluscum bodies, which are the histological hallmark of this condition.

Diagnosis and treatment

Diagnosis is usually straightforward, but an isolated lesion may not be recognized until histological examination of curettings or of a biopsy.

The aim of treatment is to stimulate an inflammatory reaction in the dermis underlying the lesion. This can be achieved by puncturing the lesions individually with a curette or forceps, and applying iodine to the area. Liquid nitrogen or carbon dioxide/acetone slush can also be used, but are less effective.

Orf

Definition

A rapidly growing solitary cutaneous lesion caused by a pox virus.

Clinical features

The infection is contracted through contact with sheep, either directly or indirectly from barbed wire, grass, or other material adjacent to the animals. It is easily and quickly recognized by agricultural workers, country dwellers, and veterinary surgeons, but may dismay and alarm a town dweller, who develops a rapidly expanding lesion on his hand 2 weeks after a visit to a farm in the country.

After an incubation period of 7–10 days a red papule develops, commonly on the sides of the fingers, rapidly grows, and finally reaches a size of 5–10 cm, with a central necrotic or bullous area (Fig. 7.14). Lymphangitis, local lymphadenopathy, and fever are not uncommon. Spontaneous recovery takes place and one attack confers subsequent immunity.

Treatment

A broad spectrum systemic antibiotic is commonly given orally for 5–7 days, for example, flucloxacillin. Topical antibiotics, such as 3% aureomycin ointment, may also be used.

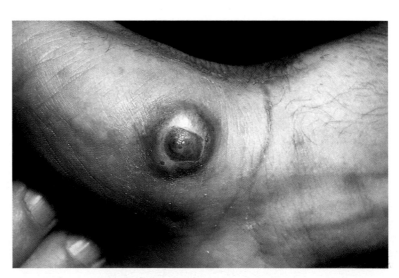

Fig. 7.14 Orf. Note large pustular lesion that has developed rapidly on the hand of a town dweller who had helped a sheep caught in barbed wire 10 days previously.

> ### Key points
>
> Primary infection with *Herpes virus hominis* type 1 is almost universal early in life.

Herpes simplex

Definition

A cutaneous infection due to *Herpes virus hominis*.

Two types of *H. hominis* virus are currently recognized. Type 1 is the variety mainly responsible for recurrent 'cold sores' in the upper lip area, and type 2 is usually associated with genital herpes lesions. Carcinoma of the cervix is commoner in women with a high titre of antibody to the type 2 virus, but no putative or proven association with malignancy has yet been reported with the type 1 virus.

Primary infection with type 1 virus is almost universal in childhood or early adult life, and is usually subclinical. Thereafter, most people have no further problems, but a few have exacerbations of *H. hominis* infection, usually on the upper lip, often in association with other viral infections. No specific immunological difference between these individuals and those without recurrent herpes simplex has yet been identified.

Clinical features

The characteristic clinical picture of an active, primary *H. hominis* type 1 infection is a miserable, febrile child, with a painful ulcerated mouth and painful enlarged local lymph nodes (Fig. 7.15). The lesions persist for 3–6 days and subside spontaneously. They consist of a group of small blisters on the skin surface, as well as on buccal mucous membrane. If the cornea is involved, immediate ophthalmological care should be instituted, as corneal scarring and ulceration are common sequelae. *Herpetic whitlow* or inoculation herpes simplex is common in hospital workers, and results from the virus entering through a small abrasion, usually on the fingers (Fig. 7.16). Frequently misdiagnosed as a pyogenic lesion, it consists of a painful, indurated, and tender area, topped by blisters, which initially are filled with clear fluid. Occasionally, primary infection on the trunk may have a linear distribution and cause confusion with herpes zoster.

> ### Key points
> Topical steroid should not be applied to herpes simplex lesions.

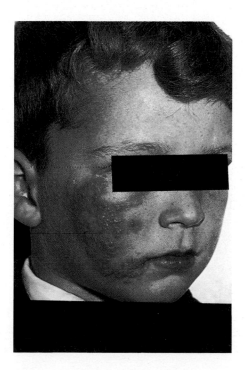

Fig. 7.15 Herpes simplex. Primary infection in an 8-year-old boy.

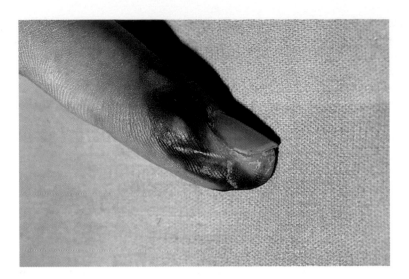

Fig. 7.16 Herpetic whitlow. Very often these lesions are regarded as bacterial and lanced. Never forget that viruses, as well as bacteria can give rise to painful fingers of this type.

Recurrent herpes simplex attacks begin with a tingling sensation and then tender, painful lesions appear, usually on the upper lip.

Patients with AIDS may develop very extensive, painful, and persistent H. simplex infections usually with herpes simplex type 2.

Pathology

The epidermis shows the significant changes. Gross intracellular oedema leads to balloon degeneration of the infected epidermal cells. The nuclei of these cells show specific intra-nuclear inclusions. Large multinucleate giant cells may also be seen in persistent infections.

Diagnosis and treatment

If there is doubt clinically, the most rapid way to confirm the diagnosis is to examine a thick smear from the surface of the lesion in the electron microscope to identify the viral particles. Blood samples can be taken both at the time of presentation and 10–14 days later to demonstrate a rise in titre of antibody to the virus. An alternative rapid diagnostic method for identifying both herpes simplex and herpes zoster is to use a specific fluorescein-labelled antibody directed against the virus in a frozen section from a skin biopsy of the lesion.

Management of severe primary infection is largely supportive, to maintain an adequate fluid balance. If necessary, systemic antibiotics can be administered to control secondary infection.

Recurrent herpes simplex lesions are difficult to prevent. Acyclovir (Zovirax) given orally in doses of 200 mg five times daily may reduce the severity of recurrent attacks, but only if introduced in the very early stages of the recurrence. In the case of patients who have already had multiple recurrences, 200 mg acyclovir given orally two or three times daily for several months may reduce the number of recurrences. Topical acyclovir preparations have, in general, been relatively ineffective.

For topical use, 10% povidone iodine paint (Betadine paint, UK) will dry the lesions and reduce secondary bacterial infection. Topical acyclovir is of doubtful value once the infection is well established. Patients with herpes simplex should be warned specifically not to use a topical steroid on the lesions and told to avoid contact with individuals who have atopic eczema.

Herpes simplex infection in the immunosuppressed and in patients with atopic dermatitis can be serious and potentially life-threatening. Hospitalization, supportive care, and full doses of acyclovir, given orally or intravenously, are matters of urgency. It is important to protect these two groups of patients from herpes simplex infection and mothers of children with atopic dermatitis should be warned that persons with cold sores are hazardous to their child.

Herpes zoster (shingles)

Definition

A cutaneous infection caused by the chickenpox virus, *Herpesvirus varicellae.*

Herpes zoster is a disease of adult life and old age, being very rare in children and healthy young adults. As with other viral infections, however, it can develop in a virulent and fulminating form in those who are immunosuppressed either by disease or by therapy. Patients with Hodgkin's disease are particularly prone to develop herpes zoster.

Pathology

As in herpes simplex, the striking histological feature of herpes zoster is balloon degeneration—the presence of grossly swollen, distorted cells in the epidermis. Direct immunofluorescence using antibodies specific for herpes simplex or herpes zoster will differentiate between the two while the infection is at a very early stage. Serology will differentiate from about 14 days after infection.

Clinical features

After prodromal pain, usually in a dermatome distribution, malaise, and sometimes fever, a linear erythematous band develops on this dermatome (Figs 7.17 and 7.18). Groups of small blisters then develop on the erythema. Some of these may become secondarily infected, and local lymphadenopathy is common. Pain may appear to be out of proportion to the other clinical signs, and when it persists and evolves into post-herpetic neuralgia, it is extremely difficult to treat.

Certain clinical varieties require special management. These include involvement of the ophthalmic division of the trigeminal nerve, leading to ocular damage and the Ramsey–Hunt syndrome when the geniculate ganglia are affected, causing pain and blistering of the external ear. Involvement of the first and second sacral ganglia may cause severe ulceration in the genital region and urinary retention. In the elderly, unfit, or immunosuppressed, more than one dermatome may be involved.

Diagnosis and treatment

The clinical appearance is usually diagnostic, but occasionally examination of a thick smear by electron microscope or immunofluorescence is required. Treatment of mild cases is symptomatic, and consists of simple analgesics, maintenance of fluid balance, and soothing topical (drying) applications of lotions such as povidone iodine or ichthyol 1% in oily calamine lotion. Topical steroids should *not* be

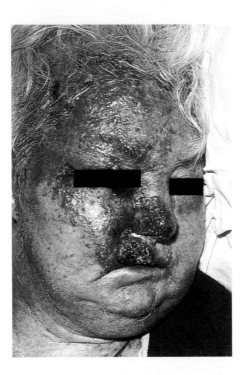

Fig. 7.17 Herpes zoster. Severe herpes zoster infection involving the trigeminal nerve.

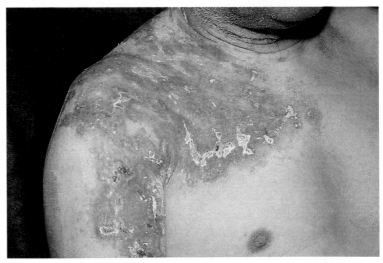

Fig. 7.18 Herpes zoster showing extensive scarring on the shoulder in the dermatomal distribution. This particular individual had extensive post-herpetic pain.

applied to this or to any other lesion in which actively growing virus is present. The lesions will clear in 7–10 days.

In patients with painful and more widespread infection or in the immunosuppressed, a full course of acyclovir 800 mg five times daily for 7 days is recommended. There is some evidence that acyclovir will reduce the incidence and severity of post-herpetic neuralgia.

The management of post-herpetic neuralgia is unsatisfactory. A 7–10-day course of systemic corticosteroids may help some otherwise healthy patients, but in others the pain is persistent and severe, and neurosurgical intervention may have to be considered.

Spirochaetal infections

Lyme Disease

Definition

A multi-system disease caused by the spirochaete borrelia and transmitted to man by the tick *Ixodes ricinus*.

Incidence and aetiology

In the early 1980s a new disease entity and its cause were recognized in the small town of Lyme, Connecticut, USA. Lyme disease develops after a bite from the tick *Ixodes ricinus*, which carries the causative organism, the spirochaete, *Borrelia burgdorferi*. These ticks are found in large numbers in the New England woods, in Scandinavia, in Austria, and in wooded parts of the UK. The exact incidence of Lyme disease is not known, but small scale population studies in countries such as Austria suggest, from serological analysis, that up to 25% of the population in these areas have had past exposure and developed an antibody response.

Clinical features

After a tick bite, which the patient may not remember, there is frequently a febrile episode and the patient then develops a red, raised, slowly changing plaque or erythema around the tick bite (Fig. 7.19). This is *erythema chronicum migrans*, the best established dermatological association of Lyme disease. A biopsy of this site and very careful search may reveal the spirochaete in the lesion. Patients will also have circulating antibodies to *Borrelia burgdorferi*, but the presence of these anti-bodies cannot be taken as proof of cause of the cutaneous lesion because of the possibility of previous exposure. A later cutaneous association with Lyme disease is acrodermatitis chronica atrophicans.

Non-dermatological manifestations of Lyme disease include musculoskeletal and neurological problems, including meningitis and isolated nerve palsies.

Treatment

Therapy for erythema chronicum migrans and any other dermatological problem thought to be associated with Lyme disease is either oral penicillin or tetracycline in full doses for a minimum of 2 weeks. Repeated courses may be required.

Fungal infections

Two main groups of fungi infect man. These are the *Candida* group of yeasts and the *dermatophytes*. *Candida albicans* is the most common species responsible for human infection and of the dermatophytes, *Trichophyton rubrum*, *Trichophyton mentagrophytes* var. *interdigitale*, *Trichophyton tonsurans*, and *Epidermophyton floccosum* are the commonest pathogens in the UK. All these dermatophytes are transmitted directly from one human host to another. However, humans can contract animal

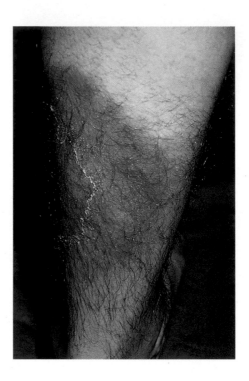

Fig. 7.19 Erythema chronicum migrans. Lower leg of a keen hill walker who had been walking in the New Forest 1 week before the development of this lesion.

ringworm from domestic animals, the usual dermatophytes responsible being *Microsporum canis* and *Trichophyton verrucosum*.

Pityriasis versicolor, due to a yeast, *Malassezia furfur*, is a superficial infection and will be discussed in this section.

Candida infections (candidosis, thrush)

Candida albicans is a normal commensal of the gastro-intestinal tract, and can be grown from apparently healthy, normal mouths and peri-anal skin. In the very young, the elderly, and in those whose natural microbiological flora has been disturbed by disease or by therapy such as antibiotics, it may become a pathogen. It can be a serious and resistant problem in those with HIV.

Clinical features

Cutaneous lesions due to *Candida albicans* present in infants as napkin candidosis and in the elderly as intertrigo affecting the submammary folds, the axillae, and the groins (Fig. 7.20). In both situations the lesions are a glazed brick-red, and are characterized by 'satellite lesions' and occasionally pustules around the main area of involvement. These are isolated individual lesions, which have the same colour and appearance as the main lesion. Painful fissures frequently develop in the affected body folds and may be resistant to therapy.

In people with occupations that involve wet work, candidal paronychia is an occupational hazard. Initially, the protective cuticle between nail and nail fold is lost, allowing Candida to invade the space thus created. The resulting inflammation produces a 'bolstered' posterior nail fold from which beads of pus can be expressed.

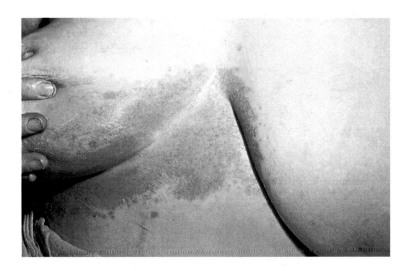

Fig. 7.20 Infra-mammary candidosis in an obese diabetic patient.

Chronic candidal granuloma, most commonly on the lips, may develop in patients who have a long history of candidosis. This consists of a firm, indurated area and must not be mistaken for a developing malignancy.

Lesions due to *Candida* on the mucous membranes may involve the mouth, the urogenital area, the oesophagus, and the alimentary tract. Oral candidosis produces adherent white patches on the tongue and inner surfaces of the cheeks. If scraped off, a raw bleeding area will be revealed. In the elderly these lesions are fairly common under dental plates and may be very difficult to cure as the plate itself is frequently colonized by the organism. Candidal vulvovaginitis causes an irritable erythema associated with a copious discharge. There is no evidence that oral contraceptives predispose to this condition, but pregnant and diabetic women are more at risk. *Candida* infecting the bronchial or alimentary mucous membranes is less common but should always be borne in mind when infants with napkin *Candida* have persistent diarrhoea.

Generalized systemic infections due to *Candida* are rare and usually associated with immunosuppression or antibiotic therapy. Chronic mucocutaneous candidosis is rare, but of great interest to dermatologists and immunologists as it is a model for establishing the relative value of cell-mediated and humoral immunity in the host response to *Candida*.

Pathology

Candida albicans exists both as yeasts and in hyphal form. In pathological conditions budding yeasts and pseudohyphae are easily seen, and best visualized by staining with periodic acid Schiff (PAS). They lie in the stratum corneum. Persistent lesions may be associated with abscess formation, acanthosis, and, in more severe cases, with a granulomatous reaction.

Diagnosis and treatment

All lesions thought to be due to *Candida* should be swabbed and examined for the presence of the organism. In typical cases this serves merely to confirm a clinical impression, but in less classic presentations it is essential. It must be remembered, however, that the presence of the organism does not automatically imply a patho-genetic role, and also that *Candida* may colonize a pre-existing skin condition such as seborrhoeic dermatitis and cause an opportunistic secondary infection, rather than primary disease.

Treatment depends firstly on altering the damp, moist, warm microclimate in which *Candida* thrives. Thus, napkin candidosis will not clear as long as the infant is wrapped in damp napkins. Similarly, obese females with pendulous breasts will retain their infra-mammary *Candida* as long as the two apposing skin surfaces remain in close contact. Soaks or swabs should therefore be used to separate skin folds in such situations.

For patients with an intact immune system, the choice of therapy lies between nystatin-containing preparations and imidazoles. Nystatin is available as an oral suspension, and in pessary, cream, gel, and ointment formulation. It has a well-established safety record and is the preparation of choice for use in infants. Imidazoles include clotrimazole (Canesten, UK; Lotrimin, USA) cream, econazole (Spectazole, US), miconazole (Daktarin), sulconazole, and ketoconazole. Ketoconazole appears to have greater activity against *Candida* than the other imidazoles.

Candida paronychia is relatively slow to respond to therapy, but good results will be achieved by instructing the patient to work nystatin ointment well into the nail fold and to keep the hands dry. If working conditions necessitate rubber gloves, a separate pair of cotton gloves should be worn next to the skin and changed frequently. 'Denture mouth' due to *Candida* requires concomitant treatment of the mouth with nystatin suspension, miconazole gel, or amphotericin B lozenges, and also nightly soaking of the dentures in an anti-fungal solution.

Infants with persistent napkin *Candida* should be given oral nystatin drops as a high proportion will have involvement of the alimentary tract.

Topical steroids are an excellent growth medium for *Candida* and are con-traindicated.

Persistent and severe candidal infection is a particular problem in patients who are therapeutically immunosuppressed or in those whose immune system is severely depressed as in HIV infection. In those situations the use of oral imida-zoles such as fluconazole (Diflucan, UK) or itraconazole (Sporanox UK) as a pro-phylactic measure appears effective and safe. Very short courses of these oral imidazoles are also extremely effective in eradicating persistent genital candidosis in otherwise healthy non-immunosuppressed individuals.

Dermatophyte infections

Definition

Cutaneous lesions due to dermatophytes, presenting most commonly as athlete's foot, nail infections, tinea corporis, and scalp ringworm.

Clinical features

Tinea pedis (athlete's foot): This common condition is found in adolescents and young adults, particularly those who use communal changing facilities, showers,

> **Key points**
>
> Persistent candidal infection is a sign of immunosuppression, not a disease *per se*. Investigate your patient for underlying problems.

> **Key points**
>
> Fungal infections are caused by yeasts and dermatophytes. Yeasts respond to nystatin, dermatophytes do not.

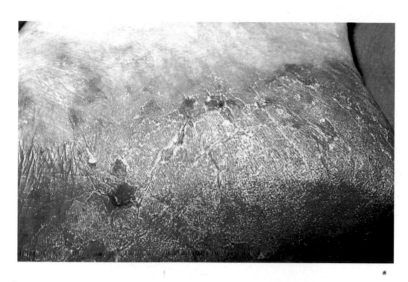

Fig. 7.21 Tinea pedis involving the instep and heel. *Trichophyton rubrum* was cultured from scrapings.

and swimming pools. The usual site of infection is the toe webs, especially the fourth, where moist, white 'blotting-paper' skin will be seen. Pruritus is common. The instep (Fig. 7.21), and in persistent cases the nails, may also be involved and therapy then poses considerable difficulties.

The organisms most commonly found are *Trichophyton rubrum, Trichophyton mentagrophytes* var. *interdigitale,* and *Epidermophyton floccosum.*

Tinea corporis (ringworm): Infection of the trunk frequently begins in the body folds such as the groins or axillae and presents as an itchy, erythematous area with a raised advancing edge. Scrapings will be most likely to yield positive results if taken from this edge.

Diagnosis is not always straightforward. Isolated scaling lesions on the trunk may resemble psoriasis (Figs 7.22 and 7.23). If tinea corporis has been treated with topical steroids, its presentation may be atypical. Persistent hand dermatitis may be due to dermatophytes, most commonly *Trichophyton rubrum,* in which case the palm is dry with itchy, scaly creases. Mycological examination should be routine in such circumstances.

Dermatophyte infection of the hair shaft

This may be on the scalp or beard area and due to *T. tonsurans, M. canis, T. rubrum,* or *T. verrucosum* (Fig. 7.24). Usually, the first sign is a well-circumscribed pruritic scaling area of hair loss, with a variable inflammatory response. Suspected hair infection should always be examined under Wood's light (ultraviolet light >365 nm) as lesions due to *M. canis* and *M. audouinii* will show a diagnostic brilliant green fluorescence. Those due to *Trichophyton* species do not give rise to this degree of fluorescence, although *T. schoenleinii* causes a dull green fluorescence and gives rise to the distinctive clinical entity called **favus**. Favus is now most common in North America, around the Mediterranean, and in the Middle East. The characteristic features are extensive—even complete—hair loss, scalp atrophy leading to permanent alopecia, and the presence of adherent scales (scutulae) on the remaining hairs.

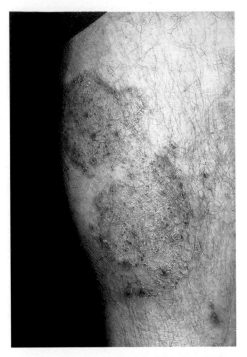

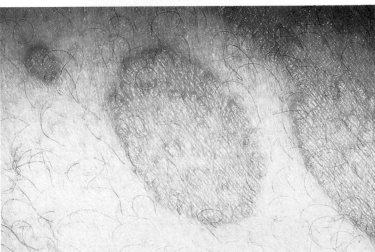

Figs 7.22 and 7.23 Scaling lesions on the trunk. Mycological examination showed both to be due to fungal infection. Note the superficial similarity to areas of psoriasis.

Infection of the hair shaft with *T. verrucosum* may cause a very brisk inflammatory reaction, termed a **kerion** (Fig. 7.25), seen commonly in children after contact with cattle or other domestic animals. There is a dramatic, acute folliculitis with pustules and swelling forming a boggy mass on the scalp. Hair loss and eventual scarring alopecia are common, but one attack usually confers subsequent immunity.

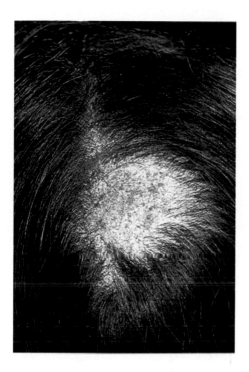

Fig. 7.24 Tinea capitis. Brilliant green fluorescence was seen under Wood's light and *Microsporum audouinii* isolated in culture.

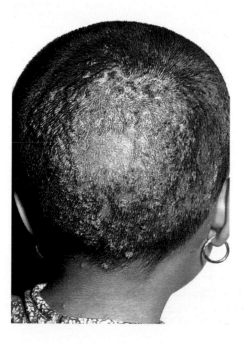

Fig. 7.25 Extensive kerion in an immigrant child.

Pathology

These pathogenic fungi inhabit the keratinized tissue of skin, hair, and nails, and generally do not invade living tissue. In active infections they are seen as branched hyphae. They grow down the pilosebaceous follicles towards the hair bulb, but are arrested before reaching the bulb itself and fan out to form multiple hyphal fronds known as **Adamson's fringe**. The hair shaft is invaded.

Dermatophytes can be seen on **direct examination** by taking skin scrapings (p. 46) or nail clippings from the affected area, and mounting them on a slide with coverslip in 10–20% potassium hydroxide, which is gently warmed and examined microscopically. To identify the particular dermatophyte present it is necessary to culture the samples for up to 3 weeks on a suitable medium such as Sabouraud's. These techniques, rather than biopsy, constitute the correct method of identifying fungi, but if it is necessary to look for fungi in a histological section it should be stained with periodic acid Schiff (PAS) or methenamine silver to show them in the stratum corneum.

Diagnosis and treatment

Direct microscopy of scrapings in potassium hydroxide and the use of Wood's light in the clinic or consulting room will immediately confirm the clinical diagnosis in a high proportion of dermatophyte infections. The remainder will require culture of skin scrapings or nail clippings. Any persistent scaling lesions should be scraped and examined in this way as atypical fungal infections may mimic psoriasis, seborrhoeic dermatitis, or mycosis fungoides. Over-diagnosis of dermatophyte infections may also occur, particularly in the case of lesions of the feet when the true cause may be simple maceration from hyperhidrosis or allergic contact dermatitis to footwear. Any persistent lesions on the feet, which do not respond to anti-fungal therapy, should be carefully reviewed, particularly if there is no involvement of the inter-digital clefts.

Cutaneous dermatophyte infections can be treated with topical or oral preparations. Topical preparations include the allylamines (terbinafine, Lamisil) and the imidazoles, which are available as creams, including sulconazole (Exelderm, UK), miconazole (Daktarin, UK), Monistat derm (USA), cicloprox (Loprox), and ketoconazole (Nizoral, UK and USA).

Oral griseofulvin and oral terbinafine (Lamisil), which are effective against dermatophytes, but not *Candida* species, should be reserved for more severe cutaneous infections involving body sites other than or in addition to the inter-digital clefts. They are, however, the treatment of choice for widespread or persistent tinea corporis, tinea capitis, and tinea unguium. The dose is 1 g of griseofulvin daily for adults. This should be give orally during a fatty meal. Duration of treatment varies with site of involvement, but in general 4–6 weeks for scalp and body lesions.

Terbinafine is fungicidal, and is effective in treating both finger and toenails that were previously resistant to therapy. It should be given in a dose of 250 mg/day for 6 weeks and the course may be repeated once. Thereafter, topical terbinafine can applied to the nail bed area as the new nail grows in.

Prevention of tinea pedis can to a large extent be achieved by simple hygiene, footbaths, and the use of an anti-fungal dusting powder after using communal baths and showers.

Pityriasis versicolor

Definition

A persistent, usually asymptomatic, fungal infection of the trunk due to *Malassezia furfur*.

This infection is relatively common in tropical countries and is seen with increased frequency in Britain during spells of hot humid weather. The causative organism is known as *Pityrosporum orbiculare* in its yeast-like form and as *Malassezia furfur* when it becomes hyphal. These hyphae and yeasts can be recognized in skin scrapings, or Scotch tape strippings, or on biopsy material using PAS stain. The hyphae are found in the horny layers and there is little underlying reaction.

Clinical features

The lesions are asymptomatic, mainly on the trunk and proximal parts of the limbs, with a fine superficial scale seen best after gently scraping the surface with a fingernail. Untanned, white, Caucasian skin shows an increase in pigmentation in the affected areas with a yellowish-brown scale, but in darker skin or heavily tanned skin there is depigmentation. The overall effect is a dappled appearance (Figs 7.26–7.28).

Diagnosis and treatment

Skin scrapings for direct microscopy and examination under Wood's light for pale yellow fluorescence can both be used to identify the organism. Vitiligo (p. 227) is frequently confused with pityriasis versicolor and scrapings should be taken from all atypical cases.

Many topical preparations have been recommended for therapy, but recurrences are common. The current treatment of choice is a topical imidazole. Clotrimazole solution, miconazole cream, and econazole cream and lotion are all effective.

In severe and persistent cases a monthly dose of itraconazole orally may prevent relapse.

Protozoal infection

Leishmaniasis

Definition

Cutaneous or systemic infection caused by the parasite leishmania and transmitted by a bite from a sand fly.

The pathology of the type of leishmania infection most commonly seen in the UK is a superficial granuloma. Careful search will reveal leishman Donovan bodies in the cells of the granuloma.

Clinical features

Leishmaniasis is a major problem in South America, Africa, and southern Mediterranean countries. The reader is advised to consult a tropical dermatology text for a detailed account. The most likely presentation in the UK is a crusted sore on the face, hand, or leg 6–8 weeks after returning from an endemic area (Fig. 7.29). Cases have recently been reported in holiday-makers after returning from Spain. The patient may not remember the sand fly bite.

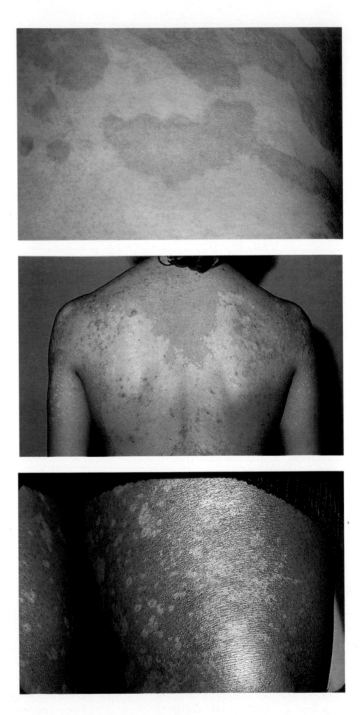

Figs 7.26–7.28 Lesions of pityriasis versicolor showing increase in pigmentation in white skinned individuals, but conversely a decrease in darker skinned individuals.

Diagnosis

Diagnosis is based on the history, histology, and, if required a positive leishmanin test, an intra-dermal injection of heat-killed organisms.

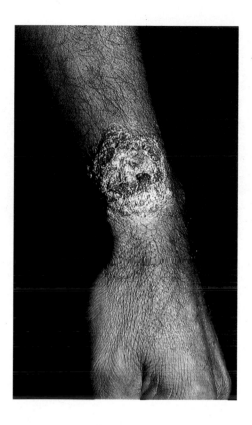

Fig. 7.29 Cutaneous leishmaniasis on the wrist in an individual normally resident in the UK 8 weeks after visiting the Middle East.

Treatment

In healthy individuals, cutaneous leishmaniasis frequently resolves spontaneously. Cryotherapy is also effective and, for persistent cases, oral pentavalent antimony (Pentostam) is required.

Cutaneous infestations

The commonest infestations in man are due to lice and scabies.

Scabies

Definition

A persistent pruritic skin eruption caused by cutaneous infestation with the mite *Sarcoptes scabei*.

The female (Fig. 7.30) inhabits a burrow in the stratum corneum and eventually dies after laying her eggs there. The eggs hatch and the new generation matures in 14 days, when the cycle is repeated.

The incidence of scabies varies on a world scale with hygiene, housing conditions, and population movements. Epidemics have been associated with world wars, and recent local increases in incidence in Europe have been attributed to changing social habits and increasing body contact. Frequently, whole households are infested, although only one member may complain of symptoms.

> ### Key points
>
> Remember that scabies infection in those who have a high standard of hygiene can be difficult to recognize.

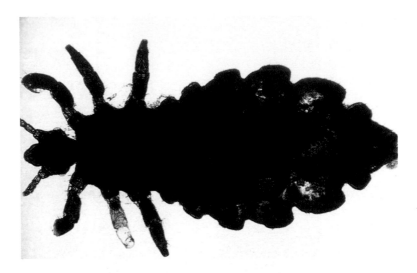

Fig. 7.30 The female scabies mite or *Acarus*.

Pathology

A local hypersensitivity reaction to the female scabies mite is assumed to cause release of inflammatory mediators, giving rise to severe and persistent itch.

If scabies lesions are biopsied, usually in error, the female mite and her eggs may be seen in a burrow high in the stratum corneum. Occasionally, nodular lesions persist long after successful therapy and these consist of a chronic inflammatory reaction with many lymphocytes in the dermis.

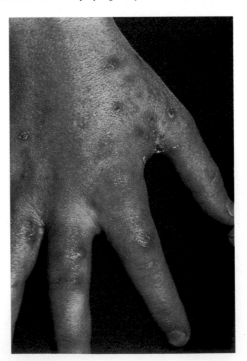

Fig. 7.31 Scabetic lesions on the hands. An acarus was extracted from the raised lesion on the third (middle) finger.

Clinical features

Patients complain bitterly of severe and persistent itch, worse after bathing and at night. In those who have a high standard of personal hygiene, lesions may be very sparse, but the classical sites of involvement are the finger webs, the sides of the fingers (Fig. 7.31), the flexor aspects of the wrists, the points of the elbows, the anterior axillary fold, the periumbilical area, the penile or scrotal skin in males (Figs 7.32 and 7.33), and the areolae of the nipple in females. In infants who are

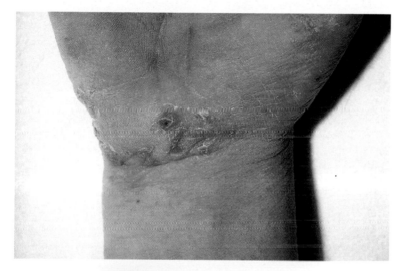

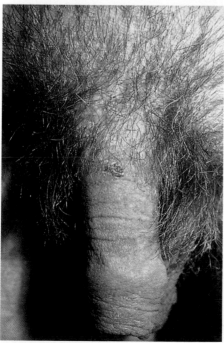

Figs 7.32 and 7.33 Scabies involving the wrists and genital area, respectively.

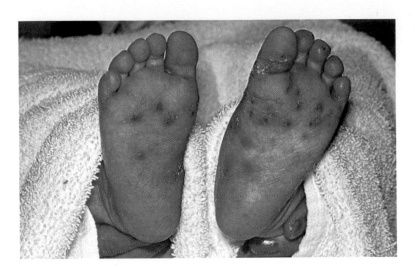

Fig. 7.34 Scabetic lesions in an infant aged 9 months. Note the striking involvement of the soles of the feet.

not yet walking, striking involvement of the soles is common (Fig. 7.34). The individual lesions may seem superficially to be excoriated papules, but on closer inspection a linear burrow may be seen extending from this papule. The mite can frequently be extracted from this burrow with a needle, and painting the area with Indian ink, then washing off the excess on the skin surface will demonstrate dramatically the extent of the burrows. In long-standing cases secondary infection with pustule formation and crusting is common. Nodular lesions that persist for months after successful therapy may be seen. These are commonest on the buttocks and the male genitalia.

A moist oozing infected dermatitis may develop on top of scabetic burrows and dermatitic lesions on scabetic sites of predilection should be very carefully examined for underlying burrows.

Diagnosis and treatment

In all cases, demonstration of the acarus by extracting it from a burrow should be attempted as this is the cardinal diagnostic test. The most common mistake is to misdiagnose scabies, either as contact dermatitis or as dermatitis herpetiformis. All cases of presumed scabies in which the acarus has not been identified and which do not respond to therapy, should be reassessed and biopsy considered.

The most useful acaricides are 1% gamma benzene hexachloride (lindane—Quellada), malathion (Derbac M, Suleo M), and permethrin (Lyclear). Sulphur preparations, such as 2.5% sulphur ointment or monosulfiram (Tetmosol), are recommended in many centres for infants because of the risk of percutaneous absorption of the first two preparations. It is essential that the entire body from the neck to the soles of the feet be treated and that the hands are re-treated during the course of the 24 hours for which the preparation should remain on the skin. A 2-inch paintbrush or cotton wool swabs are useful applicators. After 24 hours the application can be washed off in a hot bath. If it is considered necessary, this procedure can be repeated once or twice, but if instructions are properly followed, this should not be necessary. Twenty-four hours after the last application the patient should bathe, and all clothing and bed linen be washed. Boiling or fumigation is not required. Pruritus may continue for a few days even after successful therapy and crotamiton cream (Eurax, UK) will minimize this.

All household and other close contacts of a confirmed case of scabies should be warned that they are likely to be infested and should be treated at the same time as the patient, even if they are asymptomatic. The usual cause of persistent scabies is either inadequate application of topical therapy or re-infestation from contacts. Written instructions to patients on how to treat themselves and their families will increase the likelihood of the correct procedures being followed.

Pediculosis capitis

Pediculosis capitis is a relatively common problem in schoolchildren in various parts of the world, and, at present, it is prevalent in certain large cities in the UK. Pediculosis corporis is less common, and is most frequently seen in vagrants and others living in very poor social circumstances.

The well-known nit is a head-louse egg, stuck firmly to scalp hair by its capsule. Nits may look like fine adherent dandruff particles. There are no associated symptoms until the louse hatches, when an irritant dermatitis on the scalp develops. Scratching leads to secondary impetiginization, particularly at the nape of the neck and behind the ears.

Diagnosis and treatment

Identification of the nit or of the adult head louse with the naked eye is straightforward. Shaving the head is not required, but cutting the hair short will facilitate treatment and lessen the risk of reinfestation. Brushing of the hair with a fine brush will result in nits sticking to the brush (Fig. 7.35).

Malathion (Derbac M, Suleo M) and permethrin (Lyclear) are all useful preparations at present, but resistance is developing, and if a patient does not respond to one of these, an alternative should be substituted. These should be applied to the entire scalp and left for 12–24 hours, the hair should then be shampooed and

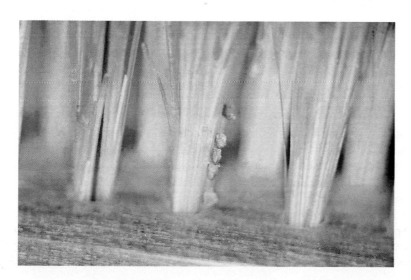

Fig. 7.35 Brushings showing nits firmly adherent to the bristles of the brush.

dead nits combed out. Treatment may have to be repeated after 7–10 days in a few cases. As with scabies, all affected family members should be examined and treated simultaneously if required. Other contacts in schools should also be checked for infestation, but a current common source of re-infection in children in the UK is from older household contacts such as grandparents.

Pediculosis corporis (body lice)

Patients infested with body lice usually present with pruritus, excoriations, and secondary infection. Weals and erythematous macules may also be seen, but the source of the problem should be sought and identified by examining the seams of clothing worn next to the skin. This is the site where lice are likely to be found. In chronic cases striking pigmentation may be observed on the trunk and limbs.

Treatment

Infested clothing should be removed and fumigated with malathion or an alternative parasiticide. The patient should be examined for concomitant infestation with scabies and head lice. One treatment with 0.5% malathion to the body is recommended, followed by the use of a topical steroid/antibiotic preparation to accelerate relief of symptoms.

Pediculosis pubis

The pubic louse is transmitted by close body contact and qualifies as a sexually transmitted disease. Patients complain of pruritus and have the characteristic blue-black 'dots' in their pubic hair. These are the pubic lice, engorged after sucking blood from their host.

Treatment

One or two applications of gamma benzene hexachloride lotion will kill the lice. Sexual partners should be treated simultaneously.

The sexually transmitted diseases

In most European countries, dermatology and venereology are combined specialties, but in the UK the two subjects are divided into separate specialties. In practice, however, patients with venereal disease may well present initially to a dermatological clinic. A brief mention of the cutaneous manifestations of syphilis and gonorrhoea is therefore included in this chapter. For a more comprehensive account the reader is referred to a specialist textbook.

Syphilis

The patient with syphilis may present with dermatological manifestations in any of the three stages of infection. In the primary stage there is a **primary chancre** at the site of sexual contact and from it the causative organism, *Treponema pallidum*, can be isolated. Local lymphadenopathy is common. Four to eight weeks after an untreated primary chancre, secondary syphilis will develop. The dermatological reaction consists of a maculopapular, sometimes lichenoid, rash, which affects the whole body including the palms, soles, and mucous membranes. It is generally asymptomatic. Tertiary syphilis is fortunately much rarer than the other stages, but may present to the dermatologist as an isolated, painless, ulcerating lesion, a **gumma**.

The primary chancre

One to four weeks after infection a moist, ulcerating lesion develops on or near genital mucosa. The ulcer has a sharply demarcated edge, and is both indurated and infiltrated. As serology does not become positive until about 4 weeks after contact, all serological studies at this stage may be negative, but *T. pallidum* can be identified by dark-field illumination of a thick smear from the ulcer. Untreated, 20–30% of these patients will develop secondary syphilis.

Secondary syphilis

As secondary syphilis develops 4–8 weeks after primary infection, the primary chancre may still be visible when secondary lesions appear (Fig. 7.36). These are small maculopapules seen on the trunk and limbs, associated with generalized lymphadenopathy, and if profuse, with **condylomata lata** on the genital mucosa. Lesions on the palms (Fig. 7.37) and soles are important in aiding clinical distinction from other dermatological disorders, such as pityriasis rosea and seborrhoeic dermatitis. Loss of scalp hair and eyebrows may be present, and the pattern of loss is described as 'moth-eaten'.

During this period all patients will have positive serology. *T. pallidum* may be identified in lesions, particularly of the mucosa, and a biopsy will show a perivascular infiltrate, often with many plasma cells, and endarteritis of the small vessels. In cases with untreated lesions, oedema is a common feature. The histological changes are non-specific, although suggestive, and therefore serology must be used for confirmation.

Tertiary syphilis

Cutaneous lesions of tertiary syphilis can appear after a latent period of many years, or even decades. At this stage serology is not reliable. Histologically, there is expansion of granulation tissue, stimulated by the presence of *T. pallidum*,

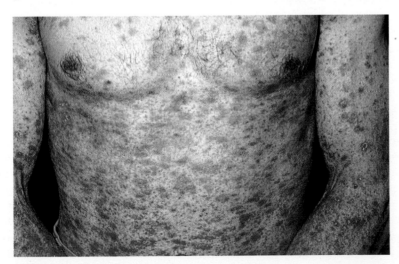

Fig. 7.36 Macular eruption of secondary syphilis. Lesions may also be seen on the palms of the hands.

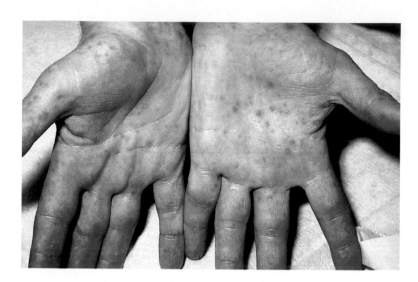

Fig. 7.37 Secondary syphilis showing typical eruption on the palms of the hands.

through the dermis and epidermis, leading to ulceration. This is seen clinically as a **gumma**, a painless lesion whose healing is slow and incomplete, with scarring. On the oral mucosa this will ulcerate the soft palate, leading to perforation.

Treatment

Patients with primary or secondary syphilis should be treated with large doses of penicillin G. Commonly, 3–5 megaunits over 3–4 days are used. Sexual contacts should be traced and treated simultaneously.

Gonorrhoea

Cutaneous manifestations of infection with *Neisseria gonorrhoeae* are most commonly superficial erosions on the genital mucous membrane. They appear up to 14 days after sexual contact, and are associated with urethritis and a urethral discharge in men. Women, however, may be asymptomatic. The organisms can be identified on thick smears from the affected area.

Treatment

High doses of penicillin and contact tracing are the important points in management.

Reiter's syndrome

The triad of arthritis, urethritis, and conjunctivitis is known as Reiter's syndrome. A proportion of patients have, in addition, gastrointestinal symptoms. Cutaneous involvement can occur and consists of heaped-up scaling lesions on the feet (termed **keratoderma blenorrhagica**) circinate balanitis and occasionally lesions on the oral mucous membrane. No causative organism has yet been identified, and there is debate as to whether it should be grouped with sexually transmitted disease or with psoriasis as the lesions on the feet are strikingly similar to psoriasis both clinically and histologically (p. 56).

Treatment

Cutaneous lesions respond to conventional topical psoriasis therapy (p. 71) and the urogenital lesions to systemic tetracycline.

Dermatological complications of infection with the human immunodeficiency virus (HIV 1)

Infection with HIV 1 can be divided into three distinct phases:

- **subclinical asymptomatic infection**;
- **ARC or Aids Related Complex** of weight loss, lymphadenopathy, and frequently one or more of the cutaneous problems listed in Table 7.1;
- **full-blown AIDS** or acquired immunodeficiency syndrome.

Several of the conditions listed in Table 7.1 may co-exist in these patients. The majority of the cutaneous complications of HIV 1 infection and their persistence are related to the loss of cell-mediated immunity associated with the condition. This is due to the affinity of the virus for the CD4+ helper T-cell subpopulation and the subsequent gross depletion of these lymphocytes.

It is important to note that, with the exception of **hairy oral leucoplakia**, none of the dermatological problems associated with HIV 1 infection are specific. However, persistent oral candidosis, or severe and recurrent genital herpes simplex infection may be the first clinical sign of HIV infection. The possibility that patients with such problems may be in one of the high-risk groups should be considered. If indicated, counselling and testing for the HIV viruses should be offered.

Patients with known established HIV infection frequently develop associated dermatological problems. Oral acyclovir may be required prophylactically to prevent recurrences of herpes simplex and oral imidazoles, such as fluconazole or itraconazole, may be needed to control or prevent candidosis.

Kaposi's sarcoma

Kaposi's sarcoma was noted in some of the earliest patients with AIDS, but is rarely seen now that triple therapy has enabled HIV associated problems to be

> **Key points**
>
> Persistent oral candidosis or recurrent genital herpes simplex infection may be the first sign of HIV infection.

Table 7.1 Dermatological complications of HIV 1 infection

Hairy oral leucoplakia
Persistent viral warts and molluscum contagiosum
Persistent or recurrent herpes simplex infection
Severe and recurrent candidosis
Seborrhoeic dermatitis-like lesions
Acute onset psoriasis
Severe adverse drug reactions, notably to Septrin
Kaposi's sarcoma

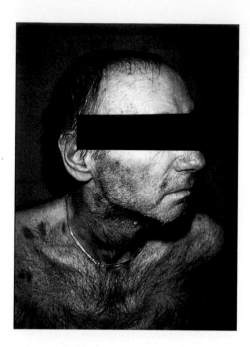

Fig. 7.38 HIV associated Kaposi's sarcoma. Bluish red nodules are seen on the right supraclavicular area. Reproduced by kind permission of Dr Dermot Kennedy.

brought under control. Kaposi's sarcoma is a multi-focal malignancy of the capillary endothelium and is recognized clinically as multiple bruise-like areas on any body site, commonly the face and the oral cavity, including the hard palate (Fig. 7.38). Temporary control of the lesions can often be achieved with either chemotherapy or localized radiotherapy but the condition tends to recur.

Newer and highly effective anti-retroviral therapy that has enabled HIV-related symptoms to be controlled may be associated with a wide range of side effects. Non-specific rashes and a partial lypodystrophy-like loss of subcutaneous fat are relatively common.

Discussion of problem cases

Case 7.1

In the child with atopic dermatitis, deterioration in his condition could be due to exacerbation of dermatitis, to secondary infection with herpes simplex causing eczema herpeticum or to secondary infection with staphylococcal impetigo. Exacerbation of atopic dermatitis would be associated, usually, with pruritus and a generalized flare. The child is not seen to be unduly itchy and the lesions on his knees are unchanged. Eczema herpeticum must be excluded in this situation, but is unlikely because the child is not generally unwell. Viral swabs should, however, be taken.

Both the history and the clinical description strongly suggest secondary staphyloccal impetigo. Bacterological swabs confirmed this diagnosis, as a very heavy growth of *Staph. aureus* was obtained on culture. Remember that a light growth of *Staph.* can be difficult to interpret as most children with atopic

Discussion of problem cases continued

dermatitis have some colonization with *Staph. aureus*, but this does not necessarily cause clinical deterioration.

The child was given systemic flucloxacillin syrup for 5 days and topical mupirocin (Bactroban) ointment. After this time, the skin on his face showed marked improvement.

Case 7.2

This history strongly suggests the viral disease orf contracted from sheep. In country families or vets, the diagnosis would be made by the patient , but town dwellers may be alarmed by the dramatic appearance and rapid growth of the lesions. The viral infection itself is self-limiting, but oral penicillin will prevent secondary bacterial infection

Case 7.3

Loss of normal pigmentation is most commonly due to vitiligo (p. 227). However, loss of pigment can cause considerable concern to those from India and Asia because of the possibility of leprosy as the depigmentation associated with tublerculoid leprosy is well recognized in these countries. This child showed no evidence of nerve hypertrophy and no loss of sensation in the depigmented area, both of which would have suggested a diagnosis of leprosy. After a discussion with the parents, a small punch biopsy was taken from the depigmented area and showed only loss of melanocytes with no evidence of granulomas in the underlying dermis. This confirmed the clinical diagnosis of vitiligo, and a moderate potency steroid was prescribed. Over a 6-month period there was no further loss of pigment at the edge of the lesion, and the parents felt there had been a slight improvement in the depigmented area with slight recovery of normal pigmentation in that site.

Case 7.4

In this situation, vigorous treatment of warts in all body sites before transplant and the necessary immunosuppression that it entails is very strongly recommended. If patients have warts at the time of receiving their transplant, the warts tend to grow exuberantly when immunosuppressive therapy of any type is introduced. Thereafter, they can be very difficult if not impossible to eradicate.

An additional reason for treating warts prior to transplantation is the possible potential for malignant change. Transplant recipients are well recognized as having a higher incidence of non-melanoma skin cancers, mainly squamous cell carcinoma, than the general population, and there is some concern that the types of human papilloma virus found in the transplant population have a higher proportion of the oncogenic types of HPV than in the normal population.

This girl had vigorous treatment with liquid nitrogen fortnightly for 6 weeks to both hand and genital warts, and was free of warts when a kidney became available for her 11 weeks later.

Case 7.5

Allergy to footware is not uncommon, but would be unlikely to be unilateral or to involve the calf, rather than the dorsum of the foot. The more likely explanation is a

Discussion of problem cases continued

bite causing secondary infection. However, the extent of the erythema and the fact that the patient was a reasonably accurate historian tells you that the area of erythema is moving day-by-day suggests the diagnosis of erythema chronicum migrans. This is the main cutaneous feature of Lyme disease or infection with *Borrelia burgdorferi*, a result of a tick bite. A biopsy was compatible with this diagnosis, although a very careful search down a microscope showed no evidence of *Borrelia*. The patient was given a 2-week course of oral tetracycline and a moderate potency steroid antibiotic combination (Trimovate). His lesion cleared within 4 weeks.

Would serology be of value here?

If the diagnosis of Lyme disease had not been made and treatment instituted, what other organs would be at risk?

Case 7.6

The history strongly suggests an infective cause. If a detergent were responsible, the entire population of the home would be likely to be affected. Instead, it is a small group of people in a close environment within the home who appear to have the problem.

Possibilities here would include a fungal infection and also scabies. Scrapings were taken from the skin of all patients complaining of itch. No fungi were seen on direct microscopy, but the scabies mite was identified in very large numbers. This suggested that the problem was an outbreak of so-called Norwegian or epidemic scabies. The lack of classic burrows on the skin of these patients may be partly due to thin skin in the elderly and partly due to the fact that the mite is proliferating on the skin surface.

All residents of the home and all staff were treated with Lindane (Quellada), and all clothing and laundry washed appropriately—a major task.

What would you plan to do about the nurse who has gone on holiday? How would you approach the problem of contact tracing relatives who visit the home?

Special study module project

Review the literature on cutaneous infection and transplant recipients. What are the risk factors? Arrange to attend clinics in your local transplant unit and ask if you can examine the skin of as many transplant recipients as possible, noting the type of lesions they have, and the duration since their transplant What advice should transplant recipients be given about skin care? Should transplant recipients have regular dermatological reviews, and if you think this is necessary, what specific points would you include in your regular reviews?

Further reading

Canizares, O. and Harman, R. (ed.) (1992) *Clinical tropical dermatology*. Blackwell Scientific Publications, Oxford.

Parish, L.C., Witowski, J.A., and Vassileva, S. (1995) *Colour atlas of cutaneous infections*. Blackwell Scientific Publications, Oxford.

Penneys, N. (1995) *Skin manifestations of AIDS*, 2nd edn. Dunitz, London.

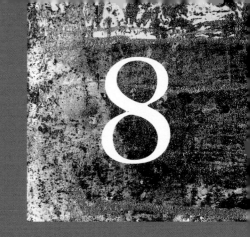

8

Autoimmune or connective tissue diseases, disorders of collagen and of elastic tissue

Autoimmune or connective tissue diseases, disorders of collagen and of elastic tissue

Problem cases

Case 8.1

A 23-year-old woman consults you about what she considers to be severe facial sunburn. She has just returned from her honeymoon on a Mediterranean island, where she was exposed to strong sunshine. Three months earlier she had started taking the oral contraceptive. On questioning she also complains of tiredness and joint pains.

What conditions would you consider in the differential diagnosis, what investigations would you carry out, and what would be your management plan?

Case 8.2

A 70-year-old male comes to your consulting room complaining of severe tiredness and weakness. He also has a red macular rash running along the dorsa of his fingers and up the backs of his hands. What diagnosis does this description suggest and how would you confirm it? What treatment would you prescribe, and are there any additional investigations which might be appropriate?

Lupus erythematosus, scleroderma, and dermatomyositis are frequently referred to as collagen or connective tissue diseases, but as there is little specific association with collagen, and all these conditions are associated with the presence of a range of circulating auto antibodies, some of which may precipitate or aggravate the disease, the term autoimmune diseases seem a more appropriate description.

The common features of these disorders is that they become clinically evident in genetically susceptible individuals as a result of environmental stimuli, such as exposure to intense ultraviolet radiation or ingestion of a range of drugs.

The term 'collagen' disease is appropriate for the Ehlers–Danlos group of disorders, as they are associated with genetically determined defects in the various types of collagen. Pseudoxanthoma elasticum is a disorder of elastic tissue.

Lupus erythematosus

This is a spectrum of disorders, ranging from a relatively benign, purely cutaneous, localized problem to a severe and life-threatening systemic disorder with minimal cutaneous involvement, but severe and progressive damage to other organs such as the kidneys.

Key points

Lupus erythematosus, scleroderma, and dermatomyositis are associated with auto-antibodies, and these are of use in confirming diagnosis.

The predominantly cutaneous variety is chronic disseminated lupus erythematosus, usually abbreviated to CDLE, and the much more serious life-threatening systemic variety is systemic lupus erythematosus (SLE). In between these two extremes there are a number of presentations of intermediate severity, such as subacute cutaneous lupus erythematosus (SCLE) chilblain lupus erythematosus and erythema multiforme-like lupus erythematosus. Children born to mothers with lupus erythematosus may have neonatal lupus erythematosus. Rarely, patients may progress from one presentation to another in the course of their disease, but it is much commoner for the type of LE to remain constant for a given individual.

All varieties of LE are commoner in females than in males

Table 8.1 lists the majority of the clinical presentations of lupus erythematosus with their usual associated auto-antibody findings.

Pathology

The dermatopathological feature common to all types of lupus erythematosus is the lichenoid tissue reaction, a pattern seen also in other skin diseases. The term lichenoid tissue reaction is used when there is a vacuolar alteration of the basal cells in the epidermis, and an underlying lymphocytic infiltrate. There is usually

Table 8.1 Clinical features of the main varieties of lupus erythematosus and rarer subsets, with commonly associated auto-antibody findings

	Clinical features	Auto-antibody profile
Systemic lupus erythematosus	Multisystem (renal, cardiac, CNS, etc.)	High-titre antinuclear antibody
	Facial photosensitivity and 'butterfly' erythema	Antibodies to double-stranded DNA
Chronic discoid lupus erythematosus	Photosensitive scaling and scarring lesions on light-exposed sites	Usually none. In 5–30% low-titre antinuclear antibody
Subacute cutaneous lupus erythematosus	Extensive erythematous macules, usually on upper trunk and arms	Anti Ro and La in 50%
Chilblain lupus	Chilblain-like lesions on hands and feet	Usually none
Erythema multiforme-like lupus erythematosus (Rowell's syndrome)		Commonly anti-La
Neonatal lupus erythematosus	Facial erythema, complete heart block	Mother has circulating anti-Ro
Systemic lupus erythematosus with thrombotic episodes and recurrent abortions	Livedo (prominent vascular) pattern in skin, CNS complications	Antiphospholipid antibodies

also epidermal hyperkeratosis and patchy thickening of the granular layer. This pattern is also seen in lichen planus (p. 78) and lichenoid drug reactions and, therefore, is not diagnostic of lupus erythematosus.

Immunopathology

Immunopathology is helpful in confirming a diagnosis of lupus erythematosus. Direct immunofluorescence of clinically involved skin shows a course band of immunoglobulin, usually IgM or IgG in association with C3 at the dermo-epidermal junction. In patients with severe systemic LE, this immunoglobulin deposit may also be seen in clinically normal skin.

The presence and type of circulating auto-antibodies is a major criterion for diagnosis of all types of LE. The non organ specific auto-antibodies likely to be present in the various types of LE are shown in Table 8.1. In CDLE circulating anti-nuclear antibody is present in about 30% of patients. It is of the speckled or homogeneous pattern, and is present in relatively low titre. In subacute LE anti-nuclear antibody (ANA) is present in up to 80% of patients who also have circulating titres of anti-Ro(SSA) and or La(SSB) auto-antibodies. All patients with SLE have circulating ANA and about one-third also have circulating Sm (extractable nuclear antigen or ENA). Patients whose SLE has been triggered by drug ingestion also commonly have circulating antibodies to histone and double-stranded DNA.

The presence of circulating anti-Ro antibodies in the mother is an important diagnostic test in suspected neonatal LE

Chronic discoid lupus erythematosus (CDLE)
Definition

A chronic, purely cutaneous disorder characterized by photosensitivity leading to the development of red scaling plaques on light exposed areas which heal with scarring.

Incidence and aetiology

Discoid LE is not a common dermatological disorder, but causes concern and referral out of proportion to its incidence because the face is the most commonly affected site, and because of permanent scarring that may be seen. Although the condition is triggered by sun exposure, the mechanisms involved are not yet understood. Females are more often affected than males.

Clinical features

CDLE usually begins in the sunny summer months as tumid, raised, red, scaling plaques on the face (Figs 8.1 and 8.2). The scales are very adherent to the underlying epidermis and run into the hair follicles, giving the so-called carpet-tack sign. This means that when a scale is pulled off a plaque, there is an obvious tack-like extension on the underside, which has come from an underlying pilosebaceous follicle opening. These plaques are usually multiple and the scalp may be involved. The plaques slowly heal with atrophy, discoloration, and scarring. (Fig. 8.3). On the scalp, this will be associated with areas of permanent alopecia

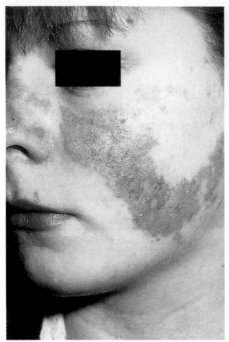 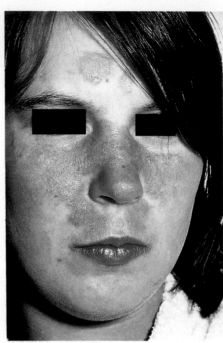

Figs 8.1 and 8.2 The facial appearance of two young girls with chronic discoid lupus erythematosus. Note the striking scaling involving the central panel of the face.

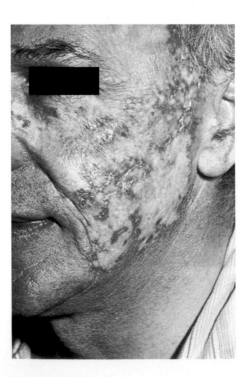

Fig. 8.3 Striking scarring on the face of a male with CDLE.

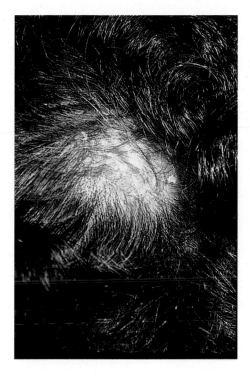

Fig. 8.4 Scalp involvement in chronic discoid lupus erythematosus. Note scarring and hair loss some of which will be permanent.

(Fig. 8.4), as the hair roots have been destroyed. There is no systemic upset. Over the winter months the problem usually becomes quiescent, but is reactivated when the skin is next exposed to sunlight. The natural history of the disease is to gradually burn out over a period of years if UV exposure is prevented. The patient may be left with a significant cosmetic disability from scarring.

Treatment

The use of protective clothing such as hats and a high SPF broad spectrum sunscreen by day will help prevent new lesions developing, and moderate to strong potency topical steroids will help reduce inflammation and scarring in lesions already present. CDLE is an exception to the rule that strong topical steroids should not be used on the face, but the necessary steroid strength should be reviewed regularly. Injection of intra-lesional steroid may also be needed in resistant cases.

If in spite of topical treatments, new CDLE plaques continue to appear, systemic anti-malarials should be considered. Chloroquine (maximum dose 150 mg/day) or hydroxychloroquine sulphate (Plaquenil, maximum dose 200 mg/day) can be helpful, usually given only over 4–6 summer months each year. If hydroxychloroquine is used, ophthalmological monitoring may be needed as this drug is deposited in the eye and can cause ocular toxicity.

Very resistant cases may require therapeutic trials of immuno-suppressives, such as azathioprine, cyclosporin A, or mycophenolate mofetil. These are usually more effective than systemic steroids in this type of LE. Oral gold and oral retinoids may also be useful in difficult cases.

Cosmetic camouflage using Covermark or Dermablend may be very helpful to those with burnt out scarred lesions of CDLE on the face.

Subacute cutaneous lupus erythematosus (SCLE)

This variant of LE is part of the spectrum between purely cutaneous discoid LE, described above, and systemic LE.

Clinical features

Patients are photosensitive, and have red, macules and plaques both on exposed skin (Fig. 8.5) and also on covered skin (Figs 8.6 and 8.7). The upper part of the trunk is often involved with diffuse and widespread lesions, which persist throughout the year. Scaling and scarring are unusual. Patients are not systemically unwell and most have no other organ involvement except mild arthropathy.

Subsets of patients in this intermediate LE category may have a clinical pattern resembling either chilblains (Fig. 8.8), or erythema multiforme. (p. 294)

The usual clinical differential diagnoses include other causes of light sensitivity such as polymorphic light eruption and photosensitive drug eruptions. Biopsy and immunofluorescence studies will be helpful, and the presence of circulating anti-Ro (SSA) antibodies in 60% of patients and anti-La (SSB) in 40% will all help confirm the diagnosis.

Treatment

These patients need both topical sunscreens and also systemic treatment. Many respond well to anti-malarials and for patients with more persistent disease which

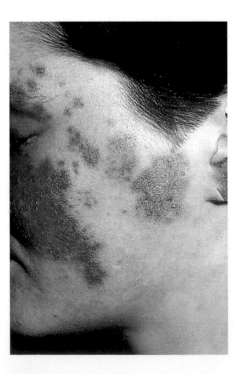

Fig. 8.5 Subacute lupus erythematosus involving the cheek. Note raised tumourous relatively non-scaling lesions.

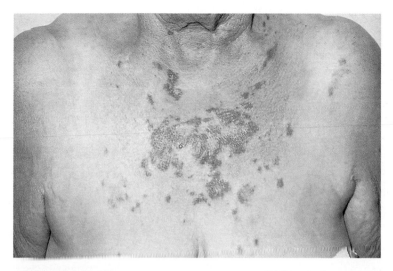

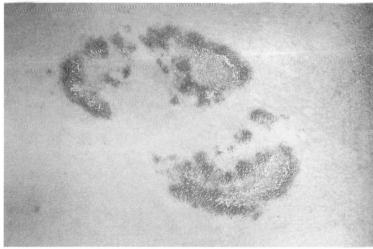

Figs 8.6 and 8.7 Lesions of subacute LE on the trunk. Note striking annular erythema in Fig. 8.7.

continues throughout the winter months, a low dose of systemic steroids (for example, prednisolone 10–20 mg/day) may be needed.

These patients are at risk of progression to multi-system SLE and should therefore be monitored carefully.

Systemic lupus erythematosus (SLE)

Women are much more often affected than men.

The classic skin lesion of SLE is a macular facial rash. While the cheeks and nose, the so-called 'butterfly area' are often heavily involved, the erythema may be rather more diffuse and generalized over the face (Fig. 8.9). This may be provoked by sun exposure. A variety of drugs, listed in Table 8.2, are known to induce SLE, sometimes in association with sunlight. The palms of the hands may show a diffuse erythema (Fig. 8.10), not unlike that seen in patients with liver disease, and

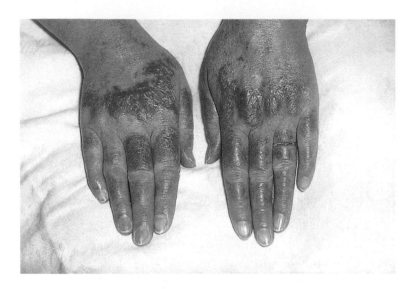

Fig. 8.8 Chilblain LE on the hands.

Table 8.2 Some of the drugs known to induce an SLE-like syndrome or SLE

Hydralazine	INAH
Methyldopa	Phenylbutazone
Griseofulvin	Procaine amide
Oral contraceptives	Sulphonamides
Penicillin	Diphenylhydantoin
Minocycline	

the backs of the hands may show a diffuse mottled pattern, particularly after sun exposure. In general, the skin lesions of SLE are much less florid than those of CDLE despite the much more serious nature of systemic LE.

Patchy, diffuse hair loss is a common feature, but as there is no scarring or permanent damage to the hair bulbs, the hair will regrow normally after successful treatment, in contrast to the permanent hair loss seen in CDLE.

These patients have potentially life-threatening multi-system disease and may therefore have symptoms such as joint pain, fatigue, breathlessness, ankle swelling, and polyuria due to involvement of the joints, respiratory system, heart, and renal system. Consequently, before they start treatment a detailed clinical and laboratory assessment is essential to establish the extent of disease involvement.

The American Rheumatism Association has published 11 criteria for the diagnosis of SLE and 4 are required to make the diagnosis.

Diagnosis and treatment

In a patient who is obviously generally unwell and who has a butterfly rash provoked by sunlight, SLE is a likely diagnosis. Anti-nuclear antibody and DNA binding determination are the most useful confirmatory laboratory tests. A care-

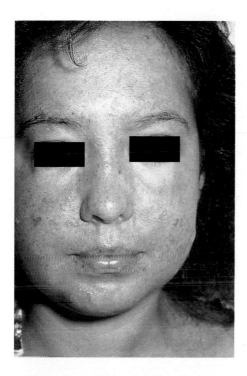

Fig. 8.9 The diffuse erythema of systemic lupus erythematosis.

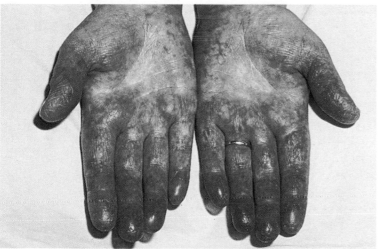

Fig. 8.10 The palms in SLE. Note the erythema and telangiectasia.

ful drug history should be taken to exclude drug-induced SLE. Occasionally, other photosensitive eruptions may mimic SLE, but in these cases there is no systemic upset and no anti-double-stranded DNA antibodies. Table 8.3 lists appropriate baseline investigations. Some more specialized investigations are also suggested, and will depend on the systems thought, on the basis of history, and clinical examination, to be involved in the disease process.

Table 8.3 Investigations in suspected systemic lupus erythematosus

Essential

> ESR and/or C reactive protein
>
> Full blood count—Hb, WBC, platelets
>
> Liver function tests
>
> Urea, electrolytes, creatinine clearance
>
> CXR
>
> ECG
>
> Urinalysis
>
> Auto-antibody profile including ANA, anti-double-stranded DNA,
>
> C_3C_4, CH50 levels
>
> Skin biopsy and immunopathology

Additional possible investigations

> Renal biopsy
>
> Pulmonary function
>
> Lumbar puncture
>
> EEG

Treatment of SLE is usually based on systemic corticosteroids together with, in some cases, an immunosuppressive drug such as cyclophosphamide, azathioprine, or chlorambucil as a steroid-sparing agent. The starting dose will depend on the patient's condition, but often a dose of 50–100 mg of prednisolone daily is required. It should be reduced as the patient's clinical condition improves. For monitoring disease activity, DNA binding may be useful and a sudden rise may give warning of a relapse. Maintenance steroid therapy should be as low as possible to limit long-term side effects and alternate day regimes are of value. The addition of immunosuppressives is also helpful in this respect and some patients can be maintained on these drugs alone. Whichever regime is found best for the individual patient, all require supervision to monitor activation of disease and to screen for treatment-induced side-effects. Azathioprine, cyclophosphamide, and chlorambucil are most likely to produce haematological or renal toxicity, while hypertension, weight gain, glycosuria, and electrolyte imbalance are the principal hazards for the steroid-treated patient.

Sun avoidance is also important. A broad spectrum high SPF sun-screen by day and a topical steroid by night may accelerate improvement of cutaneous lesions, even in patients receiving relatively high doses of systemic steroids.

Over the past decade, the prognosis for patients with SLE has steadily improved, probably due to earlier diagnosis and more effective treatment.

The anti-phospholipid antibody syndrome

This variant of LE is associated with cerebrovascular accidents, myocardial infarction, other thrombotic episodes, and in the case of females who are much more commonly affected than males, a poor obstetric history with multiple miscarriages.

A common cutaneous finding is the so-called livedo pattern—a striking accentuation of the superficial vascular patterns on the skin, usually best seen on the thighs. Ulcers, phlebitis, and even gangrene may also be present.

Affected patients have circulating anti-phospholipid antibodies, which include the lupus anticoagulant, antibodies to cardiolipin, and to phosphatidylethanolamine.

Neonatal lupus erythematosus

This is a rare LE variant, but it is important to be aware of it if working in obstetrics or neonatal paediatrics. The affected child will have red, circular, or arcuate lesions, usually on the face and upper trunk. The more serious problem is that virtually all these children have complete heart block and neonatal LE is one of the commonest causes of this condition. The mother of the child will have circulating anti-Ro antibodies and subsequent infants are also at risk. Infants born to mothers with known LE should be monitored for this problem.

Scleroderma

The term scleroderma, which literally means tight skin, describes a spectrum of diseases from the minor problem of localized morphoea to the severe life-threatening systemic sclerosis.

Morphoea

Definition

A purely cutaneous disorder seen most commonly in children or young adults, and characterized by the spontaneous appearance of a scar like band or plaque on any body site.

Clinical features

Morphoea presents as a firm, white or violet patch of skin on any body site, commonly the thighs, trunk, and upper arms (Fig. 8.11). In a developing lesion there is a well-marked red or violet margin. As the disease activity burns out, this edge assumes the same colour as the central lesion and a very firm white plaque develops with an atrophic, glazed epidermis. Calcification may develop within the lesion.

A linear variant of morphoea may occur, usually on the scalp and face and is called '*coup de sabre*' because it resembles a scar from a sword or similar weapon. This variant will cause alopecia if it involves the scalp and may cause growth irregularities of the underlying skull in a young child.

In morphoea , brown post-inflammatory melanin pigmentation may develop in 'burnt out' lesions.

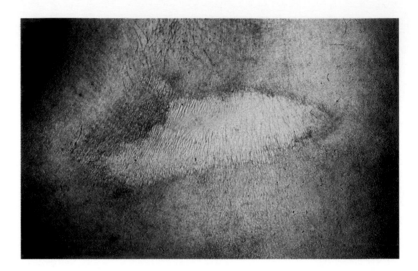

Fig. 8.11 Ivory white patch of morphea. On palpation this will be firm and indurated with a rather plaque-like feel.

Pathology

Loss of all skin appendages is the major feature in the histology of morphoea, giving a bland 'empty' look to the dermis. The collagen bundles are larger than usual and tend to run parallel to the skin surface. The normal difference between the papillary and reticular dermis is thus lost, and the overlying epidermis tends to be thin and atrophic.

Diagnosis and treatment

The clinical appearance is commonly diagnostic and biopsy is rarely required. In very early lesions, when erythema, rather than a firm white atrophic plaque is seen, the lesion may have to be observed for 2–3 months before a firm diagnosis can be made. Biopsy at this stage is not always helpful as the fully developed histological picture is not present.

At present there is no specific treatment. Topical steroids or intra-lesional corticosteroid injections into an active lesion may alter its final shape, but will not arrest its development.

Trials of very high doses of long wave ultraviolet A irradiation have been equivocal.

Systemic sclerosis (generalized scleroderma, acrosclerosis)

Definition

A systemic disease characterized by progressive accumulation of collagen, fibrosis, and loss of mobility of the skin and other organs, such as the respiratory and gastrointestinal tracts. The kidneys may also be involved and, in rare cases, this is fulminating and leads rapidly to death. Transforming growth factor beta one is currently thought to be a cytokine involved in the pathogenesis of this condition.

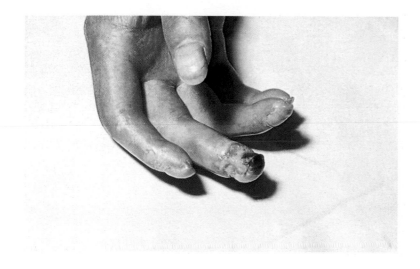

Fig. 8.12 The hand in progressive systemic sclerosis. Note the tightly bound skin, atrophy, and early gangrene in the middle finger.

Clinical features

Females are more commonly affected and many initially have severe Raynaud's phenomenon. The affected hands and feet are initially swollen and have tight shiny atrophic skin, which is bound firmly to the subcutaneous tissue (Fig. 8.12). The soft tissue of the mouth and palate are similarly affected, causing denture wearers to complain of poorly fitting plates because the mouth gradually shrinks. The face is often characteristic, with a strikingly line-free forehead, a small beaked nose, a small mouth with radial furrowing around the lips, and, in advanced cases, multiple dilated capillaries (telangiectasia; Figs 8.13 and 8.14). Small calcified nodules may develop in long-standing cases, usually in the skin of the hands and feet. A variant of this disorder has been named the CRST or CREST syndrome (c = calcification, R = Raynaud's disease, E = oesophageal dysfunction, S = sclerodactyly, and T = telangiectasia) in which extensive multi-system involvement is said to be less common than in true systemic sclerosis.

Involvement of the gastrointestinal tract causes dysphagia and malabsorption through loss of peristalsis. Pulmonary involvement presents as dyspnoea with pulmonary hypertension and cardiovascular complications may lead to heart failure. Renal involvement may also develop.

Pathology

The striking feature seen in fully developed systemic sclerosis is a reduction of the normal thickness of the dermis for the body site biopsied. Thus, the subcutaneous fat is seen to be much closer to the epidermis than is normally the case. The underlying pathological process involves both fibrosis and a vasculopathy. Endarteritis and minor inflammatory changes are found around blood vessels in the dermis. In contrast to morphoea, skin appendages are generally present in normal numbers.

Laboratory findings

Most patients with progressive systemic sclerosis have high titres of circulating antinuclear antibody, usually of the speckled variety. Antiscleroderma-70 or topoisimerase 1 and anti-centromere antibodies are also found in a high

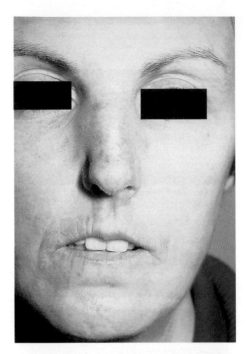

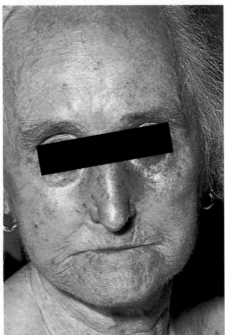

Figs 8.13 and 8.14 Facial appearance in progressive systemic sclerosis. Note loss of lines on forehead, relatively beaked nose, radial furring around the mouth, and telangiectasia.

proportion of patients. On X-ray, the jaw in dentulous patients shows a widened peridontal membrane, and the hands may show resorption of the distal phalanges and early flecks of subcutaneous calcification. On barium swallow there is loss of oesophageal peristalsis.

Pulmonary function tests show impaired diffusion and serial renal function tests may show rapid renal failure, the most serious complication of this disorder.

Diagnosis and treatment

Diagnosis is often made clinically, on the facial appearance of the patient as she enters the clinic. Confirmatory tests include an auto-antibody screen, hand and jaw X-rays, barium swallow, and respiratory function tests.

Treatment is largely symptomatic, but although there is little evidence that systemic steroids affect the course of this disease, they are certainly justified in patients with severe respiratory or renal involvement.

In general, approaches to treatment can be divided into immunosuppressive, anti-fibrotic and vasodilator. Immunosuppressive agents which have been used in addition to steroids include methotrexate, cyclophosphamide, cyclosporin A, and a technique called photopheresis. This involves extra-corporeal irradiation of the patients lymphocytes with long wave ultraviolet radiation-UVA-, and then returning the irradiated cells to the patient. Anti-fibrotic agents used with varying degrees of success include penicillamine, colchicicine, and gamma interferon. Vasodilators used include calcium channel blockers, such as nifedipine and prostacyclin infusions.

The disease tends to progress slowly, but as some cases burn themselves out, it is difficult to assess the value of any therapeutic procedure. Hands and feet should be kept warm and regular professional chiropody offered. A trial of sympathetic blockade will indicate whether or not surgical sympathectomy is likely to be of value, but this is rarely the case.

Management of Raynaud's disease and phenomenon

Three groups of drugs may be of value in the management of Raynaud's disease or Raynaud's phenomenon complicating one of the collagen disorders, usually systemic sclerosis or lupus erythematosus. These are the prostacyclins, ketanserin, and nifedipine (Adalat). The prostacyclins have been shown in small-scale double-blind studies to raise the temperatures of the hands and fingers, and bring about pain relief in patients with Raynaud's phenomenon. The 5-hydroxytryptamine receptor antagonist, ketanserin, has also been used in double-blind studies in patients with both Raynaud's phenomenon and Raynaud's disease; significant improvement has been shown in both blood flow and skin temperature measurements. The dose required is 20 mg, three times per day and no significant side-effects are recorded.

Nifedipine, the calcium channel blocker, has also been reported to be of value in patients with Raynaud's phenomenon and Raynaud's disease. As yet, there is no reported trial comparing these three approaches in the management of Raynaud's disease.

Mixed connective tissue disease

As the name of this disease entity suggests, this condition is an overlap syndrome with some features of both lupus erythematosus and some of systemic sclerosis. The specific auto-antibody present in affected patients is U1-RNP.

Treatment is symptomatic, and patients tend to have a reasonably good prognosis.

Lichen sclerosus et atrophicus (LSA) ('white spot disease')

Definition

An atrophic condition, commonly of the vulva, which may affect both children and adults, sometimes associated with morphoea on other body sites.

Clinical features

LSA and morphoea are found together more frequently than can be attributed to chance.

White, atrophic, glazed areas of skin with follicular plugging develop (Fig. 8.15), and may progress to extreme atrophy and shrinkage of genital tissue. There may also be associated dramatic increase in melanin pigmentation on the affected genital mucosa. The lesions may ulcerate, and cause pain and pruritus, although some are asymptomatic. LSA usually affects the female genitalia. It rarely affects the penis in the male, when it is called balanitis xerotica obliterans. Extra-genital lesions are most common around the neck and upper back. There is a reported incidence of 1–4% of malignant change in vulvar LSA, usually associated with severe involvement.

Children with LSA frequently complain of genital discomfort and bleeding. A number of such children have been inappropriately suspected of being victims of child sexual abuse. It is obviously important to be aware of childhood LSA and to ensure that those in other professions, such as social work, are also aware of its existence, so that such potentially serious mistakes are avoided.

Diagnosis and treatment

Diagnosis is usually made clinically, although biopsy may be required in atypical cases. This will show striking loss of all dermal appendages, epidermal atrophy, and homogenization of the dermal collagen.

Treatment is unsatisfactory and unnecessary for asymptomatic lesions. Pruritus and ulceration are helped by topical steroid preparations (for example, vioform hydrocortisone cream) or topical oestrogens (for example, Dinoestrol cream).

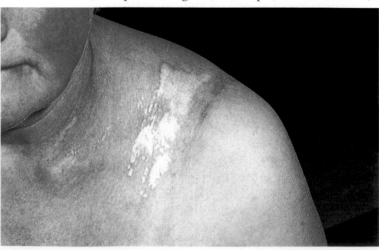

Fig. 8.15 Lichen sclerosus et atrophicus of the shoulder area. Note the atrophic white macules. Vulvar lesions are very commonly seen in patients with these extra-genital lesions.

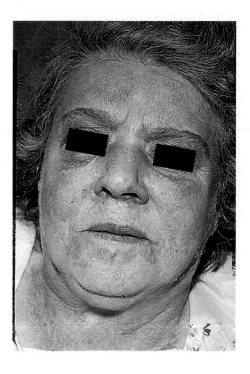

Fig. 8.16 Facial appearance of a patient with dermatomyositis showing characteristic violet discoloration around the eyes.

Long-term follow-up is required in all severe cases as malignancy may not supervene until the lesion has been present for 20 years or more.

Dermatomyositis (polymyositis)

Definition

A disorder of skin and muscle characterized by a specific skin rash and muscle weakness.

Dermatomyositis is relatively rare. There are two varieties, one affecting children, the other adults.

Clinical features

The typical rash of dermatomyositis is a macular erythema on the face, particularly marked in the peri-orbital area where it is described as heliotrope or blue violet (Fig. 8.16). The dorsa of the hands and fingers are also involved with linear erythema and nodules (Gottron's papules; Figs 8.17 and 8.18). Nail-fold haemorrhages may also be seen, but these are common to all the connective tissue disorders. Erythema can also appear on the neck and upper chest, and progress to poikiloderma (dappled skin), which consists of telangiectasia alternating with atrophy. Photosensitivity is common.

Muscle weakness is very variable. It most commonly affects the proximal muscle groups of all four limbs, so that early weakness tends to be noted on climbing stairs, or performing tasks with the hands at or above shoulder level. It may become very severe, and respiratory difficulties can result from involvement of intercostal and diaphragmatic muscles.

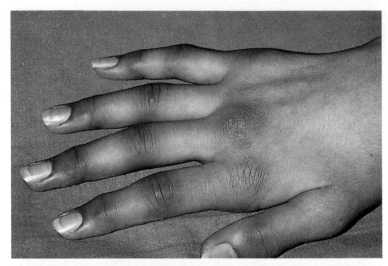

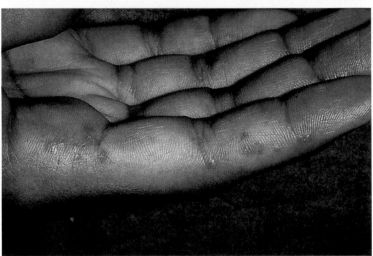

Figs 8.17 and 8.18 The hands of an Indian patient with dermatomyositis. Note erythema on the backs of the fingers and Gottrens papules on the sides.

There are also cases in which this spectrum of dermatological disease is seen, with no detectable myositis.

In childhood, dermatomyositis tends to 'burn out', but may leave severe restriction of limb movement due to calcification in and around muscles.

Pathology

The skin lesions show histological changes similar to those seen in SLE. Liquefaction degeneration of the basal layer is common, and the overlying epidermis may be thin and atrophic. In the dermis, large numbers of free melanin granules are seen due to pigmentary incontinence. Free red cells are also present, the result of capillary leakage.

The degree of muscle involvement is variable, but if affected the muscle shows fibre degeneration and internalization of the sarcolemmal nuclei.

Diagnosis and treatment

Diagnosis is usually based on the combination of a typical skin rash, muscle weakness, and raised circulating muscle enzymes (SGOT, SGPT, creatine kinase, and aldolase). If muscle biopsy is to be performed, electromyography will indicate a suitable area of involved muscle.

There is controversy over the association between dermatomyositis and detection of a previously occult malignancy. Current evidence suggests that, in at least some series, this is a significant association in older individuals, but that the malignancy will be detected by a good routine medical assessment and that extreme measures such as laparotomy are not justified in a hunt for such a malignancy. Common sites for such a malignancy include the gastrointestinal tract, the prostate, the ovaries, and the breast.

Removal of a malignancy if present may result in spontaneous, although usually temporary, improvement of the muscle weakness. If no malignancy is found, systemic steroid therapy may give symptomatic relief and a trial of prednisolone 20–60 mg/day is justified. Systemic azathioprine (150 mg/day) may also be of value either alone or as a steroid-sparing measure. Oral methotrexate may also be of value. Disease activity should be monitored by regular assays of muscle enzyme levels.

Ehlers–Danlos syndrome (cutis hyperelastica)

Definition

A group of inherited disorders characterized by defects in dermal collagen.

Clinical features

Clinically, the skin is hyperelastic (Fig. 8.19), fragile, and bruises easily. The joints have lax capsules, are hyper-extensible and readily undergo subluxation. Poor posture and hernia formation may, in part, be due to muscular hypotonia. Poor healing of minor skin trauma leaves ugly scars (Figs 8.20 and 8.21). The

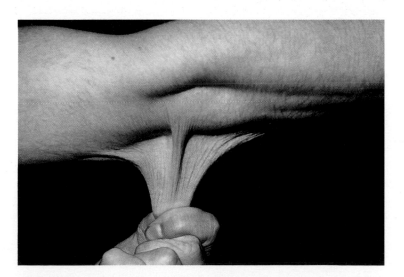

Fig. 8.19 Striking cutis hyperelastica of the Ehlers–Danlos syndrome.

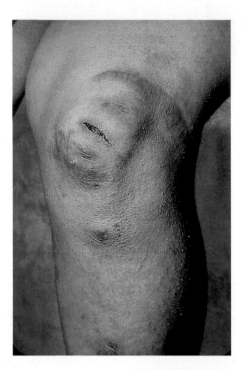

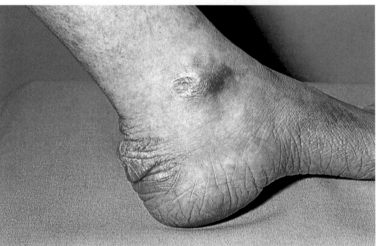

Figs 8.20 and 8.21 Poorly formed scars over the ankle and knee area in patient with Ehlers–Danlos syndrome.

patients have striking blue sclerae. In some cases, the collagen of large vessels is also affected, and death due to dissecting aneurysm or spontaneous vessel rupture is recorded. A proportion of patients also have features of pseudoxanthoma elasticum. Patients with vascular involvement may die suddenly of dissecting aortic aneurysm.

Pathology

At the present time, 11 biochemical variants of this true 'collagen' disorder are recognized. Modes of inheritance are both autosomal dominant and sex-linked recessive. The basic defects in collagen synthesis are both quantitative and qualitative, and can be accurately identified by fibroblast culture and biochemical assay. On light microscopy the collagen appears whorled and disorganized, and in some cases there is an associated increase in elastic fibres. Type 4 EDS is associated with a defect in type 3 collagen and type 5 in a deficiency in the enzyme lysyl hydroxylase. In the other variants, the exact biochemical problem has not yet been identified.

Diagnosis and treatment

Diagnosis is based on the clinical appearance and a positive family history, and should be confirmed by biochemical studies on fibroblast cultures. No treatment is yet available, but identification of the type of Ehlers–Danlos will aid genetic counselling.

Pseudoxanthoma elasticum

Definition

A hereditary disorder of elastic tissue.

Like the Ehlers–Danlos syndrome, there are genetically distinct variants. Both autosomal dominant and autosomal recessive varieties are recognized. At present, genes coding for elastin and fibrillin are considered likely candidates.

Clinical features

The cutaneous lesions are found in the axillae and groins and are soft, yellowish papules—'chamois leather' skin (Figs 8.22–8.24). Ocular lesions are common and can be seen on ophthalmoscopy as angioid streaks, haemorrhage, and choroiditis.

> ### Key points
> Involvement of the blood vessels can lead to fatal consequences in both Ehler's Danlos and Pseudoxanthoma elasticum.

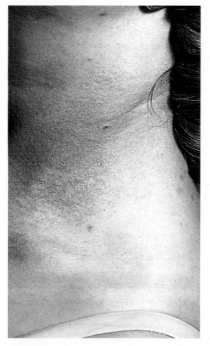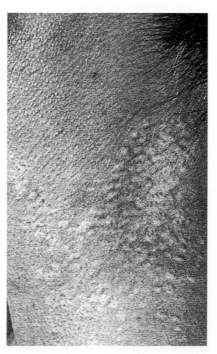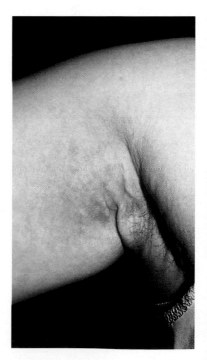

Figs 8.22–8.24 Features of the skin of the flexure areas in pseudoxanthoma elasticum.

Some degree of visual impairment is common. Involvement of major blood vessels may give rise to hypertension, angina, and haemorrhage including haematemesis.

Pathology

The characteristic pathological feature is the presence in the dermis of tangled, degenerate elastic fibres on which calcification readily occurs. This abnormality is also found in elastic tissue of the blood vessels and the heart.

Diagnosis and treatment

Diagnosis is based on the clinical appearance, a positive family history, and the histology. No specific therapy is available.

Discussion of problem cases

Case 8.1

The differential diagnosis here includes a range of photosensitive disorders, such as polymorphic light eruption, a photosensitive drug eruption, and lupus erythematosus. The history of systemic upset suggests that polymorphic light eruption is unlikely, but both SLE and photosensitive drug eruptions can cause generalized problems. As all the cutaneous erythema was on the face and mainly on the central panel, a biopsy was not carried out initially. On examination, the patient had a blood pressure of 180/120 mmHg, and electrolyte and liver function tests showed a markedly elevated serum urea and creatinine. She also had high titre circulating auto-antibodies to double stranded DNA. This last result confirms a diagnosis of systemic lupus erythematosus, possibly precipitated in a genetically predisposed individual by exogenous oestrogens in the oral contraceptive and by sun exposure.

The patient was started on high doses of oral steroids (prednisolone 80 mg/day) and the oral contraceptive withdrawn. Over the next 4 weeks her blood pressure fell, and her urea and creatinine returned to the normal range. Her facial erythema slowly cleared without scarring, and the dose of oral steroid was reduced to 15 mg on alternate days 3 months after her first presentation.

What is her prognosis? What other organs are at risk? She wishes to start a family and asks you if there are any risks to herself during pregnancy or to the baby. How will you reply?

Case 8.2

This male patient has muscle weakness and a rash. The likely diagnosis is therefore dermatomyositis. Investigations that will help confirm this diagnosis are electromyography (EMG), levels of circulating muscle enzymes in the peripheral blood, and muscle biopsy.

The patient had circulating creatine phosphokinase levels of over 20 times the upper limit of the normal range. This was considered adequate to confirm the diagnosis and the patient was given oral prednisolone 100 mg/day. There was a very rapid response with increase in muscle power. Because of the possibility of his dermatomyositis being associated with an occult malignancy, a CT scan of the thorax abdomen and pelvis was carried out, and the levels of prostate specific antigen

Discussion of problem cases continued

measured. No abnormalities were found and, over a period of 14 weeks, his prednisolone level was reduced to 20 mg/day. What will be your ongoing management
plan for this patient?

Special study module

Arrange to attend the local rheumatological, renal, and dermatological clinics that
see patients with all varieties of lupus erythematosus. Keep a clear record of each
patient seen including the clinical features, organs affected, diagnostic tests used,
and both past and current therapy.

Do patients have as much information about their disease as they require?

Further reading

Royce, P.M. and Steinmann, B. (eds) (1993) *Connective tissue and its heritable disorders.* Wiley-
Liss, Chichester.

Wallace, D.J. and Hannahs Hahn, B. (1992) *Dubous lupus erythematosus*, 4th edn. Lea and
Feibiger, Philadelphia.

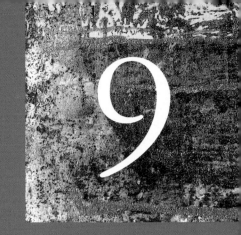

9

Disorders of the vasculature

Disorders of the vasculature

Problem cases

Case 9.1

A 62-year-old obese female consults you because of a small leg ulcer on her right ankle. She has been treating it herself with a wide range of over the counter remedies. The skin around the ulcer is very red and inflamed. What is your investigation and management plan?

Case 9.2

A 23-year-old male consults you about the regular appearance of what he describes as red weals on his skin. None are present at the consultation, but he says that they have been appearing over the past 6 months and his face is usually involved. What is the likely diagnosis, and what investigations and treatment will you suggest?

Case 9.3

Both parents come to see you with their first child, a girl now aged 6 months. She has a red, raised mark covering about 10% of her forehead. The parents are very agitated as they have been told elsewhere that no treatment is needed, but the mark is still expanding. They want to know about laser treatment and why their child is being denied this therapy. What is the likely diagnosis and what will you tell them about therapy?

Disorders of the arteries, veins, and capillaries may all present as skin lesions. Some are disorders affecting only the cutaneous vasculature, while others are more generalized, involving many systems, the skin included. In young children, the most common problem is that of vascular naevi, while in older adults the most frequent problem is lower leg ulceration, which may be due to either venous or arterial malfunction. Capillary disorders often cause a purpuric eruption and vasculitis can produce painful nodular ulcerating lesions. Vascular pathology is most commonly seen on the lower legs because of the sluggish circulation due to gravity. Biopsies from the lower leg have to be interpreted with care in older adults, as the histology of clinically normal skin of this area may show minor vascular changes due to gravity.

Vascular birthmarks

Vascular birthmarks are seen in a very high proportion of young babies. The two main types of vascular birthmarks are:

- haemangiomas;
- vascular malformations.

Haemangiomas

Definition

Benign proliferations of the vascular endothelium, seen in early infancy, which proliferate during the first year of life and then clear spontaneously.

Clinical features

About one child in 10 develops a cutaneous angioma during the first month of life. They are not usually apparent at birth. They may be superficial, deep, or mixed according to the depth of the blood vessels affected. Alternative names for the superficial haemangiomas are **strawberry angiomas** and for deep lesions **cavernous angiomas**. The superficial lesions are a bright red colour and the deeper lesions a bluish shade. The natural history of these lesions is that they expand rapidly during the first year of life, then slowly and spontaneously shrink over the next 3–4 years (Figs 9.1 and 9.2), so that by the time the child is ready for school there may only be some loose redundant skin visible. Occasionally, they are very large indeed, and there may be concern about either haemorrhage or obstruction of vision leading to blindness in the affected eye.

Treatment

As the great majority of superficial haemangiomas shrink spontaneously and this results in minimal long-term scarring, parents should be told of this and encouraged to let this happen. Showing sequential photographs of older patients whose lesions have cleared spontaneously will be helpful. Bleeding that may occur should be controlled with firm pressure. Infection may develop and should be treated with the appropriate topical antibiotic. Both bleeding and infection appear to accelerate spontaneous resolution.

The **deep cavernous angioma** has all the features described for the superficial cavernous angioma, but in addition there appears to be a proliferation of vessels

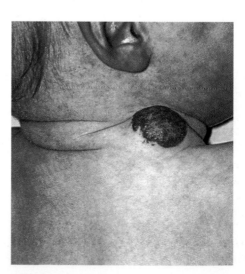

Fig. 9.1 Mixed, predominantly cavernous angioma. Child is 3 months old.

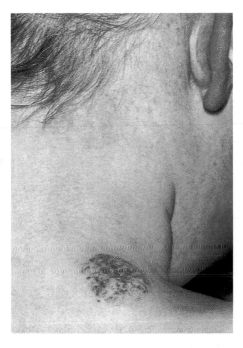

Fig. 9.2 The child in Fig. 9.1 aged 3 years, to demonstrate spontaneous resolution. Further improvement can confidently be expected.

in the deeper capillary plexus. These do not shrink as completely as the superficial vessels and resolution is usually less complete.

Rarely, with the giant lesions, treatment with either systemic steroids or intra-lesional injections of either steroids or interferon may be necessary. For this group of angiomas, there is little evidence, at present, that laser therapy gives a better long-term result than natural involution, and the main concern of the doctor involved should be to select the treatment option that will result in least long-term scarring when the child is a teenager and adult. Minor plastic surgery may be needed for the larger lesion to remove folds of redundant skin when natural shrinkage is completed.

Rare variants of cavernous angiomata can be associated with systemic abnor-malities, such as thrombocytopenic purpura, and any infant who has a very large lesion or with a family history of angiomata should be appropriately investigated.

Vascular malformations (naevus flammeus, port wine stain)

Definition

A persisting and permanent area of erythema due structural abnormalities of capillaries and other small blood vessels .

These lesions are present at birth, and the majority affect the facial skin over the area served by the trigeminal nerve (Fig. 9.3). Initially, they are deep red and macular. Here, there is no tendency for spontaneous resolution and raised nodules may develop on the naevus as the child grows. Very large port wine stains may be associated with additional vascular abnormalities of the cerebral vessels giving rise to the Sturge–Weber Syndrome.

Treatment

This can be either by cosmetic camouflage or by laser destruction of the abnormal vessels. Flash lamp pulsed dye lasers give best results with least scarring. Usually, several treatments are required and sedation of a young child will be needed to maintain the head absolutely still. Results are generally good, and current policy is to try to offer laser therapy early in life before the naevus has become raised and palpable. Clearly, there are, at present, a number of adults in the community for whom laser treatment was not an option when they were young. Results in these more mature naevi are less satisfactory, and camouflage therapy using Dermablend or Cover mark preparations may be more appropriate. In the UK, the Red Cross run an excellent cosmetic camouflage advisory and demonstration service (Figs 9.3–9.6).

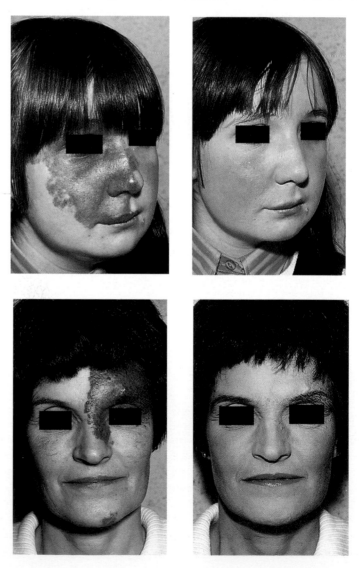

Figs 9.3–9.6 Port wine stains before and after application of camouflage cover.

Salmon patches (telangiectatic naevi, Unna's naevus, stork bite)

These faint macular lesions are seen in as many as a third of all new-born infants. They are usually on the nape of the neck or the central panel of the face. They are composed of distended and persisting foetal dermal capillaries. The majority fade spontaneously in the first few months of life, but those on the nape of the neck may persist. This is not usually a problem.

Leg ulceration

Leg ulceration is a huge burden on healthcare systems worldwide. In the UK, 3 people per 1000 have leg ulcers, rising to 20/1000 in those over 80 years, and in the US it has been calculated that 2 billion working days are lost annually because of leg ulcers. The morbidity to the individual and the cost to the health care systems is very significant. The three main types of leg ulcer are venous ulcers due to venous stasis, arterial ulcers, and neuropathic ulcers associated with diabetes.

> ### Key points
>
> Do not apply topical steroids to leg ulcers routinely. Use them sparingly, and only on the skin around inflamed ulcers.

Venous leg ulcers (stasis ulcers, gravitational ulcers)

Incidence and aetiology

Venous ulceration is very common in Britain and a common cause for referral to specialist dermatological clinics. The incidence in the community is much higher as many patients either attend their general practitioner or seek no medical assistance. Most patients are women.

Seventy to eighty per cent of ulcers on the lower legs result from venous damage, due to the increased venous pressure associated with varicose veins and past venous thrombosis.

The main at risk group for venous leg ulcers are obese females with varicose veins, who may have had past problems with venous thrombosis, perhaps during pregnancy.

Venous leg ulcers develop because of incompetent valves in the leg veins. There is secondary increase in capillary pressure, with stasis, capillary damage, fibrosis, and a poorly nourished skin, which is easily damaged by minor trauma.

Clinical features

The typical patient is an obese, middle-aged woman. A past history of a deep venous thrombosis is common and varicose veins are usually present. One or both legs may be involved. The most common site of ulceration is over the medial malleolus (Fig. 9.7) and the surrounding skin frequently shows gross fibrosis, purpura, and livedo due to extravasation of blood from damaged capillaries, an appearance termed 'atrophie blanche'. The ulcer is frequently precipitated by minor local trauma. Stasis ulcers are commonly single and although they may be extremely large they are relatively pain-free, in contrast to arterial ulcers. The surrounding skin is frequently oedematous, eczematous, and secondarily infected.

Arterial leg ulcers

Arterial leg ulcers are much less common and usually develop as a complication of a general vasculitic problem, such as systemic lupus erythematosus, rheumatoid

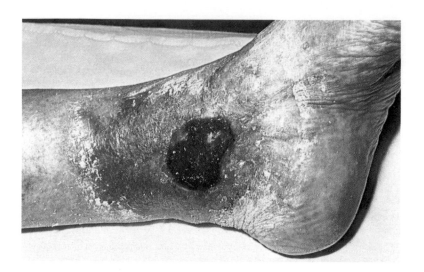

Fig. 9.7 Venous stasis ulceration. Note typical site over medial malleolus and trophic changes in surrounding skin.

arthritis, or diabetes. Affected patients often have a history of intermittent claudication, and may develop small ulcers on the toes or lower leg, which cause pain out of all proportion to the size of the ulcers. The patient has no evidence of varicose veins, but has poor peripheral pulses and multiple small painful ulcers, which have a punched-out appearance and are situated in the lower third of the leg (Fig. 9.8). As arterial leg ulcers are frequently associated with generalized arterial pathology, it is important to look for diabetes, atherosclerosis, Buerger's disease, and rheumatoid arthritis if it is not already clinically apparent. Sickle cell disease and other haemoglobinopathies must be considered in patients of Mediterranean origin.

Pain and the site of the lesion may help to differentiate an arterial from a venous ulcer, and further useful pointers are the absence of varicose veins or of a history of deep venous thrombosis.

Diabetic ulcers

Patients with diabetic leg ulcers have usually had diabetes for many years and develop their ulcers as a result of neuropathy. The foot is warm and there are easily palpated arterial pulses, but the patient has easily detectable diminished sensation.

Diagnosis

The diagnosis of a leg ulcer is self-evident. A careful history should be taken of past venous thrombosis, especially associated with pregnancy, and of other systemic disease, such as lupus erythematosus, which may be a cause of arterial ulcers. A personal or family history of diabetes should be sought. Patients with known diabetes should be investigated for sensory neuropathy

All patients with leg ulcers should have the **ankle brachial pressure index (ABPI)** measured by the Doppler technique. This simple technique will establish whether or not the arterial supply to the lower leg is impaired. A figure of 0.8 or less shows that the arterial supply to the leg is poor and pressure bandaging (see

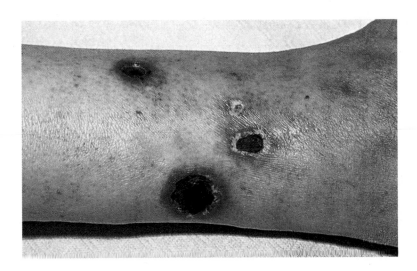

Fig. 9.8 Arterial ulceration. Note 'punched-out' quality of lesions, which are multiple and painful

below) is absolutely contra-indicated, as gangrene could result. A larger than expected number of patients with leg ulcers have circulating anti-cardiolipin antibody or lupus anti-coagulant, and the presence of these should therefore be investigated.

Any unusual looking or non-healing leg ulcer should be considered for biopsy to exclude a developing malignancy on the ulcer edge and also to exclude an unusual infective cause, such as mycobacteria.

The bacteriological results from swabs taken from leg ulcers should be interpreted with common sense. A leg ulcer is not a sterile environment and, therefore, growth of micro-organisms is not surprising, but these are often only commensals. If a leg ulcer has significant secondary bacterial infection, this will usually be clinically obvious and for this reason the routine bacterial swabbing of clinically non-infected leg ulcers is not recommended.

If the skin around a leg ulcer is inflamed and irritable, patch testing should be considered as contact dermatitis to medicaments is very common

Treatment

Treatment of an established venous leg ulcer consists of therapy designed to promote healing, and thereafter prophylaxis to reduce the risk of recurrence. These measures include surgical treatment of varicose veins, weight reduction, and the use of supportive elastic stockings and protective bandaging.

The basic principles of management of an established venous leg ulcer are the maintenance of a clean, healthy ulcer base free of infection, and protection of the surrounding skin to allow re-epithelialization to take place. Support to help reverse the effects of venous hypertension is vital. Healing can be achieved in a proportion of cases, but breakdown of the healed area after minor trauma is all too common.

A variety of astringent preparations will help to maintain a clean healthy ulcer base. These include 20% benzoyl peroxide (Benoxyl) and sodium hypochlorite 1 in 4 (Milton solution). Topical antibiotics should not be used routinely on clinically non-infected ulcer bases. For very moist exudative ulcers, 2–3 days treatment

> **Key points**
>
> Remember that redness and inflammation around the leg ulcer may be an allergic contact dermatitis to a prescribed medicament. If in doubt, patch test.

with absorbent dextranomer beads (Debrisan) will assist in drying the lesions, but this preparation should not be continued for long periods. If the ulcer is obviously infected, swabs should be sent for bacteriological sensitivities and the infection then treated with an appropriate antibiotic.

Occlusive dressings have been shown to provide a more physiological environment to allow the ulcer to heal. Although expensive, they may accelerate healing and are usually very comfortable for the patient. They include Geliperm. Granuflex, Tegasorb, and Sorbsan. These usually have a gel or colloid formulation which absorbs exudate from the ulcer and thus accelerates re-epithelialization. If the ulcer is not producing a lot of exudate, they can be left in position for up to 7 days.

The skin surrounding the actual ulcer may be erythematous and irritable with a stasis dermatitis reaction. While this is often responsive to topical steroid preparations, they must be used with caution in this situation and kept away from the ulcer base otherwise they will delay healing. They should not be used constantly on the skin around the ulcer as they will, in time, cause atrophy and possibly further extension of the ulcer. For this reason the surrounding skin is best protected with a waterproof paste such as plain zinc paste BP or zinc paste with salicylic acid (Lassar's Paste).

Adhesive bandages such as Viscopaste or Ichthopaste are also helpful, particularly for patients who have persistent stasis dermatitis around the ulcer area.

Firm support bandaging is essential in the case of venous ulcers to promote healing, but should not be used for arterial or diabetic ulcers. Four layer bandaging using an absorbent crepe next to the dressing, followed by padded support (for example, velband), followed by a firm bandage of the blue line type, followed by a final coband bandage is extremely effective and comfortable for patients with proven venous ulcers. These four layers are available as a Profore pack (Smith and Nephew).

Patients, their carers, and district or practice nurses should all be given a demonstration of how to apply these bandages. Once the ulcer is healed, patients should use an elastic stocking of appropriate grade to try to prevent recurrence.

In severe cases resistant to treatment outlined above, pinch grafting may be considered, but although this gives good initial results, there is a high recurrence rate once the patient is ambulant.

Arterial and diabetic ulcers require symptomatic treatment with control if possible of the systemic cause of the ulcer. Rest, warmth, and the avoidance of trauma such as unskilful chiropody are all important.

Vasculitis

Definition

A pathological process centred primarily on blood vessel walls (mainly small- and medium-sized vessels), resulting in purpura, nodules, and ulceration.

As the dermis has a very rich blood supply, vasculitis, which is usually a generalized systemic disease, will almost always involve the skin. There is no agreed way to classify vasculitis and the one used in this chapter is based on the cell type seen in the walls of and around the inflamed blood vessels. Thus, there are clinical conditions based on a predominantly lymphocytic, neutrophilic, or granulomatous infiltrate (see Table 9.1)

Table 9.1 The main types of vasculitis classified
according to predominant cell type in the infiltrate

Predominant cell type	Clinical conditions
Lymphocyte	Chilblains (lupus pernio)
	Lupus erythematosus
	Erythema nodosum
	Pityriasis lichenoides
Polymorph	Polyarteritis nodosa
	Allergic vasculitis
	Henoch–Schoenlein purpura
Granuloma formation	Giant cell arteritis
	Erythema induratum

Clinical presentations of lymphocytic vasculitis

Erythema nodosum

Definition

A lymphocytic vasculitis seen mainly in women (F:M = 5:1) and predominantly
affecting the lower legs.

Aetiology

Erythema nodosum is an example of a tissue reaction and may be caused by a
variety of problems. The current commonest causes in the UK are adverse drug
reactions, streptococcal infection, sarcoidosis, viral and chlamydial infections, and
tuberculosis. A common presentation with sarcoid is the development of erythema nodosum and observation of hilar adenopathy on a chest X-ray. In other
European countries, *Yersinia* infection is a relatively common precipitating factor.
However, in the majority of cases no clear cause is identified.

Clinical features

Erythema nodosum is characterized by painful, palpable, dusky blue-red lesions
on the lower legs, although occasionally the forearms are also affected. General
malaise, fever, and joint pains are common. The lesions slowly resolve over a
period of 2–6 weeks. As the lesions gradually fade they may look very similar to
simple bruises (Fig. 9.9).

Diagnosis and appropriate investigations

The clinical picture of a febrile patient with painful, non-ulcerating leg
nodules is diagnostic. Table 9.2 outlines a reasonable, appropriate plan of
investigation for cases of erythema nodosum aimed at finding the cause of the
condition.

Key points

Always take a careful drug history
in a patient with erythema
nodosum.

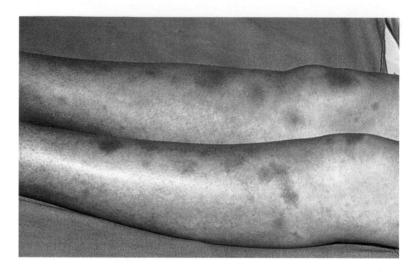

Fig. 9.9 Erythema nodosum. The lesions can be very faint, but are indurated and painful on palpation.

Treatment

This is mainly symptomatic. If the condition is thought to be drug-induced, the suspected drug should be withdrawn. Bed rest, elevation of the limb, and systemic analgesics should be prescribed. The value of topical preparations is debatable, but 10% ichthyol in water applied twice daily to acute lesions is a comfort to some patients. Steroids topically are of no value and there is little evidence that, given systemically, they change the course of the disease.

Pityriasis lichenoides

Definition

A purely cutaneous disorder of unknown aetiology characterized by multiple papules and plaques.

Clinical features

Pityriasis lichenoides presents acutely as multiple, pruritic, excoriated papules, occurring in crops on the trunk and limbs. Purpuric lesions are occasionally seen. There is rarely any systemic upset, and spontaneous remission is usual, but may take months or years to occur. Acute and chronic forms of the condition are described, and it is not clear if the one develops into the other.

Table 9.2 Investigation plan for erythema nodosum

1	History, including a careful drug history
2	E.S.R.
3	Throat swab, ASO titre
4	Chest X-ray (sarcoid, tuberculosis)
5	Mantoux test
6	Viral titres, both acute and convalescent

Diagnosis

This is based on the clinical appearance and is usually confirmed by biopsy which will show a lymphocytic vasculitis. Insect bites and atypical dermatitis herpetiformis (p. 277) are the most common causes of confusion, but the possibility of the papular form of secondary syphilis should be borne in mind. Syphilitic lesions will commonly affect the palms and soles, whereas those of pityriasis lichenoides will only do so rarely.

Treatment

This is usually based on moderate potency topical steroids. A course of ultraviolet light will benefit some patients.

Clinical presentation of polymorphonuclear vasculitis

Polyarteritis nodosa

Definition

A rare, severe, generalized disease characterized by necrosis of arterial vessel walls

Aetiology

There are many causes of neutrophilic vasculitis, but the final common pathway is thought to be an immune complex reaction based on the intermediate and small blood vessels. This can be caused for example by an adverse drug reaction or infection.

Clinical features

The patient is generally unwell and may be febrile. Subcutaneous nodules, subungual splinter haemorrhages, small purpuric lesions, and occasionally, frankly gangrenous lesions may be present. As this is a multi-system disorder, other signs and symptoms result from involvement of the renal, abdominal, cardiovascular, and CNS vasculature (Fig. 9.10).

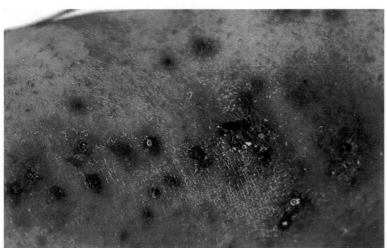

Fig. 9.10 Necrotizing (leucocytoclastic) vasculitis. Palpable lesions are surrounded by purpura and tend to break down easily.

Occasionally, a milder variant is seen, which appears to be confined to the skin and consists of a livedo pattern on the skin of the lower legs, associated with leg nodules. This has been called **cutaneous polyarteritis nodosa**.

Pathology

Histologically, there are polymorphonuclear leucocytes in the blood vessel walls and fragments of disintegrating nuclei from damaged polymorphs ('nuclear dust') will be seen.

Diagnosis

Diagnosis is based on evidence of involvement of multiple vessels and is usually confirmed by biopsy.

Treatment with systemic steroids and immunosuppressives, such as azathioprine, is required, but even so there is a significant mortality.

For patients with the cutaneous variant, low doses of systemic steroids may also be needed. Simple analgesics such as aspirin will relieve pain. Topical steroid therapy is of little value.

Pyoderma gangrenosum

Definition

The sudden appearance of large, ulcerating lesions.

Clinical features

The initial cutaneous lesions resemble indolent boils, but they rapidly expand, break down, and leave large, ulcerated, painful areas with a very characteristic undermined edge. Systemic upset, with fever and malaise, is frequent. Pyoderma gangrenosum may be the first signs of ulcerative colitis, Crohn's disease, rheumatoid arthritis, and monoclonal gammopathies or frank myeloma (Fig. 9.11).

> **Key points**
>
> Always look for an underlying cause in a patient with pyoderma gangrenosum

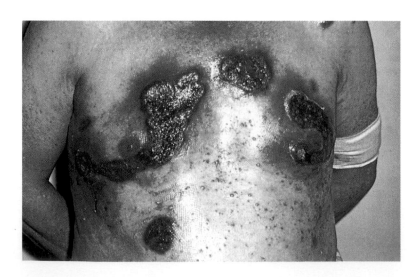

Fig. 9.11 Pyoderma gangrenosum. These large lesions can develop within 24 hours

Pathology

Pyoderma gangrenosum results from underlying thrombosis and vasculitis.

Diagnosis and treatment

The diagnosis is generally apparent on clinical grounds. An underlying systemic disease may already be obvious, but if not appropriate, clinical investigations should be carried out to identify in particular a haematological or gastroenterological cause.

Systemic steroid therapy should be prescribed in a moderately high dose (for example, 60–100 mg of prednisolone daily) and subsequently reduced as the lesions heal. If there is only one lesion, intra-lesional injection of steroid may be helpful, provided it is injected into an early lesion. A soothing non-adherent dressing should be applied (for example, Scherisorb).

Clinical presentation of granulomatous vasculitis

Temporal arteritis (giant cell arteritis)

Definition

A rapidly progressive granulomatous arteritis, which can cause blindness if not recognized and treated promptly.

Clinical features

The classic presentation of temporal arteritis is that of an elderly person complaining of severe headache and general malaise, often with some associated visual upset. There may be red palpable nodules in the temporal area.

Pathology

A biopsy will show vasculitis with granulomas around the affected vessels.

Diagnosis and treatment

These patients usually have a very high erythrocyte sedimentation rate and a temporal biopsy should be performed as a matter of urgency to confirm the diagnosis. Systemic steroids in high doses should be started without waiting for the pathology report as there is a real risk of blindness.

Erythema induratum (Bazin's disease)

Definition

A condition affecting the lower legs of young women, currently believed to be a hypersensitivity reaction to the tubercle bacillus.

Clinical presentation

This condition is relatively rare and presents as painful ulcerating nodules on the back of the lower legs of obese patients, usually female.

Pathology

The pathology is that of tuberculous granulomas around affected blood vessels.

Treatment

Treatment is difficult, but weight reduction and keeping the legs warm in appropriate trousers or tights are worthwhile. A long-term trial of full anti-tuberculous therapy should be considered, but there are no controlled comparative studies proving the value of anti-tuberculous therapy.

Urticaria

Definition

Recurrent, transient, cutaneous swellings, and erythema due to fluid transfer from the vasculature to the dermis.

Clinical features

Urticaria is common and varies from minor, but inconvenient cutaneous lesions to the severe life-threatening angio-oedema affecting the laryngeal area. A local sudden increase in capillary permeability is the common final pathway for a variety of stimuli thought to cause urticaria.

Some of the recognized types of urticaria are listed below. The majority of cases will fall into the group of unknown aetiology.

The urticarial lesion is a rapidly developing raised weal or plaque (Fig. 9.12). Lesions may be large, multiple, and appear with alarming speed. Lesions occurring around the mouth should be regarded as a dermatological emergency and the patient observed for signs of respiratory obstruction. Many patients have a chronic variety of urticaria, resistant to therapy, which persists for months or years before burning out.

> **Key points**
>
> Urticarial lesions around the mouth is an emergency condition and patients should be observed for signs of respiratory obstruction. Subcutaneous adrenaline may be required.

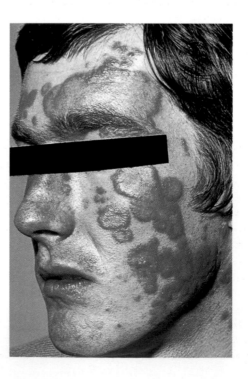

Fig. 9.12 Urticaria. Large erythematous weals are seen on the face.

Recognized varieties of urticaria

- **Due to histamine-liberating drugs:** Salicylates are the commonest group of drugs in this category and patients with chronic urticaria should be advised to use paracetamol, rather than aspirin as a simple analgesic. Codeine, morphine, and indomethacin will also release histamine, and should, therefore, be avoided.

- **Due to ingested food additives:** The two food additives known to cause or provoke urticaria are the tartrazine group of dyes, found in yellow- and orange-coloured drinks and sweets, and benzoates, used widely as preservatives.

- **Contact urticaria:** Here, the lesions develop only on actual sites of contact, for example, on the site of contact with dog hair or saliva, or on the lips after ingesting protein foods. This variety of urticaria is common in atopic patients.

- **Physical urticaria:.** In a small group of patients, pressure, heat, cold, and sunlight may provoke urticarial weals.

- **Urticaria and hereditary angio-oedema:** This rare condition is transmitted by autosomal dominant inheritance. The basic biochemical defect is in the complement pathway. The enzyme C_1 esterase inhibitor is lacking in these patients, who may present with gross and alarming swellings. They may also present as acute surgical emergencies because of sudden oedema of a part of the small intestine leading to acute pain and obstruction.

- **Related to general medical problems:** This is a miscellaneous group. Patients infested with parasites tend to develop urticaria, as do those with chronic bacterial infection in such sites as the nasal sinuses and the urinary tract. Patients with lupus erythematosus, thyrotoxicosis, and lymphomata may also present with urticaria.

- **No known or identifiable causative factor:** This comprises by far the largest group of patients.

Diagnosis, appropriate investigations, and treatment

Diagnosis is self-evident and patients frequently do not seek help until they have tried several home remedies. These should be identified in case they are histamine releasing agents, which will aggravate rather than improve the condition.

The investigation of a case of urticaria can be a time-consuming, expensive, and non-rewarding exercise, and as the disease is common, a sensible compromise is to investigate only patients who have had recurrent attacks for 6–9 months duration or longer who do not obtain relief from systemic antihistamine therapy. Patients should be told that tests will rarely reveal the cause of the urticaria and that in time the problem will resolve spontaneously. A reasonable battery of investigations to be performed as an out-patient is given in Table 9.3. A careful history should identify the rare cases of physical urticaria and may be a pointer in cases provoked by food additives. The great majority of cases will yield negative results on this screen and must be treated on a symptomatic basis.

Treatment of acute urticaria may require subcutaneous adrenalin as a life-saving measure. For less acute and chronic cases the systemic non-sedating H1 antihistamines are usually helpful. Often several need to be tried before one is found that combines symptomatic relief with minimal side-effects. Current

Table 9.3 An outline of investigations for cases of chronic persistent urticaria

Full blood count (Hb, WBC+ eosinophil count, platelets)

Liver function tests

Chest and sinus X-ray

Examination of hot stool for parasites

Examination of urine for bacteria

Complement screen including C₁ esterase inhibitor

Auto-antibody screen

popular, non-sedating antihistamines include cetirizine (Zirtek), desloratadine (Clarinex), fenoxfenadine (Telfast), and terfenadine (Triludan). All are relatively non-sedating. While there is little published evidence that the addition of an H2 inhibitor adds to the effect of the H1 inhibitor, it may be worth adding cimetidine in adequate doses in severe and persistent urticaria.

For more persistent cases, the possibility of elimination diets should be considered, and patients should be advised about avoiding tartrazine and benzoate containing food and drink. More specific dietitian elimination treatment requires expert supervision from a dietitian, particularly if provocation tests with the suspected foodstuff is part of the plan.

Very persistent cases may justify a trial of oral dapsone or cyclosporin A, and both Puva and plasmapheresis may need to be considered. In general, oral steroids are not useful, but may help delayed pressure urticaria.

Purpura

Purpura may be caused by a low platelet count, by a disease affecting capillaries, or a more general systematized disease. Common causes of purpura are ageing due to capillary fragility in which the small blood vessels of the skin lose their normal collagen support, topical, or systemic steroid therapy, which similarly increases capillary fragility, vitamin C deficiency, and side effects of drug therapy. Rarer causes include generalized amyloidosis and renal disease.

Platelet counts of 60,000/mm³ or more are unlikely to produce purpura and, in patients with platelet counts above this level, causes of non-thrombocytopenic purpura should be sought.

Henoch–Schoenlein purpura (anaphylactoid purpura)
Definition

A purpuric eruption due in some cases to an allergic reaction to bacteria or systemic drugs, associated with fever, malaise, and gastrointestinal and renal involvement.

Clinical features

Macular or papular purpuric lesions are scattered on the limbs and buttocks. General malaise and fever may be present, and also arthralgia, haematuria, and abdominal pain. The platelet count is normal. In some patients, there is a history of a streptococcal throat infection 7–14 days prior to development of purpura, and in others there is a history of systemic drug ingestion. In most cases, however, no cause can be identified.

Pathology

The underlying pathological lesion is a vasculitis affecting small vessels and the degree of systemic involvement is very variable. Children are frequently affected.

Diagnosis and treatment

Diagnosis is usually straightforward and investigations should be carried out to establish the degree of systemic involvement. The most serious complication is severe renal involvement, which can lead to the nephrotic syndrome. The disease is usually self-limiting and there is little evidence that systemic steroids will alter its course. Nevertheless, they are frequently prescribed for patients with severe multi-system involvement. Bed rest and simple analgesics may be required for arthropathy. Urinalysis should be performed and repeated to look for frank haematuria and developing proteinuria.

Discussion of problem cases

Case 9.1

The history and the patient strongly suggests that this is a venous leg ulcer, rather than an arterial ulcer. The contributing factors include the female sex, obesity, and a history of a job that involves standing for long periods of time.

This can be confirmed by the fact that the arteries around the ankle have good pulses and Doppler ultrasound would confirm the fact that the valves in the perforating veins in her legs are incompetent.

In the history it emerged that she had been treating the ulcer with a moderately potent steroid. This was withdrawn and an occlusive dressing applied to the ulcer with a weak potency steroid (1% hydrocortisone) around the ulcer. On this regime there continued to be a lot of inflammation and irritation. Patch testing was therefore arranged to establish whether or not any of the medicaments the lady was using was contributing to her problem. The patch test battery included the topical corticosteroid tixocortol and she was shown to have a topical steroid allergy. All topical steroid was, therefore, withdrawn, and copious emollients and occlusive dressings applied under four layer bandaging. On this regime, the ulcer healed in 10 weeks. During this time she was encouraged to try to lose some weight and, once the ulcer was healed, she was referred for consideration for surgery to her varicose veins.

Case 9.2

The diagnosis here strongly suggests urticaria. This has been persistent, but has not caused any general debility and the patient has lost no time from work.

A careful history has established that from time-to-time this patient does take aspirin for minor aches and pains. He was, therefore, warned against the use of aspirin and other histamine releasing drugs. A full history revealed no other possible causes of his urticaria. A blood count showed no evidence of eosinophilia. He was, therefore, started on a regime of H1 antihistamines, and returned at 3 weekly

Discussion of problem cases continued

intervals to report progress. On the third non-sedating antihistamine his urticaria improved significantly with only two minor episodes each week. These disappeared completely over the next few months.

This history illustrates the fact that most patients with urticaria have a self-limiting condition, which burns out after a period of 6 months to a year. Extensive investigations very rarely uncover the trigger for urticaria, and are expensive and time consuming for the patient.

Case 9.3

The history is that of a cavernous angioma, a vascular naevus associated with proliferation of the capillary endothelial cells. These are very common, but as they tend to grow through the first year of life, they do cause concern particularly as many of them are on the face. Many patients have read in the newspapers of the significant advances made using laser treatment for a variety of other vascular lesions and are concerned that their child is not getting state of the art treatment. At the present time, laser treatment is not the most appropriate method of managing a cavernous angioma or strawberry naevus, as natural regression of the lesion will usually produce the best result.

This was explained to the parents and photographs of older children whose lesions had regressed spontaneously were shown to encourage them. They were also given the address of the Naevus Support Group to put them in contact with other parents in the same situation. The parents departed reassured that their child was not being denied essential treatment. Eighteen months later there had been very significant reduction in the size of the lesion and by the time the child was three the lesion was virtually invisible.

Further reading

Falanga, V. and Eaglestein, W. (1995) *Leg and foot ulcers, a clinicians guide*. Martin Dunitz, London.

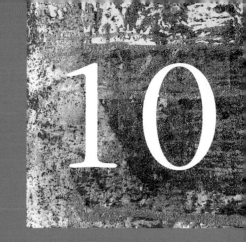

10

Problems of skin pigmentation

- Problem cases

- Albinism

- Vitiligo

- Physiological and age-related changes in skin pigmentation

- Actinic lentigines (PUVA or UVA freckles)

- Benign melanocytic naevi (moles)

- Chloasma

- Addison's disease

- Discussion of problem cases

Problems of skin pigmentation

Problem cases

Case 10.1

A 38-year-old, fair-skinned, auburn-haired woman comes to consult you about two irregular macules on her shoulder. She was born in South Africa and lived in that country until she came to the UK as a student aged 19. She has large numbers of freckles and also large numbers of naevi, mainly on her trunk and limbs. She misses the warm South African sunshine and uses a sunbed regularly at home.

What investigations will you carry out on the two lesions on her shoulder, which are both about a centimetre in diameter and irregular in outline?

What advice will you offer her in general?

Case 10.2

An Asian student at the local technical college consults you about patchy depigmentation on her trunk. She is reluctant to undress completely, but the lesions are asymptomatic and you make a diagnosis of vitiligo. You tell her there is little that can be done. She returns 3 months later to tell you that the depigmented areas are now itchy and that her two younger sisters have developed the same problem. What action do you take?

The structure and melanin-producing function of the epidermal melanocyte network has already been described (p. 26). Differences in activity, rather than numbers of melanocytes explain skin colour differences in different ethnic groups. In addition, one of the evolutionary functions of epidermal melanocytes is considered to have been the production of a protective pigment layer in response to exposure to sunlight as a protection against damaging wavelengths of solar radiation.

Problems may arise from an absence of melanocytes or of functioning melanocytes as in albinism, a disease that is a severe handicap in normally dark-skinned races in a tropical climate. Other problems such as vitiligo may appear merely cosmetic to the non-sufferer, but may cause great social and psychological distress. An increase in skin pigmentation, usually only visible in white-skinned races, may be the first signs of endocrinological problems such as Addison's disease, and temporary localized increase in skin pigmentation may be seen during pregnancy as chloasma due to endocrine stimulation of melanocyte activity.

Lentigines or freckles are common on the exposed skin, usually facial, of red-haired individuals. Benign melanocytic naevi or moles are not a skin disease, but a physiological variant, found in skin of all colours, although usually only visible on pale skinned individuals. The first signs of excessive sun exposure on older pale skin may be the development of actinic lentigines.

Malignant melanoma, the malignancy arising from the melanocyte is discussed in Chapter 15 with other skin tumours.

Key points

The presence of a large number of melanocytic naevi is a risk factor for melanoma.

Table 10.1 Melanocyte abnormalities and their clinical manifestations

Melanocyte abnormality	Clinical manifestation
Non-function or poor function of melanocytes	Albinism
Localized loss of melanocytes	Vitiligo
Localized increase in melanogenesis	Freckles (ephelides)
Hormonally-mediated increase in melanogenesis	Chloasma
Localized increase in numbers of epidermal and dermal melanocytes	Junctional and compound naevi
Localized increase in numbers of dermal melanocytes	Blue naevus
Localized increase in both epidermal and dermal melanocytes and naevus cells	Giant pigmented hairy naevus
Malignant change in epidermal melanocytes	Malignant melanoma (see Chapter 15)

Albinism

Definition

An autosomal recessive disorder, characterized by a lack of pigment production by melanocytes in the epidermis, hair bulb, and eye.

Clinical features

Albino children are diagnosed at or shortly after birth when the absence of any melanin pigmentation in the skin and hair is obvious. The skin is white or pink and the hair pale blonde. The eyes are also involved due to lack of activity of the ocular melanocytes, so the iris will be translucent. Sunlight is very poorly tolerated, and sunburn and photophobia are common symptoms. Nystagmus may also be present. Albinism is a serious condition that may shorten life if the sufferer is exposed to tropical or subtropical sunlight. Their skin ages prematurely and they have a high incidence of malignant skin tumours, mainly squamous carcinoma. In temperate climates, as in the UK, the main problems that arise are usually ocular due to poor vision.

Pathology and genetics

Melanocytes are present in the basal layer of the epidermis, but are not performing their normal function. The melanocyte either totally lacks tyrosinase necessary for melanin pigment synthesis (tyrosinase negative albinism) or has tyrosinase present, but poorly functional (tyrosinase positive). These two varieties of albinism can be differentiated by incubating plucked hair bulbs *in vitro* with tyrosine or DOPA. The hair bulbs with functionally normal tyrosinase will show a black deposit, but in those without the enzyme there will be no pigment deposit. The gene for tyrosinase positive albinism is on chromosome 15q11.2-q12 and the gene for tyrosinase negative albinism is on chromosome 11q14-q21.

Key points

In albinism the melanocytes either lack tyrosinase or have poor enzyme function.

Diagnosis and treatment

Diagnosis is based on clinical examination and if necessary genetic studies.

Prevention of sun damage to both skin and eyes is essential. Sun avoidance should be practised with appropriate clothing and hats. Where sunlight exposure is inevitable a total sunblock should be used. Regular clinical review is essential for early diagnosis of skin tumours. Children with ocular albinism may have learning difficulties due to poor vision and require specialist ophthalmological supervision.

Vitiligo

Definition

An area of acquired cutaneous depigmentation due to loss of normal melanocytes.

Incidence and aetiology

Vitiligo affects around 0.4% of the European population, and prevalence figures for genetically dark-skinned races suggest that it is commoner among them. As has been discussed in Chapter 2, it is currently one of the commoner conditions referred for specialist dermatological assessment. A high proportion of affected patients have a positive family history, suggesting a genetic aetiological component.

There is a significant association with autoimmune diseases, such as pernicious anaemia, thyroid disease, and Addison's disease, and anti-melanocyte antibodies can be detected in a proportion of vitiligo patients suggesting that autoimmune destruction of melanocytes may be involved in the pathogenesis.

Clinical features

Patients present with irregular white patches due to slowly extending acquired loss of normal melanin pigment on any body site (Figs 10.1 and 10.2). In white-skinned

> ### *Key points*
> Vitiligo is associated with other autoimmune diseases.

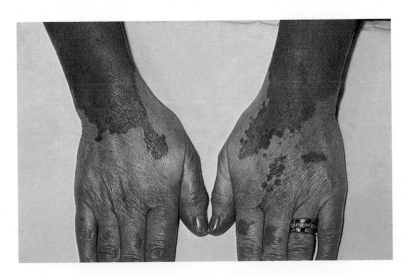

Fig. 10.1 Vitiligo. The areas in which melanin pigment has been lost are particularly prone to sunburn.

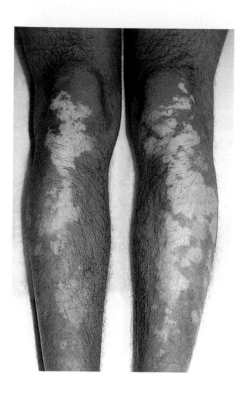

Fig. 10.2 Vitiligo appearing on coloured skin. Note very striking depigmentation.

individuals this can be of little cosmetic or medical concern, but the appearance can be very unacceptable on exposed areas of darker skinned individuals.

Vitiligo demonstrates the Koebner phenomenon as it is provoked by minor trauma and may develop on the site of even a mild scratch.

Pathology

Dopa or silver staining techniques show that there are no epidermal melanocytes in the basal layer of the epidermis.

Diagnosis and treatment

Diagnosis is usually self-evident, but in darker skin pityriasis versicolor (p. 161) can be confusing, so scrapings should be taken for mycological examination. Leprosy is a very much rarer possibility, but can worry the patient greatly, particularly if he or she comes from a part of the world where leprosy is endemic. In leprosy the hypopigmented macules are usually anaesthetic, while in vitiligo normal sensation is present. In cases of doubt a biopsy should be performed.

Treatment is unsatisfactory. Some patients achieve a reasonable cosmetic result with topical artificial tanning creams containing dihydroxyacetone, but those with a dark skin rarely find these preparations satisfactory. Preparations containing a topical steroid, hydroquinone, and tretinoin are available (e.g. Tri Luma cream), and appear to be effective in some patients. Photochemotherapy (psoralens + UVA = PUVA) is of some value in a very small proportion of patients, but is

Key points

Remember that patients from dark-skinned races with vitiligo may be very concerned about leprosy, which also causes loss of pigment. Be aware of this and offer reassurance.

time-consuming and may carry a long-term risk of skin cancer. Grafting of autologous melanocytes, after taking a small biopsy from pigmented skin of the patient and expanding the melanocytes in tissue culture, can be effective for small areas, but is time consuming, not always successful, and only available in a limited number of centres.

Patients must be warned that the depigmented skin is easily sunburned and that they should use a topical sunscreen.

The prognosis for vitiligo is very varied. In some individuals only a small area of skin is affected and some spontaneous repigmentation occurs, but in others there is continuing and extensive loss. This can cause great distress, particularly if the affected areas are mainly exposed sites and the patient is dark skinned.

The Vitiligo Society is a very active patient support group, which raises funds for research and runs useful conferences. Many patients with vitiligo find membership useful (website: www.vitiligosociety.org.uk).

Physiological and age-related changes in skin pigmentation

Freckles (lentigines)

Freckles or lentigines are simple areas of over activity of an increased number of melanocytes, which are confined to the basal layer of the epidermis (Fig. 10.3). They are found in large numbers on the skin of fair- or red-haired individuals of

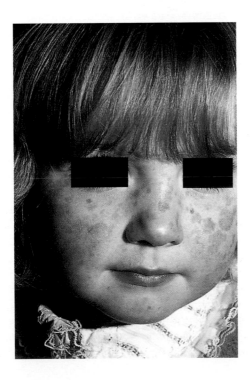

Fig. 10.3 Freckles or lentigines on the face of a young girl.

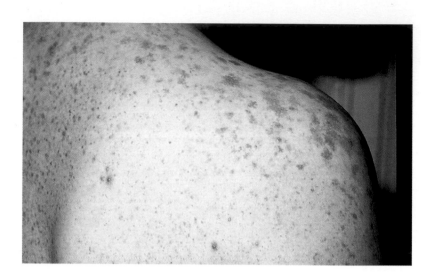

Fig. 10.4 Actinic lentigos following sunburn on the shoulder of a young boy.

Celtic descent. Their development is stimulated by sun exposure in genetically predisposed individuals. Their importance lies in the fact that they are a marker of an individual with relatively sun sensitive skin and an increased risk of future skin cancer who should receive advice about rationing sun exposure.

Actinic lentigines (PUVA or UVA freckles)

These are large (1 cm diameter or more), macular, brown lesions, which develop in individuals who have received a lot of natural sunlight as young adults after severe sunburn, or UVA from sun beds, or PUVA therapy. The shoulders are a common site and large actinic freckles may develop on the shoulders of young adults after only one severe sunburn (Fig. 10.4). They are a physiological marker of skin that cannot tolerate intense UV exposure and indicate an increased future skin cancer risk.

Benign melanocytic naevi (moles)

Pigmented melanocytic naevi or moles are extremely common. Despite this, they are a common cause for specialist referral, mainly because of concern that they might be early malignant melanoma (p. 345). It is therefore very useful for those working in primary care to be able to differentiate totally benign naevi for which reassurance is the only treatment required from potentially more serious problems that do require specialist referral.

The majority of naevi first appear on the skin during the second decade of life and the average young white-skinned adult has 20–50 such naevi. After the age of about 50, many of these naevi disappear spontaneously.

Individuals who have had a lot of natural sunlight exposure tend to have more naevi than those who have not had such exposure, and a large number of naevi is the strongest risk factor for malignant melanoma, so individuals with an excess of 100 naevi should be warned of this, and taught to recognize the signs of early melanoma.

Clinical types of pigmented naevi

- Banal acquired naevi, which may be described by the pathologist as junctional, compound, or intra-dermal—by far the largest group (Fig. 10.5);

- halo naevi;

- Spitz naevi, previously called juvenile melanoma;

- clinically atypical or dysplastic naevi

- congenital naevi, including the rare giant garment or bathing trunk congenital naevus;

- blue naevi, arising from dermal melanocytes.

Banal or acquired melanocytic naevi

These lesions are very common and the average young Caucasian adult in the UK has between 20 and 40 naevi. They are small (usually 2–3 mm in diameter) and a uniform brown (Fig. 10.6). In younger patients these naevi are a pale brown, but as the patient and the naevus matures it frequently becomes darker and may become elevated. With further ageing, many of these naevi, particularly on the face, lose their pigment completely and appear as flesh-coloured skin tags (Fig. 10.7), often with an outgrowth of one or two terminal hairs.

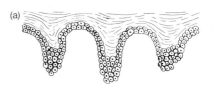
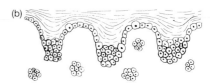
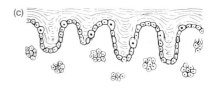

Fig. 10.5 Patterns of naevus cell distribution in melanocytic naevi. (a) Junctional naevus, (b) compound naevus; (c) intra-dermal naevus.

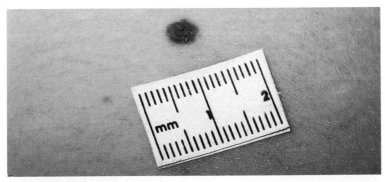

Fig. 10.6 Compound naevus on the neck of a young woman. The lesion is a uniform brown, slightly raised, and about 4 mm in the largest diameter.

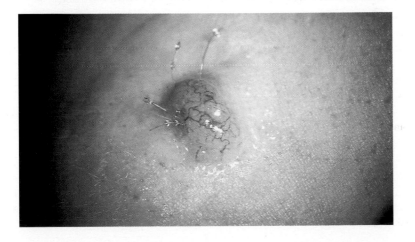

Fig. 10.7 Intra-dermal naevus on the face of a 45-year-old woman. Note the lack of pigment, the visible capillaries, and terminal hair growth.

Banal melanocytic naevi very rarely give rise to skin cancer, although in excess they are a marker of skin on which melanoma is more likely to develop, but not necessarily on a pre-existing mole. Apparently, benign naevi need only be excised if they have changed in shape, size, or colour, or if there are any other grounds for concern about malignant change. The chances of malignant change in any one naevus are very small, indeed, and there is no logic in extensive preventive excision. **If a naevus is excised, always send it for pathological examination.**

Halo naevi

These are common and harmless. They are usually compound naevi with a halo of surrounding depigmentation. They are frequently seen on the backs of teenagers during the summer months, and are much more easily seen on darker skin than on pale skin (Figs 10.8 and 10.9). Over a period of months, the central naevus will disappear, leaving a flat pale area, which may take years to repigment. While this is happening, the area should be protected from strong sunlight as there are no melanocytes present and severe burning can occur.

Excision is not necessary.

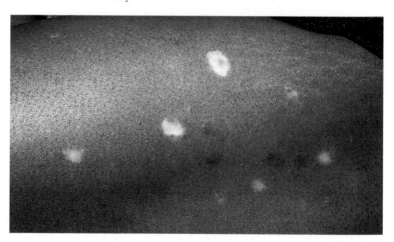

Fig. 10.8 Halo naevi on coloured skin, note very striking depigmentation.

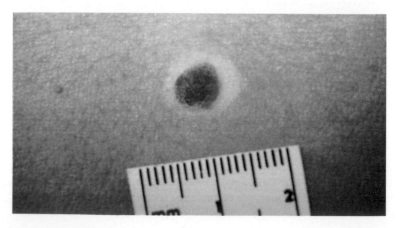

Fig. 10.9 Halo naevus on Caucasian skin, note much less dramatic appearance.

Spitz naevi (formerly called juvenile melanoma)

These naevi are most commonly seen on the faces of children, but can occur at any age. They are variants of compound naevi and their importance lies in the fact that, if excised, they can be difficult for the pathologist to distinguish from malignant melanoma without a clear history of the age of the patient and the clinical appearance of the lesion. They usually present as a growing, pink or pale brown lesion on the cheek (Fig. 10.10) in a child, but may be darker and more worrying in an adult.

Excision is rarely required in children, but may be necessary in adults to rule out developing melanoma.

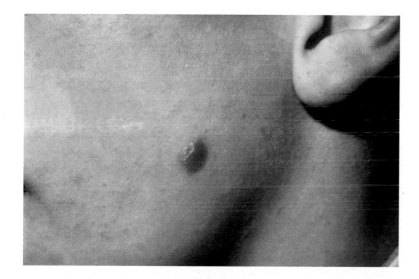

Fig. 10.10 Spitz naevus or juvenile melanoma, typical site on the cheek of a child.

Clinically atypical or dysplastic naevi

These melanocytic naevi are defined as naevi that are larger than banal naevi (>4 mm in diameter), and have, in addition, an irregular outline, irregular colour, and/or inflammation. They can be cosmetically unattractive, but their real importance is that larger numbers of such naevi are found on the skin of melanoma patients than would be expected by chance, so individual with large numbers of these naevi should also receive advice about rationing sun exposure and recognizing early melanoma.

Atypical naevi are found on all body sites, but are commoner on the male back and the female leg (Figs 10.11–10.13).

Many atypical naevi have clinical features that make them difficult to distinguish from early malignant melanoma and excision with a narrow margin of surrounding normal epidermis is therefore necessary. Some patients have large numbers of such naevi and large-scale excision is not practical. These patients should be referred to specialist centres that will manage them with a mixture of photography, regular review, and excision of any changing lesions.

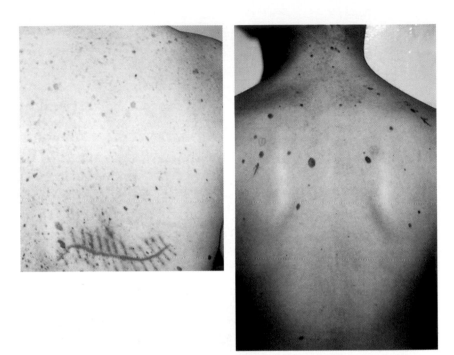

Figs 10.11 **and** 10.12 Clinically atypical naevi on the back of young males showing striking increase in normal numbers of naevi and in their size.

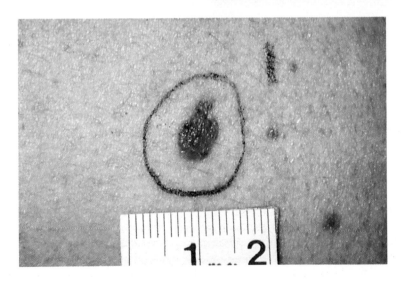

Fig. 10.13 Close up of a clinically atypical naevus showing irregular outline and irregular pigmentation.

Congenital melanocytic naevi

These are usually defined by size as small, medium, or giant. Three per cent of all newborn babies have a small, congenital, pigmented melanocytic naevus. This is usually small (less than 5 cm in diameter; Fig. 10.14) and only pale brown at birth, although it may darken with time and also develop coarse terminal hair. The pathology of these lesions usually shows naevus cells infiltrating into the skin appendages in a pattern not seen in acquired naevi.

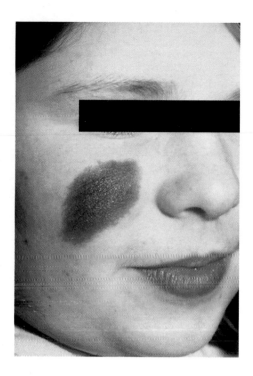

Fig. 10.14 Relatively small congenital naevus on the face of a young girl.

The giant congenital naevus (bathing trunk or garment naevus) is fortunately extremely rare (Fig. 10.15, see overleaf). This is a very large naevus usually covering a large part of the trunk and sometimes also associated with several smaller congenital naevi. There is an increased life-time risk of developing malignant melanoma in these giant naevi, and this may occur either in the skin or in associated involvement of the melanocytes in the central nervous system. For this reason, early and complete removal of giant pigmented naevi is theoretically ideal, but in practice the size and site of these giant naevi makes this very difficult.

Children born with a giant congenital melanocytic naevus should be referred to a local specialist in this field with no delay. There is no universally agreed method of managing what is a serious and distressing problem for the family involved. Some authorities believe that the lesions should be surgically excised as far as possible in very early infancy, and others prefer to wait until the baby is older and the risks of a general anaesthetic are less. The use of tissue expanders by inserting inflatable balloons under normal skin to expand the surface area of normal skin and so create 'spare' epidermis, which can then be used for definitive excision and grafting procedures is a common procedure.

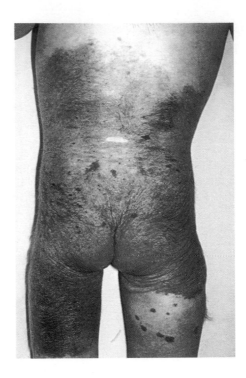

Fig. 10.15 Giant pigmented hairy naevus. These lesions are also termed bathing trunk or garment naevi. There is a significant incidence of development of malignant melanoma in this type of lesion.

Blue naevi

These naevi arise from dermal melanocytes. They are usually first identified in late childhood as deep-blue or black lesions, commonly on the face, hands, or feet (Fig. 10.16). A variant of the blue naevus is seen on the sacral area of dark-skinned babies as the so-called Mongolian spot.

Blue naevi are frequently excised both for cosmetic reasons and also to rule out melanoma.

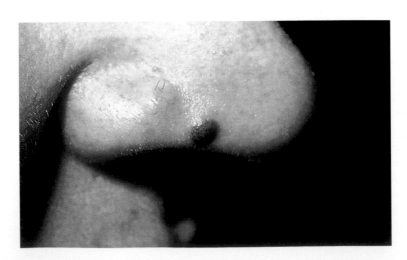

Fig. 10.16 Blue naevus on the nostril.

Pathology of naevi

The majority of melanocytic naevi arise from the basal layer melanocytes and are junctional, compound, or intra-dermal (Fig. 10.15). Junctional means that all the benign, proliferating melanocyte, or naevus cells, which comprise the naevus, are in contact with the overlying epidermis. Compound means that there are, in addition, small clusters of naevus cells lying free in the underlying epidermis and intra-dermal means that all the naevus cells are lying in the dermis in small clusters under a completely normal epidermis.

Halo naevi are usually compound naevi with an associated infiltrate of lymphocytes. Spitz naevi and dysplastic naevi are usually compound naevi with some unusual and worrying features for the pathologist. Congenital naevi have features of a compound naevus with evidence of the presence of both epidermal and dermal melanocytes, and blue naevi arise exclusively from dermal melanocytes.

Chloasma

Definition

A hormonally-stimulated increase in melanogenesis, which mainly affects the face, and may be seen in pregnant women and those on the contraceptive pill.

Both oestrogens and progesterone can affect melanogenesis and cause in pregnancy a mask-like increase in facial melanin pigment—chloasma uterinum (Fig. 10.17). This is commonest in females with naturally dark colouring and

> **Key points**
>
> Chloasma is a hormonally stimulated increase in melanogenesis.

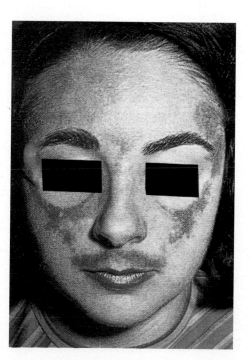

Fig. 10.17 Chloasma. This is seen both in pregnancy and in some users of the oral contraceptive pill. It can persist for some time after parturition or discontinuing the pill.

may take months to resolve after the birth of the child. A similar appearance is seen in some women on oral contraception. Sunlight increases the depth of pigmentation. Circulating levels of melanocyte stimulating hormone are normal.

While most women find that the pigmentation clears after delivery, it can persist in some cases. These women should be advised that the oral contraceptive will aggravate the situation and warned that the problem will almost certainly recur in future pregnancies. A high SPF sunscreen should be used.

Addison's disease

One of the early signs of Addison's disease may be excessive grey brown pigment, particularly of the mucous membranes. It is often best seen on the inside of the mouth. This is because ACTH, which is present in excess in Addison's disease, has a structure very similar to melanocyte stimulating hormone and can stimulate melanocyte to produce more melanin pigment.

Discussion of problem cases

Case 10.1

This description indicates that this patient is genetically at risk of sunlight induced skin damage because of her hair colour, fair skin, and freckles. This risk has been increased by her upbringing in a country where exposure to strong sunlight for long periods of the year is virtually unavoidable.

The possibilities, therefore, are that the two brown lesions on her shoulder area are actinic lentigos, or even frank, early skin cancer, possibly early malignant melanoma.

Biopsies showed that both lesion were actinic lentigos and in the report the pathologist commented, without being given a full history, on the severe actinic damage seen in the dermal collagen surrounding the lesions.

The two lesions for which she sought help have therefore been removed, but she also needs advice on reducing further actinic damage. The first step is to strongly recommend that she give up sunbed sessions. Sunbeds mainly emit UVA or long-wave ultraviolet radiation (320–360 nm), and this contributes significantly to age changes of photo-ageing. Sunbeds may also contribute to skin cancer risk.

Early childhood natural sun exposure, as has been experienced by this patient, also increases the risk of both melanoma and non-melanoma skin cancer (see Chapter 15). This patient should, therefore, be advised to avoid excessive sunlight exposure and be given a leaflet illustrating the features of early skin cancers of all types—melanoma, basal cell carcinoma, and squamous cell carcinoma—with advice to seek medical help if she notices any similar changes on her own skin. She also should be advised to avoid mid-day sun, and use a high SPF broad spectrum sunscreen in sunny weather. In many parts of the world she would also be offered annual skin cancer checks by a dermatologist.

Discussion of problem cases continued

Case 10.2

Vitiligo is relatively common in the Asian population and would be a likely diagnosis. There is a genetic component to vitiligo, so more than one family member may well be involved. However, rapid onset of pruritic depigmentation in three family members almost simultaneously does not suggest vitiligo. These girls must be examined properly. This was done by a female doctor at their request, when it became clear that the pattern of depigmentation suggested pityriasis versicolor (p. 161), rather than vitiligo. Pityriasis versicolor is frequently slightly pruritic. Scrapings were taken from all three girls for mycological examination and these confirmed the presence of *M. furfur*, the causative organism of pityriasis versicolor. All three patients were treated with a topical imidazole cream with relief of symptoms and slow repigmentation.

Further reading

Ortonne, J.P., Mosher, J.B., and Fitzpatrick, T.B. (1983) *Vitiligo and other hypomelanoses of the hair and skin*. Plenum Publishing Co, New York.

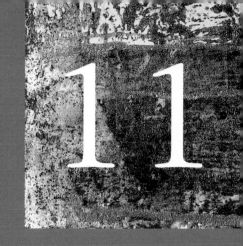

11

Acne, hair problems, and other disorders of the skin appendages

Acne, hair problems, and other disorders of the skin appendages

Problem cases

Case 11.1

A female in her late twenties consults you about easy flushing and papules on her face. She has a job that involves meeting the public, and finds the development of these lesions distressing and unacceptable. She is on no regular medication other than the oral contraceptive, and thinks herself that the problem is due to an allergy to makeup. She tells you that, until this point in time, she has always had an exceptionally good skin. What is the likely diagnosis, and what are the appropriate investigations and management plans for this patient?

Case 11.2

The mother of an 8-year-old boy who lives on a farm consults you about her son's recent hair loss. The boy has striking loss of hair, mainly on the crown in regular, circular areas. The underlying scalp looks healthy. What condition does this description suggest and what is the differential diagnosis? What treatment would you recommend? What factors might affect the prognosis?

Case 11.3

A colleague asks your advice on the diagnosis and management of a male in his late twenties who has recurrent abscesses in both axillae. These began about 10 years ago and have persisted ever since. Several courses of systemic antibiotics have had little effect. Your colleague is concerned about the possibility that the patient has an immunodeficiency problem. What is the likely diagnosis and what treatments might be of value?

Disorders of the pilosebaceous follicle

Acne vulgaris

Definition

A disorder of the pilosebaceous follicles causing comedones (blackheads), papules, and pustules on the face, chest, and upper back.

Epidemiology and aetiology

Mild acne vulgaris is almost universal at some time during the second decade. Surveys of teenage school children suggest that girls develop acne 2–3 years earlier than boys, but that boys have rather more persistent lesions. Most acne sufferers have a mild form of the disease, which can be managed with topical preparations, but a small proportion require oral antibiotics from their general practitioner, and an even smaller group require specialist referral and consideration for oral retinoid therapy. There appears to be a growing number of older patients, usually women, in the third decade who have mild, but stubborn acne persisting for over 10 years.

The four factors that contribute to development of the acne lesion are:

- production of excessive sebaceous gland secretion;
- obstruction to outflow of this sebum at the mouth of the pilosebaceous canal;
- inflammation arising as a result of leakage of contents of the pilosebaceous follicle into the surrounding dermis;
- excessive colonization or infection of the pilosebaceous ducts with *P. acnes.*

Sebaceous gland secretion is partly controlled by androgen stimulation. In the neonate small visible sebaceous glands are often seen on the central panel of the face due to stimulation by maternal androgens. After the first few days of life, these become vestigial until puberty when the individual's own androgen levels rise, causing expansion of the sebaceous glands, and in many cases temporary overproduction of sebum.

Clinical features of classical acne vulgaris

The early lesions are open and closed comedones (blackheads and whiteheads), which develop into papules and pustules, mainly on the forehead, nose, and chin (Figs 11.1–11.5). In more severe cases the entire face with the exception of the peri-orbital skin may be affected, often with additional involvement of the upper chest and back. These sites are most densely populated with well developed sebaceous glands. Generally, acne is associated with clinical signs of excessive sebaceous secretion, and a greasy facial skin and scalp. This inter-relationship is

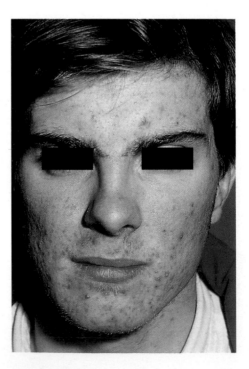

Fig. 11.1 Relatively mild acne vulgaris.

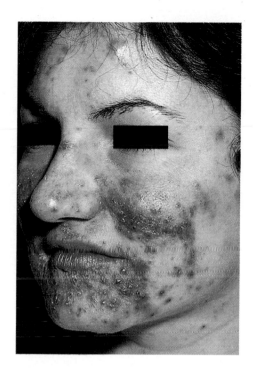

Fig. 11.2 More severe acne vulgaris, involving the cheeks and chin.

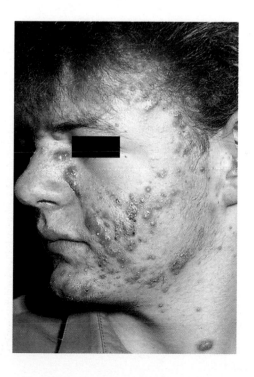

Fig. 11.3 Severe pustular acne vulgaris. This young man already has scarring.

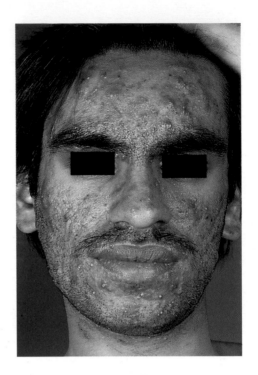

Fig. 11.4 Acne vulgaris in an Indian showing extensive involvement of the face.

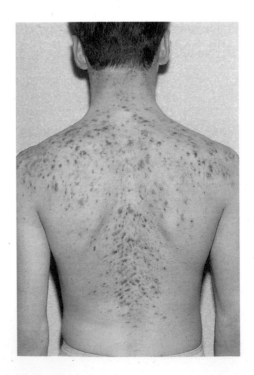

Fig. 11.5 Acne vulgaris of the back showing typical distribution.

not, however, exclusive because in conditions, such as Parkinson's disease also associated with excessive sebaceous secretion there are no accompanying acne lesions. Many females with acne notice premenstrual deterioration of their lesions. If acne has been severe and persisted for some time leading to rupture of pilosebaceous follicles, there may be scarring. With modern methods of treating acne, scarring should totally preventable by prompt treatment.

Variants

- **Tropical acne** affects young Caucasians in a hot, humid environment such as the Far East. They develop gross acne lesions, mainly on the trunk, which can be disabling and resistant to all therapy other than return to a temperate climate.

- **Steroid acne** appears in some patients on systemic steroid therapy. This acneiform eruption tends to affect the trunk, rather more than the face and, although papules and pustules are present, comedones are usually absent.

- **Chemical acne** is due to cutting oils and chlorinated hydrocarbons. This acneiform eruption is usually seen in those who handle these substances at work. They develop some lesions on atypical sites, such as the legs, due to protracted contact with oil in saturated working clothes.

- **Chloracne**, a very disfiguring disorder, is rare. Dioxin and chlorinated hydrocarbons are absorbed in the body, and cause an acneiform eruption, characterized by large numbers of occluded whiteheads (Fig. 11.6) and inflamed cysts. These may persist for very many months after only transient exposure.

- **Infantile acne** is a rare variant in which acne lesions are seen in male infants, usually between the age of 3 and 12 months. If severe, endocrine studies should

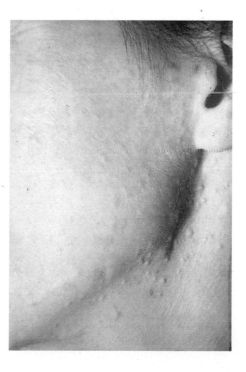

Fig. 11.6 Chloracne of the side of the face showing typical closed comedones.

be undertaken to exclude an androgen-secreting lesion. There is some evidence that infants affected with acne are prone to develop severe acne again when they reach puberty.

Differential diagnosis

The clinical diagnosis of acne is usually simple and is normally made by the patient prior to seeking advice. Acneiform drug eruptions should be considered, particularly in any patient presenting outwith the normal age range. Anti-tuberculous and anti-epileptic drugs are both responsible not only for aggravating pre-existing acne, but also for provoking an acneiform eruption. Rosacea may give rise to confusion, but generally it is seen in an older age group. Although pustules may be present in rosacea, there are no comedones and there is associated erythema.

Pathology

Classical acne is not normally biopsied. The picture is that of a distended pilosebaceous follicle with a surrounding cellular infiltrate in the dermis. If there has been rupture of the duct with leakage of its contents into the surrounding dermis, granuloma formation, foreign body giant cells, granulation tissue, and scar formation may also be seen.

Therapy

Acne therapy can be divided into topical therapy, which may be all that is needed for mild acne, systemic therapy (including oral antibiotics and anti-androgens) that are needed for most acne patients referred for specialist opinion, and oral retinoids for patients with severe persistent acne who have not responded to first line systemic treatment.

Topical treatment for acne includes:

- benzoyl peroxide-containing preparations;
- topical antibiotics—erythromycin and tetracycline;
- topical retinoids-tazarotene;
- topical vitamin A acid—tretinoin;
- antiseptics and keratolytics;
- azaleic acid preparations—Skinoren

Systemic therapy for acne includes:

- antibiotics—tetracycline or erythromycin;
- hormonal therapy—Dianette
- in severe or persistent cases, isotretinoin (Roaccutane, UK; Accutane, USA).

Experimental therapy includes:

- photodynamic therapy
- laser treatment for acne scarring

Table 11.1 outlines the range of acne therapies currently available.

Mild acne

Useful and effective preparations for mild acne include 5–10% benzoyl peroxide in a clear gel base (for example, Panoxyl 5 and 10, Quinoderm, Benoxyl). These

Table 11.1 Management strategies for varying types of acne

Type	Management
Mild teenage acne	Topical benzoyl peroxide or tretinoin
	Advice about non-greasy cosmetics
	Add systemic tetracycline or erythromycin if persistent after 3 months topical therapy
Moderately severe acne	Topical benzoyl peroxide
	Tetracycline or erythromycin 1 g/day for a minimum of 3 months
	If no response to full doses of antibiotics for 3–6 months, refer for consideration for isotretinoin
Persistent acne in mature females	Consider for hormonal therapy (Dianette)
Severe acne	Oral retinoids with oral contraception in females

preparations are clear and odourless, and therefore acceptable by both sexes. There may well be some initial mild redness and scaling, particularly in fair-skinned patients. They should be warned of this and encouraged to persevere. True contact dermatitis to benzoyl peroxide is rare, but has been recorded. Topical tetracycline (for example, Topicycline, USA and UK) and topical erythromycin (for example, Eryderm, USA; Stiemycin, UK) are both cosmetically acceptable and effective.

Topical vitamin A-containing preparations (for example, Retin-A gel) are particularly useful if the main problem is closed comedones (whiteheads). Here, again, some inflammation and irritation is very common.

Topical isotretinoin (Isotrex) and tazarotene are also useful for moderate inflammatory acne, but full contraceptive precautions as for oral retinoids (see below) must be taken in case of systemic absorption. Topical adapalene (Differin) is a similar retinoid like drug

Topical preparations containing azaleic acid (Skinoren) may help some cases of relatively mild acne.

Moderate acne

Patients with acne who have not responded to topical therapy, should have a 4–6-month trial of a systemic antibiotic taken in adequate doses. The two antibiotics of choice are tetracycline and erythromycin. Tetracycline or erythromycin should be given in full doses of 1 g/day for at least 3 months. Much the commonest reason for apparent non-response of acne to systemic antibiotic therapy is the prescription of too low a dose for too short a period of time. Tetracycline should be given 30 minutes before meals on an empty stomach and should be washed down with water, not milk, which interferes with absorption. Tetracycline should not be given concomitantly with oral iron, which will also hinder absorption. Although more expensive than tetracycline, doxycycline (Vibramycin, UK) 50 or 100 mg daily is worth considering. It may be used successfully even when conventional tetracycline has failed, possibly due to better absorption and a simpler dosage schedule.

The mode of action of systemic antibiotics in acne is not understood. While a part of their action may be in reducing the *P. acnes* colonization of pilosebaceous follicles, it is also postulated that they may affect chemotaxis of polymorphonuclear leucocytes and thus reduce the inflammatory response.

Side-effects of long-term antibiotic therapy for acne are rare, possibly due to the fact that the patients are otherwise healthy. Over growth with *Candida* is unusual. Girls should be warned that tetracycline will be deposited in bones and teeth of a foetus, should they become pregnant. For this reason, erythromycin should be given in preference to other antibiotics to women who require acne therapy during pregnancy.

For women whose acne persists into their late twenties and thirties, despite adequate topical therapy and repeated courses of systemic antibiotics, a trial of hormonal therapy may be beneficial. Cyproterone acetate is currently available in a dose of 2 mg combined with ethinyl oestradiol as an essential contraceptive (Dianette). If there is no response to a 6-month course of Dianette, these patients should also be considered for retinoid therapy.

Severe acne

Severe or persistent acne can now be well controlled in almost all cases by the use of isotretinoin, a synthetic retinoid, which is given systemically. In the UK, this drug is available only on hospital prescription. Isotretinoin (Roaccutane, UK; Accutane, USA) appears to have a very specific effect on the pilosebaceous gland and measurements of sebum excretion in patients on isotretinoin show a dramatic reduction in outflow of sebum, which persists for up to 12 months after withdrawal of the drug. If the acne-bearing skin is biopsied, the pilosebaceous follicles will be seen to have shrunk to the size seen prior to puberty. Isotretinoin is usually prescribed in a dose of 1.0 mg/kg body-weight daily for 4 months, but some patients, usually males with severe back lesions, may need a longer course.

Minor side effects include dry skin, cheilitis, and in some cases, a temporary elevation of serum lipids which revert to normal at the end of the course. A few patients on therapy for varying periods of time have been found to have bony abnormalities in the form of hyperostoses, and the development of bony spurs around the wrists and ankle areas.

By far the most serious problem, however, in the use of isotretinoin is its teratogenicity. **It is essential if isotretinoin is to be prescribed that females understand that pregnancy is absolutely contra-indicated.** There are reports of foetal abnormalities in children born to women who only took the drug for 1 or 2 weeks. A pregnancy test should therefore be done prior to starting therapy and the patient started on oral contraceptives 1 month before she starts oral retinoid therapy. This should be continued for at least 1 month after stopping retinoid therapy.

There is currently some concern that isotretinoin may provoke depression in predisposed individuals and there have been sad cases of teenage suicides while on oral retinoid for acne. While there is no strong statistical evidence for a causative relationship between oral retinoids and severe teenage depression, it is wise to discuss this tactfully with the patient or a parent when the possibility of prescribing oral retinoid is being considered.

> ### *Key points*
> Occasionally acne may persist in women into the second and third decades.

Most patients only need one 4-month course of treatment, but if necessary this can be extended or repeated after 12 months or so.

Acne scarring

The aim of modern acne therapy is to prevent scarring, but in some patients scarring has developed before the patient seeks medical advice. In such cases, once all acne activity has ceased, it may be possible to reduce scarring by chemical peeling techniques or dermabrasion, but good results cannot be guaranteed. Laser treatment of acne scars is available in some centres and appears to be of value in a proportion of cases.

Rosacea

Epidemiology and aetiology

Rosacea is relatively common and affects 1% of dermatological out-patients in the UK. It is commoner in women, although men tend to have more severe facial lesions, and a higher incidence of the associated complications of keratitis and rhinophyma.

The cause of rosacea is unknown. There appears to be a hyper-responsive blood supply to the pilosebaceous follicle, and most patients complain of easy flushing and blushing. Large numbers of the mite *Demodex folliculorum* can be found in the pilosebaceous follicles, but their role in the pathogenesis of rosacea is unknown.

Clinical features

Most patients first develop rosacea in the third and fourth decades. Flushing and erythema begin typically on the forehead, the bridge of the nose, and cheeks—the so-called butterfly area of the face (Fig.11.7). It may, however, be more widespread and spread to the neck, and occasionally beyond the face and neck areas. Over a period of months or years transient flushing is replaced by persistent erythema on which papules and pustules develop. Unlike acne, there are neither comedones nor seborrhoea.

In severe chronic cases, particularly in males, the sebaceous gland hypertrophy is concentrated on the nose, and produces gross soft tissue overgrowth and hypertrophy. The resulting appearance, termed **rhinophyma,** can be disfiguring and at times grotesque (Fig. 11.8).

Ocular involvement is a potentially serious complication. It presents as a sense of 'grittiness' or other discomfort in the eyes. Clinically, there may be a mild blepharitis and conjunctivitis. If keratitis develops, corneal ulceration, vascularization, and visual impairment may also become problems. Rosacea keratitis may develop in those with relatively mild cutaneous lesions.

Pathology

Dilatation of the vessels in the papillary dermis and sebaceous gland hyperplasia are hallmarks. A granulomatous dermal inflammatory infiltrate containing giant cells may be seen in chronic cases.

Differential diagnosis

The commoner facial dermatoses to be considered in the differential diagnosis of rosacea include acne vulgaris, light sensitivity, contact dermatitis, lupus

Key points

The aim of acne treatment is to prevent scarring.

Key points

Complications of rosacea are rhinophyma and keratitis.

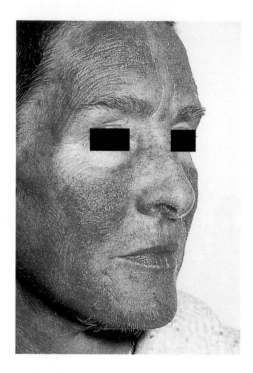

Fig. 11.7 Extensive rosacea.

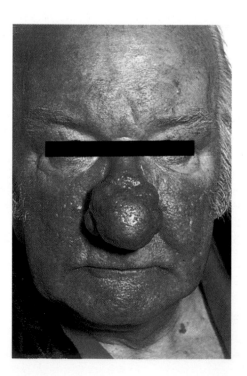

Fig. 11.8 Classic rhinophyma complicating rosacea in an elderly male.

erythematosus, and peri-oral dermatitis. Acne usually affects younger patients and is distinguished by comedones. Both facial photosensitivity and contact dermatitis are more rapid in onset than rosacea, and lack pustules. Chronic discoid lupus erythematosus is characterized by discrete scaly lesions leading to scarring, and in the systemic variety of lupus erythematosus the rash has a rapid onset and the patient is generally unwell.

Treatment

Long-term systemic antibiotics, commonly tetracycline, should be prescribed. Oxytetracycline, 250 mg four times per day for 2 months, reducing to twice daily 30–60 minutes before food for 3–6 months, is usually effective (Figs 11.9 and 11.10). Topical metronidazole (Metrogel) is also useful, but rarely effective alone. Oral retinoids have been used in rosacea, but in general the results are disappointing.

Moderate and potent topical steroids are positively contra-indicated, as they will aggravate the condition

Severe rhinophyma should be treated surgically. Shaving or excision of the excess soft tissue on the nose and skin grafting can be most effective. This should be done while the patient is receiving systemic tetracycline to reduce the chance of recurrence.

Any patient with rosacea and ocular symptoms, however mild, should be referred to an ophthalmologist without delay. As there is no clear relationship between the severity of cutaneous lesions and the risk of developing ocular lesions, all patients without exception should be asked about ocular symptoms.

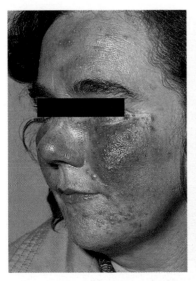 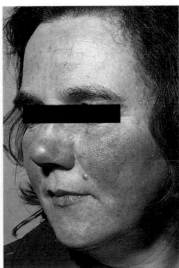

Figs 11.9 and 11.10 Patient with rosacea before and after 4 months treatment with systemic tetracycline.

Peri-oral dermatitis

It is likely that the condition peri-oral dermatitis is a variant of rosacea, mainly affecting the chin and cheek area around the mouth. It was relatively common in the 1970s when strong steroids were used inappropriately on the face. Over the past 30 years it has become much less common.

Excessive loss of hair

The normal structure and growth cycle of hair are detailed on p. 35. When dealing with alopecia, it is useful to remember that normally 80% of scalp hairs are in the anagen phase, and 20% in catagen or telogen, and that new follicles cannot be formed in the adult, so that a scarred scalp with irreversible damage to hair follicles will have permanent alopecia.

Hair loss on the scalp may be diffuse or patchy, and the commoner causes are listed in Tables 11.2 and 11.3. Patients rarely complain of hair loss from other sites, although it does occur, both in isolation and in association with scalp disorders.

Alopecia areata

Definition aetiology and incidence

A condition characterized by either generalized or localized sudden hair loss from the scalp or other body sites.

In some patients there appears to be an underlying genetic predisposition, but in others the cause is not yet known. Certain subgroups are recognized, including one associated with atopy and one with 'autoimmune' disorders, such as thyroid

> ### Key points
>
> At present the prospects for hair regrowth in persistent alopecia areata are poor. Do not build up false hopes in your patient prior to hospital referral.

Table 11.2 Common causes of diffuse hair loss

Male pattern baldness (androgen-dependent baldness)
Telogen effluvium (post-partum, fever, 'stress')
Syphilis
Systemic lupus erythematosus
Endocrine causes: hypothyroidism, hypopituitarism
Nutritional (iron deficiency)
Drug-induced (cytotoxics, anticoagulants, vitamin A, and analogues)
Hair shaft defects (pili torti and monilethrix)
Trichotillomania
Alopecia areata (may be diffuse or localized)

Table 11.3 Common causes of localized patch hair loss

Alopecia areata
Naevoid abnormalities
Fungal infections, including kerion
Chronic discoid lupus erythematosus
Follicular lichen planus
Traction ('ponytail' hair styles, the use of harsh setting implements)

disorders, vitiligo, and diabetes. Alopecia areata is commoner in children with Downs syndrome.

Alopecia areata is common and accounts for approximately 2% of new cases seen as dermatological out-patients.

Clinical features

Most cases are in children or young adults, and the commonest initial sign is one or more well-demarcated, completely bald areas. The affected scalp is normal with no sign of inflammation, scaling, or scarring, but hairs plucked from the margin of the area are often 'club hairs', that is in telogen, and broken hairs in this area resembling exclamation marks (!) are diagnostic (Fig. 11.11).

Complete loss of scalp hair is referred to as **alopecia totalis** and, when all body hair also is lost, the term **alopecia universalis** is applied.

It is not unusual in alopecia areata for the nails to be pitted and ridged.

Spontaneous regrowth takes place after an interval of 2–6 months in the majority of cases, but repeated episodes of hair loss are by no means uncommon. Features suggesting that the prognosis must be guarded include associated atopy, loss of eyebrows and lashes, nail change, and multiple lesions at the scalp margins—the so-called ophiasic type.

Diagnosis and treatment

The diagnosis is usually evident on clinical examination, but atypical or scaly lesions require mycological examination of scrapings, and hair samples to exclude a fungal infection. The use of Wood's light (p. 46) will exclude fungal infection due to most *Microsporum* species and to *Trichophyton schoenleinii*, but not to other species of fungi.

Scalp biopsy is rarely necessary, although the histology is characteristic. There is no loss of hair follicles, but the bulbs lie high in the dermis, are surrounded by lymphoid cells, and produce imperfectly keratinized hair.

As most cases of alopecia areata are self-limiting, the best plan is to reassure the patient and to encourage patience. Sometimes topical steroids or a course of ultra-violet light (UVB) is helpful. Corticosteroids (for example, triamcinolone)

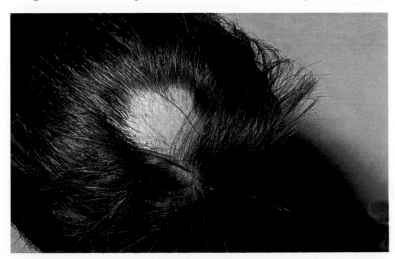

Fig. 11.11 Alopecia areata. Regular circular lesions appear rapidly. The underlying scalp appears smooth and healthy.

intra-lesionally may stimulate the regrowth of a tuft of hair adjacent to the needle track, but the cosmetic result is no improvement on the pre-existing alopecia. Trials of application of topical dinitrochlorobenzene (DNCB), which induces both irritation and an allergic contact dermatitis have shown variable results. DNCB can be very irritant and should not be used by those who lack experience.

In severe and extensive cases prescription of a wig is indicated.

Male pattern baldness (androgenic alopecia)

Androgen-dependent loss of scalp hair is physiological in men and increases with age. There is a genetic component determining the age of onset and severity of the process. A small proportion of post-menopausal women are similarly affected. The main area of loss in men is the crown, with some frontal recession, whereas in women there is fronto-vertical thinning, but retention of the frontal hair margin.

In otherwise healthy young men, one can only reassure them that there is no underlying disease. The anti-hypertensive drug minoxidil has been used topically, usually as a 2% solution, in various types of alopecia. In male pattern baldness it does appear in some patients to retard hair loss, but only as long as the topical application continues. In the UK, it is available only on private prescription, and individuals who wish to use it should be informed that it will reduce the rate of hair loss, but that it is not a cure.

Topical finasteride, a selective 5 alpha reductase inhibitor (Propecia) has been introduced for use in males only and also requires to be taken continuously to maintain affect.

For women with androgenic alopecia, a wig will be helpful, once endocrine, drug-induced, and iron deficiency alopecia have been excluded (see below). In the UK, however, there are clear-cut regulations governing the prescription on the National Health Service of either human or synthetic hair wigs. Artificial hair wigs are relatively inexpensive and, unlike those made of human hair, they can be easily washed at home.

Telogen effluvium

During pregnancy when blood oestrogen is raised, the percentage of hair follicles in anagen rises. As a result, there is a luxuriant head of hair, but after delivery, the follicles held in anagen all enter telogen, and these hairs are therefore shed. This can give rise to significant hair thinning, commonly seen 4–9 months after delivery, but the situation is self-limiting. The diffuse loss of hair which follows high fever, severe illness, or 'stress' results from a similar disturbance of the hair cycle. No specific treatment is available, and after 3–4 months hair follicles resume their normal synchronization.

Miscellaneous causes of hair loss

Syphilis

Some patients with secondary syphilis present with a diffuse 'moth-eaten' pattern of hair loss, but its relationship to the other signs and symptoms at this stage is unclear. Serology is positive. Hair regrowth follows adequate antibiotic therapy (p. 170).

Always consider checking syphilis serology in unusual patterns of hair loss.

Systemic lupus erythematosus

Patients with active, usually severe, systemic lupus erythematosus and multi-system involvement may have diffuse generalized hair loss. Unlike the patchy alopecia seen in chronic discoid LE, it is temporary, as there is no scarring destroying the hair follicles and good regrowth will follow successful systemic therapy.

Endocrine alopecia

Hair loss can accompany hypofunction of the thyroid and pituitary glands. In hypothyroidism hair growth is poor, and the hair shaft is coarse and wire-like. In hypopituitarism total loss of scalp, eyebrow, and secondary sexual hair is frequently seen. This type of alopecia does not always recover after adequate endocrine replacement.

Nutritional alopecia

Chronic iron deficiency anaemia is associated with thin fragile scalp hair (Fig. 11.12). Severe, generalized malnutrition also causes hair loss and premature greying of remaining hair. Always check serum iron, ferritin, and iron binding capacity in a female complaining of hair thinning.

Drug-induced alopecia

A large number of cytotoxic drugs cause alopecia and those responsible are listed in Table 11.4. Patients tolerate this form of iatrogenic alopecia much more easily if they are warned beforehand. A well-made wig should be prescribed well in advance.

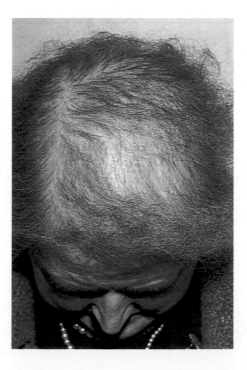

Fig. 11.12 Hair loss coincident with hypochromic anaemia. Good regrowth was achieved after correction of iron deficiency.

Table 11.4 Drugs that commonly cause alopecia

Drug type	Drug
Cytotoxic drugs	Cyclophosphamide
	Mercaptopurine derivatives
	Colchicine
	Adriamycin
	Vinca alkaloids
Anticoagulants	Heparin
	Coumarins
Anti-thyroid drugs	Thiouracil
	Carbimazole
Anti-tuberculous drug	Ethionamide

Heparin and warfarin occasionally cause hair loss, and large doses of vitamin A and the newer synthetic retinoids cause generalized diffuse alopecia in some patients.

Topical applications have, as far as is known, only a placebo effect in the above disorders. All patients presenting with generalized hair loss should be investigated for a remediable cause. In a small proportion, usually female, no obvious cause is found and the condition fits no recognized pattern. In these cases, the label 'idiopathic diffuse hair loss' is applied.

Hair shaft defects

A variety of congenital abnormalities of the hair shaft causing undue fragility have been described. Children present with short broken hair and patchy alopecia. The most common are **monilethrix** (beaded hair) and **pili torti** (twisted hair; Fig. 11.13). Both of these, and also rarer abnormalities, can be diagnosed on light microscopy of the hair. No topical treatment is available, but gentle handling and a short hair style can be of some value.

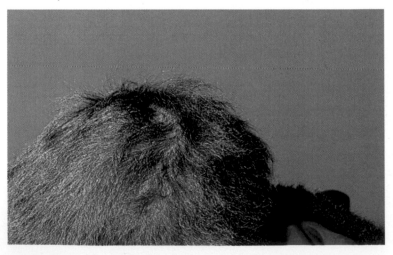

Fig. 11.13 Pili torti. Note the 'spangled' appearance and dry, brittle hair.

Trichotillomania

This condition is a compulsive desire to pull, twist, and tug at scalp hair. Extreme forms may be seen in the mentally subnormal and bizarre patterns of hair loss, often unilateral, with clearly visible broken hairs, will suggest the diagnosis.

Naevoid abnormalities

Infants and very young children with a well-demarcated patch of complete alopecia, and with neither scaling nor fragility of the surrounding hair may have a naevoid abnormality, such as **aplasia cutis**, but histological confirmation of this diagnosis is needed.

Fungal scalp infections

The patient is usually a child who has had contact with animals . There is patchy, scaly alopecia, and siblings may also be affected. All suspected cases and contacts should be examined under Wood's light (long UV wavelength 365 nm). However, only lesions due to *Microsporum canis* or *M. audouini* will show bright, blue-green fluorescence. Other fungi which commonly cause tinea capitis, such as *Trichophyton verrucosum* and *T. tonsurans*, will not fluoresce in this manner. Scalp scrapings and hairs should be examined microscopically, and cultured to demonstrate the fungus.

Sometimes the fungus stimulates an intense inflammatory reaction that forms a large boggy lesion with hair loss and a purulent discharge from the follicles. This constitutes a **kerion**, and is usually due to *T. verrucosum* or *T. mentagrophytes* (animal ringworm; p. 158).

Proven scalp ringworm is treated with full doses of oral griseofulvin or lamisil (p. 160). Hair regrows normally unless a kerion has led to scarring.

Chronic discoid lupus erythematosus

Patients with facial lesions of CDLE may have similar lesions on the scalp. The alopecia resulting from these lesions is patchy and scaly, and has follicles plugged by scales and an erythematous advancing margin. As it is a scarring process, permanent alopecia will result. Treatment of early lesions and attempts to prevent new lesions developing are discussed on p. 183.

Lichen planus

Occasionally, lichen planus affects the scalp and causes permanent, scarring alopecia (p. 78).

Traction alopecia

Localized hair loss and broken hairs, particularly round the hair margin, may be caused mechanically by tight hair styles, such as ponytails, or tight plaits, or the use of harsh hair-setting equipment.

Excessive growth of hair

Two terms are applied to excessive hair growth. Hirsutes refers to excess growth of androgen-dependent hair in a male pattern, whereas hypertrichosis is an excess growth of hair in a non-androgenic pattern. Hypertrichosis is seen in both sexes, but hirsutes is restricted to females for, although men are quick to seek help for baldness, they do not complain of excessive growth of hair in a normal distribution.

Hirsutism

Fine vellus hair covers much of the body in both sexes and can be induced by androgens to transform into coarse terminal hair. The causes of hirsutism can be grouped under general headings as in Table 11.5.

Women with hirsutism complain of hair growth in the beard area (Fig. 11.14), around the nipples, and in a male pattern on the abdomen. They are more likely to be dark-haired and the problem appears to be commoner in certain racial groups, for example, those of Mediterranean origin. Hirsutism can cause great distress to a healthy woman and lead to psychological disturbance with depression, even those in whom the condition is relatively mild.

Investigation and treatment

The aim in investigating the hirsute patient is to exclude an underlying, treatable endocrine cause. Although many tests of adrenal, ovarian, and pituitary function are available, the young woman who is menstruating regularly, and has had one or more successful pregnancies, requires little endocrine assessment and is likely

Table 11.5 Causes of hirsutism

Adrenal: Cushing's syndrome, virilizing tumours, congenital adrenal hyperplasia
Pituitary: acromegaly
Ovarian: polycystic ovaries, virilizing tumours, gonadal dysgenesis
Turner's syndrome
Iatrogenic: due to androgenic drugs
Idiopathic: target or end-organ hypersensitivity—much the commonest cause

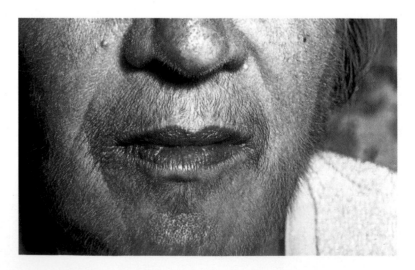

Fig. 11.14 Hirsuties. Excessive growth of facial hair on the chin of a female.

to fall into the idiopathic group, in which, to date, only marginally elevated levels of plasma testosterone have been found. It would appear that the fault in this group, by far the largest, lies in the hypersensitivity of the hair follicle as an end-organ of androgen stimulation.

Full endocrine assessment is, however, essential in patients with amenorrhoea, scanty, irregular periods, or other signs of excess androgen stimulation. This assessment should include estimation of plasma cortisol, free testosterone, of sex hormone binding globulin, FSH, LH, and ultrasound of ovaries and adrenals. Polycystic ovaries are relatively common in these women and may respond to gynaecological treatment

Treatment for those with no endocrine cause consists of physical methods of hair removal. Shaving, bleaching, and depilatory creams are all used, but the most satisfactory method is waxing as it also removes a large part of the hair shaft lying under the skin surface. Laser epilation is also useful and may require to be repeated. If systemic therapy is considered, Dianette may be effective, but must be used for at least 6 months before any response can be anticipated.

Hypertrichosis

Hypertrichosis may be either congenital or acquired.

Congenital varieties are frequently associated with melanocytic naevi, while lumbosacral hypertrichosis ('faun tail') should alert the paediatrician or obstetrician to the possibility of spina bifida occulta.

Acquired hypertrichosis is most commonly drug induced, although porphyria (p. 312) and endocrine disorders (thyroid dysfunction and anorexia nervosa) are recognized causes. Drugs in current use that can cause hypertrichosis include diazoxide, diphenylhydantoin, penicillamine, and the psoralens. If the offending drug is withdrawn, the excessive hair growth will cease.

Disorders of the nails

The normal anatomy of the nail is described on p. 36. Factors controlling nail growth are poorly understood, but the average time taken for a finger-nail to grow out is 6–12 months and for a toe-nail 18–24 months. These figures increase with age and there is seasonal variation, with some acceleration in the summer months. Individual nails also vary in their growth rates, with the thumb nail growing relatively rapidly.

Nail involvement is common in many skin diseases: for example, onycholysis and pitting in psoriasis, discoloration, and crumbling in fungal infections, pitting and ridging in chronic dermatitis, and a more severe dystrophy in lichen planus. These are all discussed with the relevant diseases.

Nail disorders can, however, occur in isolation, and can be either congenital or acquired.

Although nail biopsy through both nail and nail bed is feasible, it is much more traumatic than a skin biopsy, so fewer histological specimens from nail disorders than from other sites have been studied. Diagnosis is, therefore, commonly based on clinical appearances.

Congenital nail disorders

The nail-patella syndrome

This condition is transmitted by autosomal dominant inheritance and the gene is on chromosome 9q34. The patellae and some of the nails are rudimentary or absent. The thumb nails are usually involved. Affected patients have a 25% chance of developing a nephropathy. Children with a congenital thumbnail abnormality should therefore have the patellar region X-rayed to establish the diagnosis

Pachyonychia congenita

Misshapen, hypertrophic nails are present from birth and there may also be associated mucous membrane abnormalities. The condition is inherited by autosomal dominant transmission. In some cases, the gene has been mapped to chromosome 17q (Fig. 11.15).

Acquired nail defects

Beau's lines

Transverse ridges on the nails due to temporary interference with nail formation.

These lines are commonly seen during convalescence from a variety of severe disease states, for example, pneumonia and other conditions causing prolonged fever. The condition is self-limiting.

Koilonychia

Loss of the normal nail contour resulting in a flat or even depressed surface.

Nails of this shape are commonly slow-growing and brittle. They are most commonly associated with hypochromic anaemia and correction of iron deficiency may be followed by return to normal growth of the nails.

Finger clubbing

An exaggeration of the normal nail curve associated with loss of the normal angle between nail and posterior nail fold.

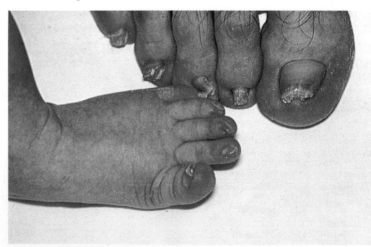

Fig. 11.15 Pachyonychia congenita. Note the gross abnormality of all toenails in both father and son. Finger-nails were similarly affected.

In adults this appearance is commonly seen in those with pulmonary pathology. If of slow onset, chronic respiratory infection, and bronchiectasis is a likely cause, and if of more rapid onset, the possibility of carcinoma of the lung must be considered. In young people, clubbing and nail changes may be seen in association with cyanotic congenital heart disease.

The mechanisms giving rise to these conformational changes of the finger tips are not understood. The resultant lesions may be both disfiguring and painful.

Paronychia

Acute paronychia is commonly due to staphylococcal infection and consists of an acutely inflamed posterior nail fold with a purulent discharge. There is frequently a history of trauma. Response to an appropriate systemic antibiotic is prompt.

Chronic paronychia is more persistent and troublesome. Usually, several nails are affected and show striking loss of the cuticle with tender, bolstered, posterior nail folds. If bacterial in origin, the likely organisms are *Pseudomonas pyocanea* and *Proteus vulgaris*, but frequently the cause is *Candida*, usually *C. albicans*. Persistent immersion of the hands in water is a common predisposing factor, so that housewives and barmaids are particularly at risk.

Treatment should be directed at organisms identified on culture. *Candida albicans* usually responds well to nystatin suspension or amphotericin B lotion. A useful paint is freshly prepared sulphacetamide 15% in 50% ethanol applied four times daily. Griseofulvin is not of value in these cases.

If the paronychia is shown to be due to *Candida,* and does not respond to topical therapy, a 2–4-week course of ketoconazole (Nizoral) 200 mg/day is justified. The drug must not be given to pregnant women and liver function must be monitored.

If wet work must be done, cotton gloves under rubber gloves must be worn and changed frequently.

Herpetic whitlow

Acute paronychia due to herpes simplex is an occupational hazard in doctors and nurses. It is discussed and illustrated on p. 150.

Paronychial tumours

Warts are frequently found around the nails and may be extremely painful due to pressure on the nail bed. They respond slowly to conventional therapy (p. 145).

Malignant tumours may also occur in this site, the most serious being a malignant melanoma. Any patient with a bleeding or pigmented nodule in the region of a nail should be referred without delay for a diagnostic biopsy and definitive treatment (p. 349).

Iatrogenic nail abnormalities

Systemic drug therapy can cause a variety of nail changes. Tetracycline-induced photosensitivity can lead to nail loss and long-term ingestion of tetracyclines may cause yellow nails. Anti-malarial drugs cause blue and blue-black discoloration of the nail beds.

Disorders of the sweat glands

The sweat glands are of two sorts. The **eccrine glands** are concerned with thermoregulation and are distributed over the entire body surface. The **apocrine glands**, found chiefly in the axillae and groins, have no apparent function in man, but appear to be stimulated by emotional stress and contribute to axillary odour.

Eccrine gland disorders

Miliaria (prickly heat)

In the UK, miliaria is a rarity, except in a heat wave or the tropical environment of a neonatal nursery. In subtropical or tropical climates it is common, especially in recent arrivals who have not yet acclimatized. Sweat duct obstruction due to high humidity is the cause.

Clinically, there is an acute papulo-vesicular eruption, usually on the trunk. It is itchy, and scratching often leads to crusting and secondary infection.

Treatment is palliative, unless the humidity can be adequately reduced. This is feasible, desirable, and effective in the nursery, but less so in the tropics if no air conditioning is available. A shake lotion, such as calamine lotion BP, can be soothing.

Hyperhidrosis

Over-production of eccrine sweat can be due to heat or to emotional stimuli, but is rarely due to endocrinological or neurological disorders. The nature of the stimulus determines whether the hyperhidrosis is localized or generalized. When localized, the palms, soles, and axillae are the usual sites. Malodour of the feet and axillae due to bacterial overgrowth is common and distressing. Hyperhidrosis of the palms can incapacitate those whose work involves writing and handling of paper.

In generalized hyperhidrosis it is important first to exclude underlying systemic disease. Propranolol 20–40 mg four times per day may be useful.

For localized hyperhidrosis, topical preparations are generally more effective, but may require supplementation with systemic therapy. A paint consisting of 20% aluminium chloride hexahydrate made up in 70% alcohol applied overnight to clean, dry palms, soles, and axillae is effective, mainly in the axillae.

Intra-dermal injections of botulinum toxin have been shown in randomized clinical trials to reduce sweating and may require to be repeated at varying intervals.

If the axillae only are affected, surgical excision of ellipses of skin 2–4 inches long from the vault of the axilla can be dramatically effective. The areas of maximum sweat production should be removed and they can be identified prior to surgery by starch-iodine application. This entire procedure can be done as an outpatient under local anaesthesia.

Chemical or surgical sympathectomy are also helpful in some cases, and a trial of chemical sympathectomy is recommended.

Apocrine gland disorder

Hidradenitis suppurativa

Deep-seated inflammatory lesions chiefly in the axillae and groins (Fig. 11.16).

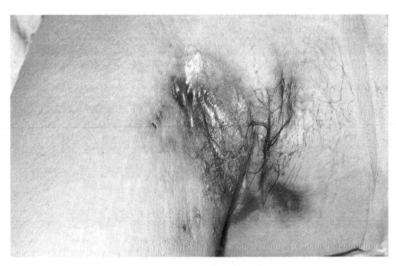

Fig. 11.16 Hidradenitis suppurativa. Recurrent infection in the apocrine glands causes development of fibrotic scar tissue.

A functional and structural abnormality of apocrine sweat glands is the cause. Patients do not have normal communication between the secretory and excretory components of the gland. They present with multiple, deeply-situated pustules and abscesses that, in time, damage the dermis and lead to deep scarring. Deep, cord-like fibrotic lesions may restrict movement.

Long-term systemic antibiotic therapy given for a minimum of 3–6 months may give temporary relief. In some patients hidradenitis suppurativa is associated with severe acne. In patients with this combination the use of oral isotretinoin (Roaccutane) given orally in a dose of 1 mg/kg/day for 3 months may be of therapeutic value. In women of child-bearing age adequate contraception is essential.

Surgical excision of the affected area with skin grafting, if required, is the most useful method of permanently eradicating this difficult problem.

Discussion of problem cases

Case 11.1

This young woman is older than the normal age for presentation with acne vulgaris, although late onset acne is becoming commoner especially in females. Cosmetic allergies do not usually present with papules. Erythema and itch would be more common presenting features of a cosmetic allergy.

The description suggests rosacea, and on questioning the patient she agrees that she flushes easily when in a warm room and after eating spicy foods. Careful examination establishes that she has papules, and one or two pustules, but no comedones (blackheads) are present.

This patient, therefore, requires treatment with a systemic antibiotic, probably tetracycline, for 3–6 months. If there is any possibility of her wishing to start a family, an alternative antibiotic should be used because of the fact that tetracycline will stain the developing teeth of the foetus. She should also be given topical metronidazole gel and she should be specifically asked not to use any topical steroids on her face.

On this regime this patient's papules cleared although she continues to flush easily in a warm environment.

Discussion of problem cases continued

Case 11.2

Conditions to be considered in the differential diagnosis of hair loss in children are fungal infections, alopecia areata, and trichotillomania. Tinea capitis (p. 157) must be excluded particularly if the child has had contact with animals and if there is any scaling or itch on the scalp. Neither of these were present in this boy's case, but taking some clippings and scrapings for mycological assessment is good practice in this type of presentation. The pattern of hair loss, with several circular patches involved, does not suggest trichotillomania, where the usual presentation is of one area of hair loss with broken hairs around the area of visible alopecia. The pattern strongly suggests alopecia areata.

Treatment of alopecia areata is difficult. Both the boy and his mother should be told that the hair will re-grow in time, but that it is impossible to predict when this will occur. This may be accelerated by use of a moderately potent topical steroid or by a course of ultraviolet radiation.

The prognosis for re-growth following a first attack of alopecia areata is good, but after the second or subsequent episodes, it is wise to be rather more cautious about the likelihood of complete re-growth. Patients who have atopy in addition to alopecia areata have a poorer prognosis for re-growth.

This boy had no history of atopy and his hair re-grew well over a period of 6 months.

Case 11.3

Persistent, recurrent infection is one of the presenting features of several of the immunodeficiency syndromes, but these infections usually start in early childhood, not after puberty as has been the case with this young man. This patient is otherwise fit, and has no lesions on any other body site. This anatomic distribution suggests an apocrine gland abnormality, and the age at onset and clinical description suggest hidradenitis suppurativa. The patient should have full doses of an appropriate systemic antibiotic, determined on bacteriological sensitivity tests, for at least 3–4 months or until complete clearance of the lesions. If this is not effective, then he should be considered for surgical excision of the areas with skin grafting if necessary.

Nine months later, after a further unsuccessful trial of systemic antibiotics, this young man had the worst affected axilla surgically treated with an excellent result. He himself requested surgery for the second axilla, and is currently relatively free of problems.

Further reading

Berker, D., Baran, R., and Dawber, R.P.R. (1995) *Diseases of the nails and their management*. Blackwells, Oxford.

Cunliffe, W.J. (1989) *Acne*. Martin Dunitz, London.

Sinclair, R.D., Banfield, C.C., and Dawber, R.P.R. (1999) *Handbook of diseases of the hair and scalp*. Blackwells, Oxford.

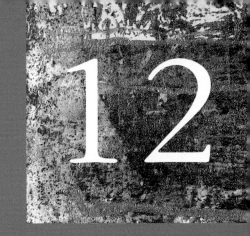

12

Blistering diseases

Blistering diseases

Problem cases

Case 12.1

You are doing a 6-month obstetrics post prior to entering general practice. One Saturday night a young woman is admitted to the labour ward and delivers a female child who is otherwise healthy, but who has small blisters on both feet and one hand. What conditions must be considered in the differential diagnosis of blistering in a neonate and what investigations should be carried out? What is the likely diagnosis in this situation?

Case 12.2

You are asked to visit a retirement home because an 86-year-old female has an itchy eruption on her limbs, which has not settled with topical 1% hydrocortisone cream. Because of the pressure of other commitments, you do not manage to visit the home until 48 hours later, by which time the patient has developed blisters on inflamed skin of her upper arms and thighs. She is on multiple drugs including anti-hypertensives, non-steroidal anti-inflammatories, regular laxatives, and hypnotics. What is the likely diagnosis and how would you confirm it?

Introduction

Many skin problems may be associated with the development of blisters at some stage. Common examples are bullous impetigo, burns, and severe contact dermatitis. Skin diseases in which blisters are the main or presenting lesion are relatively rare, but important, because in both children and adults they may be the first sign of a severe and potentially fatal problem. In adults, the main group of blistering problems is associated with auto-antibody formation, while in children, the rare, but important group of genodermatoses, epidermolysis bullosa is associated mainly with mechanical defects in and around the basement membrane zone.

Blisters may arise either because of disruption of the desmosomes between keratinocytes in the epidermis, causing an intra-epidermal blister, or because of a defect in the basement membrane zone between the epidermis and dermis, leading to a sub-epidermal blister.

Accurate pathological diagnosis of blistering problems requires a biopsy of a small, newly-formed lesion and also a piece of perilesional skin frozen for immunopathological studies. In the case of blisters in infants electron microscopy may be required and DNA for genetic studies may also be necessary for an accurate diagnosis.

Key points

Blistering diseases are rare, but important as they may be a sign of a severe and potentially fatal problem.

Pemphigus
Definition

A group of disorders characterized by the development of auto-antibodies against desmocollins and desmogleins in the epidermis, giving rise to superficial erosions and blisters on both epidermal and mucosal surfaces. Desmocollins and desmogleins are transmembrane desmosomal glycoproteins and are members of the cadherin gene superfamily.

There are four main clinical varieties of pemphigus:

- **Pemphigus vulgaris** is the commonest variety of pemphigus, and usually begins with shallow erosions and easily ruptured blisters on mucosal surfaces (Figs 12.1 and 12.2).

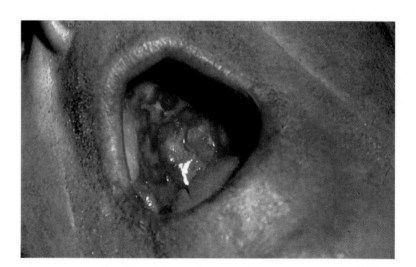

Fig. 12.1 Oral lesions in a case of early pemphigus vulgaris.

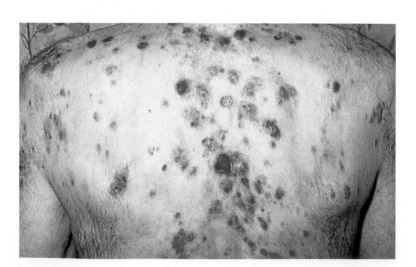

Fig. 12.2 Lesions on the back of a patient with pemphigus vulgaris. Shallow erosions are see and healing lesions show some increase in pigmentation.

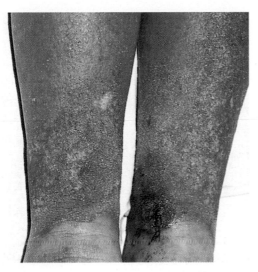

Fig. 12.3 Pemphigus vegetans. Note warty lesions with minimal blister on lower legs.

- **Pemphigus vegetans** is characterized by striking papillomatous proliferations in the flexures (Fig. 12.3).

- **Pemphigus foliaceus** in Europe and North America is a mild, superficial variant (Fig. 12.4). It is endemic in parts of South America, where it is called fogo selvagem, and there is evidence that in this form it may be caused by an infective agent. This form of pemphigus does not affect children.

- **Pemphigus erythematosus** shares some of the features of both pemphigus and of lupus erythematosus. Blisters tend to form on sun-exposed sites, and the patient has both pemphigus-associated and anti-nuclear antibodies.

Key points
Think of pemphigus in severe persistent oral ulcers not due to candida or herpes.

Clinical features

Pemphigus vulgaris frequently begins insidiously with the slow development of raw areas and shallow erosions on the mucous membranes (Fig. 12.1).

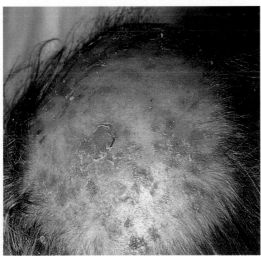

Fig. 12.4 Pemphigus foliaceus. Note very superficial blistering with scaling on light exposed site.

Involvement of the skin tends to come later (Fig. 12.2). The patient may, therefore, complain first of mouth ulcers or genital discomfort. The lesions do not itch, but can be very painful. Blisters on mucous membrane and skin, are quickly ruptured by friction or pressure, leaving a raw surface. This feature reflects the thin blister roof of the intra-epidermal blister in pemphigus, in contrast to the greater resilience of the sub-epidermal blister in bullous pemphigoid and dermatitis herpetiformis (see below). Clinically normal skin may display the **Nikolsky sign**—if lateral pressure is put on the skin surface with the thumb the epidermis literally slides over the underlying dermis—do this test gently or you may leave the patient with a large raw area.

Secondary infection and disturbance of fluid and electrolyte balance are common complications of untreated pemphigus that, prior to the introduction of corticosteroid therapy, was regularly fatal.

Pathology and immunopathology

The main pathological feature of all types of pemphigus is the presence of a superficial, fluid-filled blister within the epidermis.

In pemphigus vulgaris the base of this blister is formed by the basal cells of the epidermis, which remain attached to the basement membrane zone; in the other varieties the blister may be even more superficial, forming just under the stratum corneum. Individual keratinocytes detach from their neighbours and float free in the blister, a process called **acantholysis**.

Immunopathology shows the presence of auto-antibodies directed against the epidermal intercellular material. These auto-antibodies are both tissue-fixed—on the patient's perilesional skin—and circulating in the patient's serum. This antibody is tissue-specific, but not species-specific, and thus the substrate used for detecting auto-antibodies in the patient's serum need not be human tissue, but any source of stratified squamous epithelium, such as guinea-pig lip or primate oesophagus. The auto-antibody is usually an IgG, and complement is also fixed at the site (Fig. 12.5).

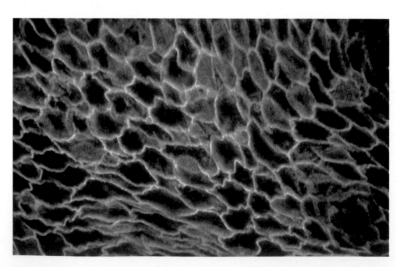

Fig. 12.5 Indirect immunofluorescence test in pemphigus vulgaris. The patient's serum has been layered on mucous membrane substrate and subsequently treated with fluorescein-conjugated antihuman IgG. Specific staining of the intercellular substance is observed.

Circulating pemphigus antibody titres correlate with disease activity, and high-titre serum can induce pemphigus-like lesions both in experimental animals and in organ culture. These observations are supporting evidence that pemphigus is an autoimmune disease, and that the auto-antibody causes the disease, and is not just a secondary development.

Commercial kits are now available to measure circulating antibodies to desmoglein 1 and 3 as an aid to diagnosis and treatment in pemphigus. In pemphigus vulgaris the main circulating auto-antibody is desmoglein 3, while in the more superficial forms of pemphigus the main form is desmoglein 1. It is likely that this approach will replace the older labour intensive indirect immunofluorescence technique as a diagnostic and monitoring aid.

Diagnosis and treatment

The diagnosis should be confirmed and treatment started without delay. Table 12.1 lists conditions that may cause diagnostic confusion. Systemic steroids will be needed. The exact dose depends on the patient's size and disease severity, but the range is 60–100 mg of prednisolone or equivalent per day. Once control has been achieved and no fresh blisters are developing, the dose can be slowly reduced by 20–30 mg/week. A maintenance dose is usually necessary, possibly for life, to prevent recurrence. This should be kept as low as possible, preferably using an alternate-day regime to minimize steroid side-effects. In some patients the addition of an immunosuppressive agent, such as azathioprine cyclophosphamide or mycophenolate mofetil will allow further reduction of the steroid dose. Oral cyclosporin may also be useful. Plasmapheresis is occasionally needed in severe cases and the use of intravenous immunoglobulin can be effective, but is mainly used in experimental situations. In the USA, use of intravenous immunoglobulin in pemphigus does not yet have FDA approval.

Topical therapy is mainly symptomatic, and aimed at protecting the raw areas and decreasing the incidence of secondary infection. Vaseline-impregnated gauze dressings are kind to the patient and the lesions should be managed in the same way as burns. As the disease comes under control, the use of moderate or potent topical steroids to limited body areas may enable more rapid reduction of the systemic steroid dose.

Although the disease is usually controllable, it rarely remits spontaneously. Consequently, the patient will probably have to remain on systemic steroids for life and will therefore require careful surveillance for steroid-induced side effects.

Bullous pemphigoid
Definition

A blistering disorder characterized by large, tense blisters on an erythematous base.

Bullous pemphigoid is found mainly in those aged 60 or older. It is therefore becoming a commoner disease in Europe and North America as the average age of the population increases. All those who are involved in caring for the elderly should be aware of the presenting features.

> ### Key points
> Blisters arising on an inflamed base in an elderly patient-think of bullous pemphigoid.

Table 12.1 The differential diagnosis of blistering diseases in the adult

	Site	History	Histology	Immunology	Other tests
Pemphigus	Mucous membranes, and trunk	Insidious onset	Intra-epidermal blister	Direct IgG C_3 Circulating IgG	
Pemphigoid	Upper arms and thighs	Blisters on eczematous base	Sub-epidermal blister	Fixed Ig and C_3 at dermo-epidermal junction. Circulating IgG	
Dermatitis herpetiformis	Scalp, scapular area, elbows, buttocks	Pruritus + + +	Sub-epidermal blister	IgA in papillary dermis	Subtotal villous atrophy on jejunal biopsy
Erythema multiforme	Hands and feet	Target lesions blister	Sub-epidermal	Negative	Occasionally drug or viral history
Mechanical blisters	Site of trauma	Friction, e.g. marching, poorly fitting shoes	Sub-epidermal blister	Negative	
Atypical herpes simplex or zoster	Variable	Prodromal pain and tingling	Balloon degeneration within the epidermis	Rising specific antibody titre	Electron microscopy to demonstrate virus particles
Herpes zoster	Linear dermatome distribution	Pain and tingling: may be severe	Intra-epidermal balloon degeneration	Rising specific antibody titre	
Porphyria cutanea tarda	Sun-exposed sites	Sun exposure, minor friction, and trauma	Sub-epidermal blister	Autofluo-rescence of porphyrins	Raised uroporphyrin levels

Clinical features

Patients are usually elderly and present with large, tense blisters, mainly on the upper arms and thighs (Figs 12.6 and 12.7). These arise on an eczematous base and there is itch, rather than pain. There is frequently a prodromal phase when the skin on which the blisters subsequently develop is inflamed and itchy, and at this stage the diagnosis of contact dermatitis may be considered. Some spontaneous haemorrhage into the blisters is not uncommon. Oral lesions are less frequent than in pemphigus.

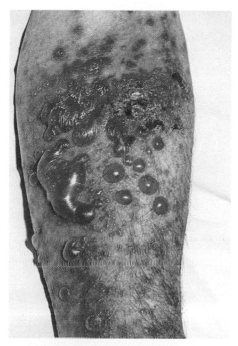

Fig. 12.6 Blisters of bullous pemphigoid. Large, tense, raised lesions are seen on an erythematous eczematized base.

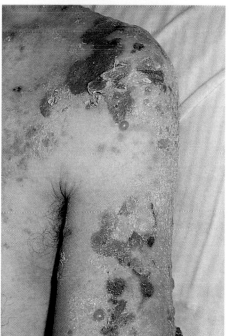

Fig. 12.7 Bullous pemphigoid showing typical involvement of upper limb.

Pathology

The blister is sub-epidermal, formed between the dermis and epidermis. As the entire thickness of the epidermis forms the roof of the blisters, they are relatively resilient and may remain intact for several days.

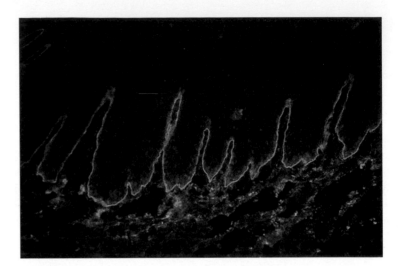

Fig. 12.8 Indirect immunofluorescence test using bullous pemphigoid serum on primate oesophagus as a substrate. A clear band of IgG is seen in the basement membrane zone.

As with pemphigus, tissue-fixed and circulating auto-antibodies have been demonstrated, suggesting that the disease has an autoimmune pathogenesis. To date, two bullous pemphigoid antigens have been identified BP 1 and BP 2. In bullous pemphigoid, immunoglobulin and complement are deposited in the lamina lucida of the basement membrane in a linear band, and there is a circulating antibody specific to this site (Fig. 12.8).

Commercial kits are now available to quantitate levels of circulating bullous pemphigoid antigens 1 and 2, and are likely time to replace more traditional, but labour intensive immunopathological methods of confirming the diagnosis.

Treatment

Steroid therapy is required. In the case of severe pemphigoid, this will be systemic, but unlike pemphigus, it may be possible to discontinue this after 2–3 years. A recent systematic review of treatments for bullous pemphigoid suggest no advantage in increasing the starting dose of prednisolone above 0.75 mg/kg/day, but a definite increase in side effects at higher doses. The addition of either azathioprine or of plasma exchange to oral steroids were shown in this review to enable the oral steroid dose to be reduced more rapidly.

In milder cases oral dapsone in doses of 50–150 mg/day may be effective therapy. Milder may also respond very well to potent or moderately potent topical steroids alone.

Although bullous pemphigoid does not carry as high an immediate morbidity and mortality as pemphigus, the elderly do not tolerate oral steroid or cytotoxic therapy well, and there is a high incidence of treatment-induced complications in bullous pemphigoid patients, some of them fatal. Mortality figures related to bullous pemphigoid show higher figures for complications of therapy than for direct effects of the disease itself. These patients therefore need very careful supervision.

Dermatitis herpetiformis

Definition

An intensely itchy, blistering skin condition associated with gluten-sensitive enteropathy.

Clinical features

Dermatitis herpetiformis (DH) affects a younger age group than pemphigus and bullous pemphigoid. Patients present in the third and fourth decade, and males are more commonly affected.

Patients complain of an intense, burning itch on the affected sites, commonly the scalp, shoulders, buttocks, and elbows (Figs 12.9 and 12.10). Very small blisters may be found, but as they are quickly scratched, raw bleeding areas may be

> ### *Key points*
>
> Dermatitis herpetiformis can be misdiagnosed as scabies. Think of it if only one family member is affected and does not respond to anti-scabetic therapy.

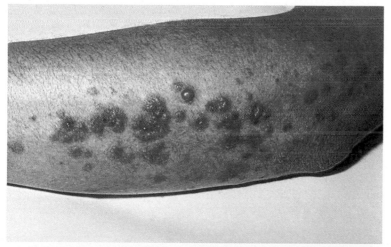

Fig. 12.9 Dermatitis herpetiformis. Small grouped blisters are seen.

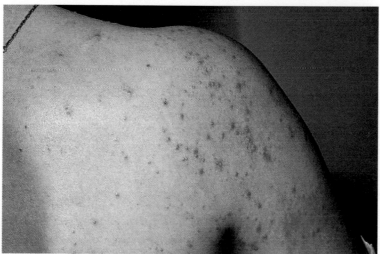

Fig. 12.10 Dermatitis herpetiformis showing intensely itchy vesicles and blisters on the shoulder area.

the only lesions seen. As these heal small scars will develop due to disruption of the dermis by scratching.

Most patients will have no obvious evidence of malabsorption and opinion is divided as to whether or not a jejunal biopsy should be performed in this situation. There is a morbidity associated with this procedure that should only be carried out by those trained in the technique and performing it regularly. If pathological evidence of subtotal villous atrophy is seen in a jejunal biopsy, the patient may be more easily persuaded both to try and thereafter to stick to a gluten-free diet

Pathology

The blisters are sub-epidermal and are small by comparison with the larger lesions in bullous pemphigoid. There are frequently aggregates of leucocytes in so-called 'micro-abscesses' at tips of the dermal papillae flanking the blister.

No circulating antibody has yet been consistently found in DH patients, but direct immunofluorescence of the skin around lesions will reveal the presence of granular deposits of IgA and sometimes complement in the dermal papillae (Fig. 12.11). This is used as a confirmatory diagnostic test.

Treatment

Dermatitis herpetiformis does not respond to systemic steroids. Itch will be controlled by dapsone in doses of 50–150 mg/day, but careful haematological monitoring is necessary, as a haemolytic anaemia may develop. Patients starting dapsone should have a full blood count twice in the first month of treatment to detect excessive haemolysis usually preceded by a high reticulocyte count. This is essential as a small number of patients have a hypersensitivity reaction to dapsone leading to a very severe haemolysis. In these patients, the dapsone must be stopped immediately and alternative therapy used.

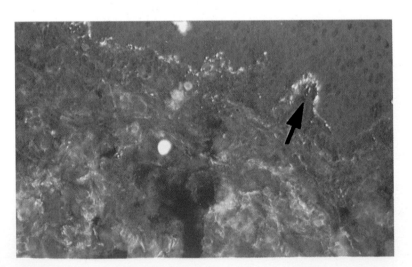

Fig. 12.11 Immunopathology of dermatitis herpetiformis. This section of perilesional skin has been treated with FITC-labelled antihuman IgG. Note fluorescence marked with arrow in dermal papilla.

A gluten-free diet should be discussed, and all patients advised to consider a 6–12 month trial period of such a diet. Both those who have pathological evidence of gluten sensitive enteropathy and also those who do not appear to benefit. The disadvantages are that any benefit is slow to appear, that the diet is not particularly palatable, and that even small amounts of gluten taken may cancel out any benefit. The obvious advantage is that it is non-toxic.

Topical steroid-antibiotic combinations (for example, vioform-hydrocortisone, *b*-methasone 17-valerate with chinoform, or aureomycin) are useful supplements to systemic therapy.

As this is a chronic disease, treatment may need to be life-long.

The epidermolysis bullosa group of blistering disorders

This group of blistering genodermatoses comprise the rare, but serious group of mechanobullous disorders. They usually present at birth or in infancy, but continue to cause problems throughout life. They are a large group of diseases, and range from localized relatively mild problems with trauma induced blisters to life threatening and life ruining conditions. As prenatal diagnosis is now available for couples known to be at risk, it is essential to be aware of the features of these diseases, so that if a neonate presents with blisters an accurate pathological diagnosis can be made on which future genetic counselling can be based.

The main subsets (Table 12.2) are:

- **epidermolysis bullosa simplex**—mainly autosomal dominant;
- **junctional epidermolysis bullosa**—autosomal recessive;
- **dystrophic epidermolysis bullosa**—both autosomal dominant, and autosomal recessive varieties.

A tentative diagnosis can be made on the basis of a family history, clinical examination, and light microscopic examination of a skin biopsy, but a definitive diagnosis is essential for genetic counselling, and for this both electron microscopy

> *Key points*
>
> Blisters in the newborn may be the first sign of life ruining epidermolysis bullosa. Seek expert help early.

Table 12.2 Current major subdivisions of the epidermolysis bullosa group of disorders

Type	Number of varieties	Inheritance	Site of blister	Specific defect	Clinical features
Simplex	12	Mainly autosomal dominant	Basal cells	Keratins 5 and 14	Mainly friction induced blisters on hands and feet
Junctional	7	All autosomal recessive	Lamina lucida	Hemidesmosomes	Extensive blistering of skin. Mucosal involvement
Dystrophic	11	Dominant and recessive	Below basement membrane	Anchoring fibrils Type 7 collagen	Varied loss of nails and scarring

and molecular studies are required. Our understanding of the genetics of this group of disorders is continuing to expand rapidly. At least 20 phenotypes are currently recognized, 10 of which are those most frequently seen.

Epidermolysis bullosa simplex

Four main variants of EB simplex are currently recognized, the majority inherited by autosomal dominant transmission. The pathological damage in this variety lies within the epidermis and consists of a split through the cytoplasm of the basal cells. Thus, there is true cell lysis. In three of the main types of EBS the molecular defect lies in defective genes coding for keratins 5 and 14, which are found preferentially in the basal layer. In the fourth, the defect lies in the plectin gene.

Blisters may be present at birth, but often the disease first becomes apparent when the child starts to walk or crawl, and develops mild blistering and desquamation on knees, hands, feet, and other sites of friction (Fig. 12.12). These blisters quickly rupture and heal with no subsequent scarring. Other ectodermal structures (hair, teeth, and nails) are unaffected and mucous membranes, although occasionally involved, do not show gross changes. There is little tendency to remission in later childhood or adult life.

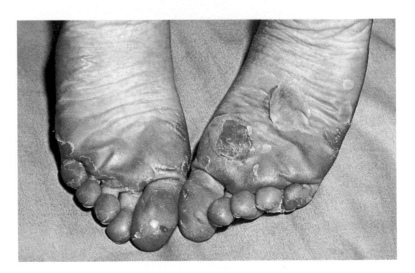

Fig. 12.12 Epidermolysis bullosa simplex. This child develops blisters on sites of friction. Healing is rapid without scarring.

Junctional epidermolysis bullosa (Herlitz type, epidermolysis bullosa letalis)

There are currently three main recognized variants of this type, all inherited by autosomal recessive transmission. The protein/gene system, which is abnormal, is laminin 5 in two types of junctional EB, and alpha 6 beta 4 integrin in the third. This results in the development of a split at the level of the lamina lucida. The overlying epidermis appears normal and there is no obvious loss of cohesion between the cells. The base of the blister is formed by an intact basal lamina still firmly adherent to the dermis.

Clinical abnormalities may be present at birth either as blisters, often around the nails, or raw denuded areas, with little tendency to heal. Mucous membranes

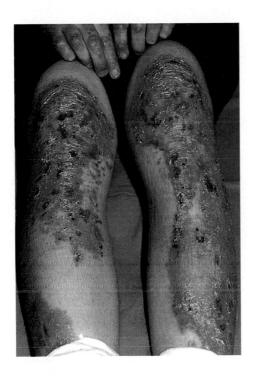

Fig. 12.13 Epidermolysis bullosa of the dominant dystrophic type. Note extensive blistering with scarring on knees and shins.

may be severely involved and the teeth are commonly abnormal. A high proportion of these children die in infancy.

Dystrophic epidermolysis bullosa

There are three main variants and inheritance can be either autosomal dominant or autosomal recessive. All are associated with defects in the type 7 collagen gene. This causes defective anchoring fibrils connecting the basal lamina to the dermis and a sub-epidermal blister results. In the dominant varieties, blisters develop in later infancy or early childhood on friction sites and heal with scarring. Milia may be seen in these scars, which tend to become keloidal or hyperplastic (Fig 12.13). Hair and teeth develop normally.

In the recessive types, there is also a defect of anchoring fibrils, due to defects in the type 7 collagen gene. Large bullae are present at birth, and they heal with scarring, which is associated with the formation of webs between fingers and eventually a useless fist Mucous membranes, hair, nails (Fig. 12.14), and teeth may all be abnormal, and squamous carcinoma may develop on the scar sites.

Treatment and prenatal diagnosis of epidermolysis bullosa

Children with epidermolysis bullosa should be managed by a team with experience of the problem. An accurate diagnosis is essential to enable the parents to be offered genetic counselling. This will involve careful selection of sites for biopsy and ultrastructural studies, and also molecular genetic studies. Protective measures should be taken in all cases to prevent friction bullae. Infants who are still crawling should have padded trousers and special soft footwear will be needed. A

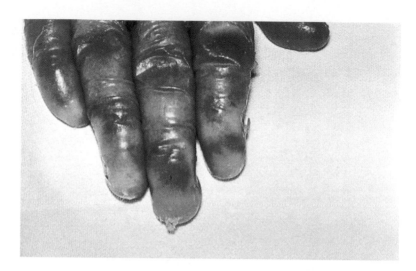

Fig. 12.14 Dystrophic epidermolysis bullosa. Note the loss of finger-nails. This 5-year-old child already has web formation between the digits.

trial of systemic steroids is worthwhile in the junctional and dystrophic varieties. Specialist dental care will be needed for children with oral lesions. Occupational therapy may delay the development of contractures or webs in the autosomal recessive dystrophic variety, but the prognosis for both survival and the ability to lead an independent adult life must be guarded in these varieties of the disorder.

The technique of foetal skin biopsy to diagnose epidermolysis bullosa in mothers who are at risk is now relatively well established. Chorionic villus biopsy is taken at around 9 weeks gestation and DNA analysis performed. If the test is positive for one of the more severe types of epidermolysis bullosa, the parents can decide whether or not the pregnancy should proceed.

Skilled nursing care is vital for the more severe forms and membership of Debra, the patient support group, is very worthwhile (website www. debra org.uk).

Erythema multiforme

Definition

An erythematous disorder characterized by annular, target lesions, which may develop into frank blisters.

Aetiology

Erythema multiforme (EM) is a cutaneous reaction pattern, which may be provoked by many stimuli. These include viral infection, commonly herpes simplex, bacterial infection, and adverse drug reactions. In many cases, however, no aetiological or precipitating factor can be identified. In the bullous lesions of EM, the blister forms at the dermo-epidermal junction, and there is necrosis and destruction of the overlying epidermis.

Clinical features

The lesions are most commonly seen on the hands and feet and initially present as raised erythematous plaques which expand laterally to give the classic 'iris lesion' or 'target lesion' appearance (Fig. 12.15).

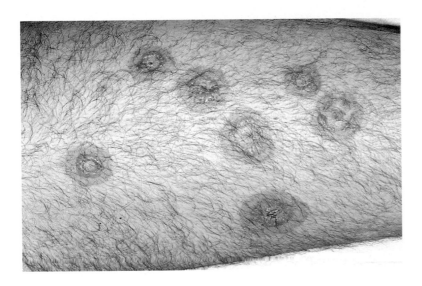

Fig. 12.15 Erythema multiforme on the leg, note the presence of target lesions.

Severe involvement of the eyes and mucosal surfaces is termed the **Stevens–Johnson syndrome**.

Toxic epidermal necrolysis (TEN; Fig. 12.16) is also a severe variant of EM with extensive shedding of epidermis, but less mucosal involvement. Identification and removal of the cause is important, and all suspect drugs should be withdrawn.

Treatment

A search should be made for the precipitating factor, which should be withdrawn in the case of a suspected drug or treated in the case of a suspected viral infection. Patients should, thereafter, be treated symptomatically with bed rest and topical dressings as required.

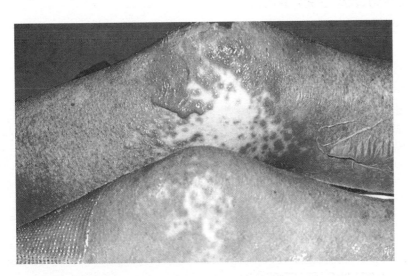

Fig. 12.16 Toxic epidermal necrolysis. Note extensive erythema and early development of blisters and raw areas on the legs.

In severe cases the use of systemic steroids may be considered, but there is controversy as to whether or not steroid treated patients actually have a higher mortality. Those who disagree with this view argue that it is the more severe cases who are considered for steroid therapy in the first place.

Key points

Superficial staphylococcal infection is easy to mistake for non-accidental injury

Staphylococcal scalded skin syndrome

Staphylococcal scalded skin syndrome is a blistering disorder caused by an epidermolytic toxin of certain phage types of *Staphylococcus aureus*, which splits the epidermis at the level of the granular layer, by cleaving desmoglein 1. The condition is commoner in children than in adults and is seen as rapidly expanding, very shallow blisters, which quickly rupture, leaving painful, raw areas (Figs 12.17 and 12.18). The condition as its name suggests can look very like a scald caused by boiling water, and it may therefore be necessary in the case of affected children to consider non accidental injury.

All patients should be swabbed for bacteriological sensitivities and should then be started on a systemic anti-staphylococcal antibiotic. This can be changed, if necessary, once bacteriological sensitivities are known. Non-adhesive topical dressings will accelerate healing of the affected areas. Parents can be assured that there is unlikely to be any scarring because of the superficial nature of the blisters.

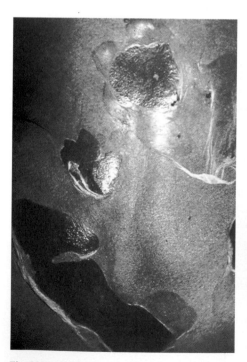

Fig. 12.17 Staphylococcal scalded skin syndrome. Note the shearing of the epidermis and lack of inflammation of the surrounding skin.

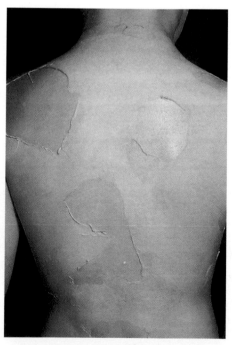

Fig. 12.18 Staphylococcal scalded skin syndrome. Note superficial peeling that is due to the high level blistering.

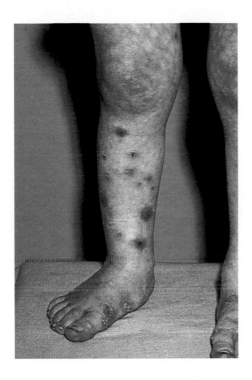

Fig. 12.19 Papular urticaria. Crops of papules are seen most commonly on the lower legs.

Papular urticaria (bites)

Although papular urticaria is frequently seen in paediatric skin clinics, a high proportion of affected children are managed either by parents or the family doctor.

Characteristically, the lesions are grouped and occur in crops (Fig. 12.19). Morphologically, they are tender, erythematous papules or small blisters. They are quickly scratched and subsequently become secondarily infected.

In a high proportion of cases, fleas or mites are to blame, possibly from the family pet, but tact must be used when persuading parents that this is so.

Suitable treatment of established lesions is a topical antipruritic, such as crotamiton or 2% menthol in calamine cream. Prevention of further crops is difficult and depends on eliminating the causative factor. The child's bedding and family pets should be treated with an insecticidal dusting powder.

Urticaria pigmentosa

Definition

Blisters due to release of histamine from focal aggregation of mast cells in the dermis, seen usually in infancy.

Although both children and adults are affected, urticaria pigmentosa is most often seen in infancy. The lesions are multiple erythematous weals, which may blister and are provoked by minor trauma or a warm bath. The lesions resolve, leaving some melanin pigmentation (Fig. 12.20). Rare familial cases are recorded.

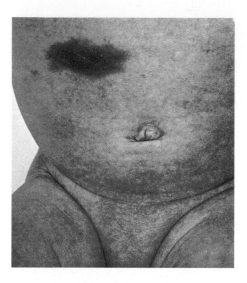

Fig. 12.20 Urticaria pigmentosa. This 2-year-old child had three lesions that urticated on pressure and left surrounding pigmentation as seen here.

Biopsy will reveal foci of mast cells: these degranulate on trauma, releasing vasoactive substances, which elicit the lesion.

Spontaneous improvement throughout infancy and childhood is usual. Treatment consists of avoiding trauma until remission occurs. Antihistamines are not indicated.

In severe cases of urticaria pigmentosa, a trial of oral sodium cromoglycate (Nalcrom) is justified as there are reports of a good response, presumably due to mast cell stabilization.

Discussion of problem cases

Case 12.1

The differential diagnosis of blisters in the newborn range from benign and transient to serious life-threatening problems. The minor problems include trauma from the pressure of delivery, particularly if forceps have been applied, and low grade infection, either staphylococcal or viral. More serious concern is that of epidermolysis bullosa group of disorders, some of which are potentially lethal. The majority of these present as blisters at birth.

The blisters in this child's case persisted and extended over the first few days of life, and bacteriological and virological culture showed no growth. A biopsy of a small fresh blister with immunopathology and electron microscopy was therefore arranged. The ultrastructural findings showed that the child had a blister that was forming as a result of a split through the basal cells of the epidermis. This pattern confirms the diagnosis of the most benign type of epidermolysis bullosa, EB simplex. The clinical pattern suggested an autosomal dominant variety of this condition. What genetic counselling can be offered in this situation? What management plan would you devise for this baby? What is the prognosis?

Discussion of problem cases continued

Case 12.2

Pruritus in the elderly is common. The majority of patients have so called senile pruritus and no clear cause is identified other than dry elderly skin. This diagnosis would not be appropriate here as the patient has obvious erythema. An irritant dermatitis or drug eruption would, therefore, be a possible diagnosis. However, the changing clinical picture with the development of obvious blisters on inflamed skin strongly suggests that the clinical diagnosis is bullous pemphigoid, although a bullous adverse drug reaction would still have to be excluded.

The patient had a biopsy of the small, early, new blister, and both pathology and immunopathology were requested. The blister was sub-epidermal, and there was a linear band of IgG and also of C3 deposited at the dermal/epidermal junction (p. 276), confirming the clinical diagnosis of bullous pemphigoid.

The patient was, therefore, commenced on prednisolone 40 mg orally per day, and over the next 7 days the erythema and blisters cleared. The steroid dose was reduced over 2 weeks to 10 mg a day, and over the following 4 months was discontinued completely.

Special study module

- Carry out a literature search on current knowledge of the genetic variants of epidermolysis bullosa.
- Try to see one or two cases in your local specialist paediatric dermatology clinic.
- Review the literature produced by the patient support group Debra.
- Consider the implications of a diagnosis of any type of epidermolysis bullosa for a single parent in poor financial circumstances.

Further reading

Wojnarowska, F. and Briggeman, R.A. (ed.) (1990) *Management of blistering diseases*. Chapman and Hall Medical, London.

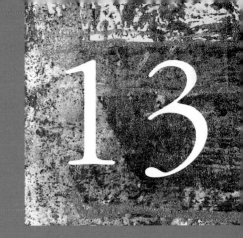

Drug eruptions

- Problem cases

- The mechanisms of cutaneous reactions to systemic drugs

- Commonly used systemic drugs in dermatology, and their possible side effects and interactions

- Adverse reactions to topical applications

- Discussion of problem cases

- Special study module project

Drug eruptions

Problem cases

Case 13.1

You are asked to see an elderly male with chronic obstructive airways disease on the respiratory wards. He has been admitted with an exacerbation due to infection and was started on an oral antibiotic 7 days ago. He is now erythrodermic with blisters on his trunk. He is also febrile and anuric. What are the likely diagnosis, the likely cause, and the prognosis?

Case 13.2

A 20-year-old college student home for the vacation consults you about a generalized macular rash and a general feeling of lethargy. She consulted the college medical officer about a sore throat last week and was given an antibiotic. She has not brought the remainder of the antibiotic capsules home with her and does not know the name of the antibiotic.

What diagnosis does this presentation suggest and why?

There are three aspects of adverse drug reactions of particular importance to dermatologists:

- The first is that the commonest request for a dermatologist to visit in-patients in other hospital wards is to advise on suspected adverse reactions to systemically administered drugs.

- The second is the need for dermatologists to be aware of undesirable side effects and drug interactions of the systemic drugs commonly used in dermatology, such as methotrexate, dapsone, and cyclosporin. There is also a growing need to be aware of the side effects of the newer immunomodulating agents coming into use in severe psoriasis.

- The third is that topical therapy may also give rise to undesirable side effects, as is the case with relatively potent topical steroid preparations. These are largely preventable.

The mechanisms of cutaneous reactions to systemic drugs

The majority of skin rashes induced by systemic medication are the result of immunological sensitization to the medicament. Ideally, it should be possible to classify them types of immunological reaction, namely:

Type I	anaphylactic reactions
Type II	cytotoxic reactions
Type III	Arthus or immune complex mediated reactions

Type IV   delayed hypersensitivity or cell-mediated reactions.

In practice, many adverse drug reactions are probably admixtures of two or more of these mechanisms.

History

The most important factor in establishing the likely precipitating agent in a suspected drug rash is a good history. However, the patients' notions of a 'drug' may be surprisingly variable, and laxatives, hypnotics, and simple analgesics are often regarded as part of a normal diet. Similarly, any medicament taken for a long period of time (for example, a diuretic for the past year) tends to be forgotten, as both doctor and patient may assume that a drug taken for 3 or more months has proved its safety.

The most useful approach is to ask the patient to bring samples of all medication, both systemic and topical used in the month prior to development of the problem. A relative or carer will often be invaluable in presenting a complete collection. A list from the family doctor is frequently incomplete, but should also be obtained. He may not be aware, however, of patent medicines and other over-the-counter preparations used by the patient.

Patients with rheumatological diseases seem relatively more susceptible to adverse drug reactions, probably due either to the nature of the medicaments or to brisk immunological responses. It should also be remembered that patients on multiple medication for general medical disorders can have quite unrelated coincidental dermatological disorders. Both pemphigoid and scabies, for example, may cause confusion with adverse drug reactions in elderly people on multiple medications.

Clinical features

Table 13.1 lists drugs relatively frequently incriminated as causing drug eruptions and Table 13.2 lists some of the cutaneous reaction patterns associated with drug reactions.

Table 13.1 Common causes of drug eruptions and likely patterns

Medicament	Pattern of eruption
Sulphonamides, pencillins	Morbilliform eruption, erythema multiforme, systemic lupus erythematosus
Phenylbutazone	Purpuric eruption
Beta-blockers	Psoriasiform
Barbiturates and tranquillizer over-dosage	Blistering eruption of lower limbs
Pencillamine	Pemphigus-like eruption
Phenothiazines	Light-sensitive dermatosis
Anti-malarials	Lichen planus-like eruption
Iodides and bromides	Acneiform eruption
Salicylates	Urticaria, angio-oedema

> ***Key points***
>
> It is important to obtain a complete history of medicaments, including any long-term drugs, 'natural remedies', and over-the-counter preparations that the patient may not consider important.

Table 13.2 Cutaneous reaction patterns, which may be due to drug reactions

Reaction pattern	Likely drugs
Toxic erythema	Antibiotics (ampicillin), sulphonamides, barbiturates, anti-rheumatics
Erythema multiforme and Stevens–Johnson syndrome	Sulphonamides, antibiotics, anti-rheumatic drugs
Erythema nodosum	Sulphonamides, contraceptive pill
Erythroderma	Antibiotics and anti-rheumatic drugs
Vasculitic and purpuric eruptions	Carbromal, phenytoin, indomethacin
Psoriasiform eruptions or aggravation of psoriasis	Beta-blockers, lithium
Very severe blistering eruption (toxic epidermal necrolysis)	Sulphonamides, allopurinol, phenylbutazone
Photosensitivity	Tetracyclines, phenothiazines
Alopecia	Coumarin anticoagulants, cytotoxics, anti-thyroid drugs
Acne, gingival hyperplasia	Phenytoin
SLE-like syndrome	Classically hydralazine. Also penicillin, sulphonamides, and, rarely, many others
Exfoliative dermatitis	Gold, isoniazid, phenylbutazone

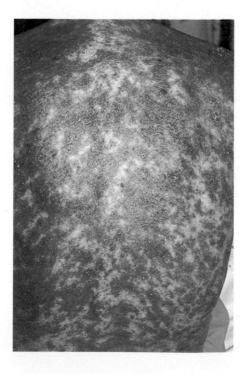

Fig. 13.1 Toxic erythema. This patient developed a morbilliform eruption 10 days after commencing a course of phenylbutazone.

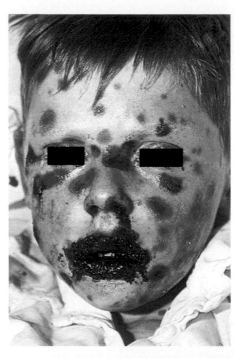

Fig. 13.2 Mucous membrane and skin involvement in a child with drug-induced Stevens–Johnson syndrome.

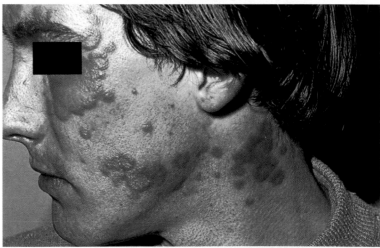

Fig. 13.3 Acute urticaria developing 4 hours after administration of systemic penicillin.

A common pattern of drug eruption is that of toxic erythema (Fig. 13.1). This is a widespread erythematous and morbilliform eruption, which tends to affect the trunk more than the extremities. It appears 5–10 days after first introduction of the causative drug, but only 2–3 days after introduction if the drug has been given previously. Malaise, fever, and lymphadenopathy are common.

Other cutaneous reaction patterns associated with adverse drug reactions are erythema multiforme and its more severe form, the Stevens–Johnson syndrome (Fig. 13.2), erythema nodosum, vasculitic lesions and purpura, hair loss, pigmentation, exfoliative dermatitis, lichen planus-like eruptions, and urticaria (Figs 13.3–13.7).

Once a drug is strongly suspected it should, if at all possible, be discontinued. If it has been the cause, the reaction can be expected to subside within the following 4–7 days. Confirmation by laboratory tests is not yet feasible, as available *in vitro* immunological tests will yield both false-positive and false-negative results. No safe or satisfactory provocation test is available and challenge tests based on re-introduction of the drug are *not* recommended. Indeed, patients should be warned about the drugs incriminated, and relevant notes made in case sheets or practice notes as subsequent exposure is likely to provoke more severe reactions. The one exception to this rule is the morbilliform rash produced by ampicillin in patients with infectious mononucleosis (Fig. 13.8). For reasons that are not understood, this is a time-limited hypersensitivity and, once the infectious mononucleosis has resolved, the patient is unlikely to show an adverse reaction to ampicillin.

Penicillamine is used as a chelating agent and as an anti-rheumatic, and in a proportion of patients it causes a blistering eruption that is clinically, histologi-

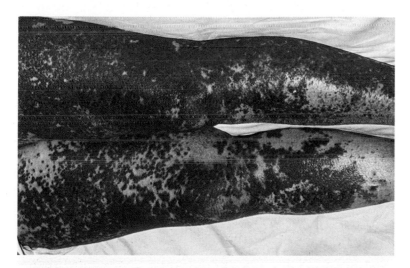

Fig. 13.4 Purpuric lesions developing days after initial administration of oxyphenbutazone. The platelet count was normal.

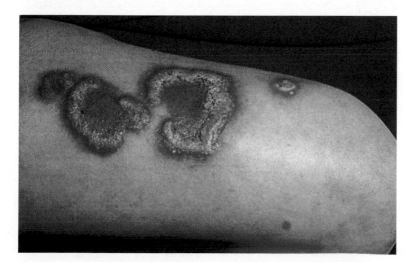

Fig. 13.5 Pustular drug eruption due to bromide administration. Acneiform lesions are also seen.

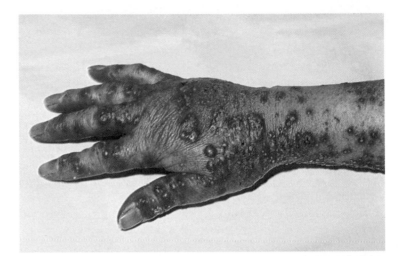

Fig. 13.6 Vesiculo-pustular drug eruption due to trimethoprim-sulphamethoxazole.

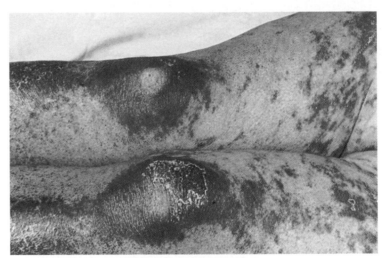

Fig. 13.7 Psoriasiform lesions developing for the first time 3 months after commencement of b-blocker therapy.

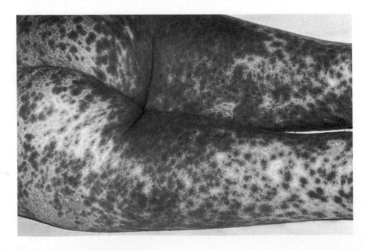

Fig. 13.8 Morbilliform eruption caused by administration of ampicillin to a patient with infectious mononucleosis.

cally, and immunologically identical to pemphigus vulgaris. The blistering eruption does not always subside after withdrawal of penicillamine.

Remember also that, while the general public considers natural herbal remedies safe, they too may have side effects. Herbal concoctions marketed for use in atopic dermatitis, for example, have been found to be hepatotoxic in some cases and others have been found to contain unexpected quantities of potent steroids.

Treatment

Withdrawal of the likely drug is frequently all that is required, followed by careful instructions to the patient concerning future avoidance. In very severe anaphylactic reactions, emergency administration of subcutaneous adrenaline (0.5 ml of a 1:1000 solution given slowly over 2–3 minutes) may be life-saving. Systemic antihistamines will relieve itch, but there is little evidence that they accelerate spontaneous clearance of drug-induced lesions. Topical steroids will relieve itch if present.

Commonly used systemic drugs in dermatology, and their possible side effects and interaction

Systemic drugs needed on occasion for difficult psoriasis include methotrexate, retinoids, and cyclosporin.

With **methotrexate** the commonest problems are drug interactions, liver toxicity, and renal toxicity.

The main problems associated with **retinoid** therapy are treatogenicity and elevation of triglycerides.

Cyclosporin may be used in severe psoriasis, dermatitis, and experimentally in other conditions. Here, the most serious potential problem is irreversible renal toxicity and careful monitoring is essential.

Patients with dermatitis herpetiformis are commonly treated with **dapsone**. This can cause a haemolytic anaemia, commonest at the start of treatment, and patients should be carefully monitored during the first month of therapy.

Patients on **systemic steroids** for dermatological problems should be monitored for hypertension, glycosuria, osteoporosis, and excessive weight gain.

Mycophenolate mofetil has been used for many years in transplant recipients as an immunosuppressive and, more recently, has been used in a wide range of dermatological conditions, including severe psoriasis and bullous disorders . Common problems include marrow suppression and severe nausea.

Drug induced lupus erythematosus may be provoked by a wide range of drugs including long term use of **minocycline** in acne and **terbinafine** for fungal infection.

There are currently a large number of immunomodulating agents in use in studies or on a named patient basis for severe psoriasis. These include anti-TNF alpha preparations, **etanercept, infliximab**, and **alefacept**. Experience to date is limited, but there are reports of reactivation of latent tuberculosis, as well as immunosuppression.

Tacrolimus and similar drugs are also potent immunosuppressives with a mode of action similar to cyclosporin A. The main use for these drugs at present in dermatology are as topical preparations for atopic dermatitis, but good

> ### *Key points*
>
> Common problems with systemic drugs used in dermatology
> Methotrexate: drug interactions
> Retinoids: elevation of
>   triglycerides
> Cyclosporin: renal toxicity
> Dapsone: haemolytic
>   anaemia

responses have been reported when used systemically in patients with severe and resistant lupus erythematosus, and pyoderma gangrenosum. Side effects include renal toxicity and neurotoxocity. As with other immunosuppressives, there is an increased risk of lymphoproliferative disorders if used long term.

It is wise when starting any new systemic drug in a patient who is already on medication for other problems to check possible drug interactions and, if necessary, amend prescribing plans. Local drug information centres, Regional and District Medicines Information Services in England Wales and Scotland, Martindales Pharmacopia, and the American Academy of Dermatology's Derminfonet are all useful sources of such information.

Adverse reactions to topical applications

Adverse reactions to topical applications are relatively common, especially to those containing antihistamines, anaesthetics, and antibiotics.

Antihistamines, if required, should only be given systemically as they are potent sensitizers when administered topically. The same applies to many topical anaesthetics, and antibiotics such as neomycin and sulphonamides are equally troublesome. An important reason for avoiding their use topically is that, once sensitized, these patients will react subsequently to systemic, as well as topical administration of the causative drug.

Adverse effects of topical corticosteroids

Sensibly used, topical steroids are a valuable part of the treatment for a wide range of inflammatory dermatoses. However, as with any potent and effective form of therapy, they must be prescribed with care, bearing in mind that percutaneous absorption, particularly through inflamed and excoriated skin, can be significant. If large quantities of a potent steroid are applied continuously to damaged skin, all the classic side effects associated with systemic steroid administration can occur, particularly in children. Much commoner, however, are the adverse effects on the skin itself. These are frequent, and include thin and fragile skin, spontaneous bruising, striae, and telangiectasia (Figs 13.9 and 13.10). The skin thinning, which is due to loss of dermal collagen, is reversible on withdrawal of the steroid, but striae and telangiectasia are permanent.

The speed of onset of such changes will depend on the site of application, the frequency of use, and the potency of the preparation. They develop rapidly in the warm humid microclimate of the body flexures.

Other complications of topical steroid therapy include tinea incognito, a term used to describe an atypical presentation of fungal infection on the skin due to unchecked growth of fungi on the steroid-treated skin. If simple scabies is not diagnosed or incorrectly treated with steroids, the presentation may be confusing and atypical.

Sensitization to topical steroids leading to an allergic contact dermatitis is now well recognized, but may be difficult to identify in the early stages, as topical steroids are often prescribed for a dermatitis thought to be due to another cause. Patch testing using tixocortol pivalate and budesonide should be arranged if there is any suspicion.

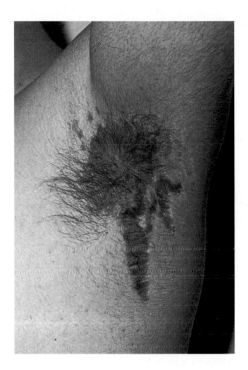

Fig. 13.9 Striae on the axilla caused by topical steroid therapy.

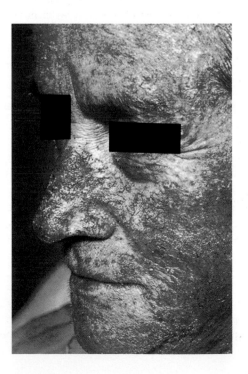

Fig. 13.10 Facial erythema and telangiectasia caused by application of potent topical steroid preparations.

The sensible approach to topical steroid usage is to prescribe the weakest effective preparation for as brief a spell as possible and to review the patient regularly. This is particularly important in paediatric practice. However, many parents of children with chronic atopic dermatitis are now very well aware of topical steroid side effects and are very reluctant to use prescribed moderately potent steroids. In these families it is important to strike a sensible balance between well controlled use of appropriate potency topical steroids and possibly more hazardous approaches, such as severe dietary restrictions, which some parents view as much safer than topical steroids.

The choice of topical steroid preparation requires care. Table 13.3 divides a representative list of topical steroid preparations into very strong, strong, medium, and mild categories. Very much more extensive tables will be found in MIMS and the British National Formulary, and it is wise to consult these.

It is good practice only to prescribe preparations in the mild category for the face and flexures, and to avoid using the very strong preparations in children. It is possible to weaken a strong steroid by dilution, but the correct diluent must be used, otherwise all potency may be lost through the molecular change in the steroid molecule.

Table 13.3 Relative strengths of some topical steroid preparations

Very strong	Medium
	Hydrocortisone 17 butyrate 0/1% (Locoid)
Clobetasol propionate 0.05%	Clobetasone butyrate 0.05% (Eumovate)
(Dermovate, Removate)	Flurandrenolone 0.0125% (Haelan)
Strong	**Mild**
Bethamethasone 17-valerate 0.1% (Betnovate)	Hydrocortisone 0.1%, 1.0%, 2.5% (Efcortelan)
Beclomethaone dipropionate 0.25% (Propaderm)	Fluocinolone acetonide 0.01% (Synadone)
Betamethasone dipropionate Diprosone	Mild steroids are now available without prescription in the UK
Budesonide. Preferid	
Fluticasone propionate. Cutivate	

Discussion of problem cases

Case 13.1

The two most important conditions to consider here in the differential diagnosis are bullous pemphigoid and an adverse drug reaction. Patients with bullous pemphigoid

Discussion of problem cases continued

generally are not unwell, despite large blisters, so the fever and renal problems would be unusual. The clinical picture and the timing of its appearance both suggest that an adverse drug reaction to the antibiotic prescribed 7 days earlier is the likely diagnosis. The features suggest toxic epidermal necrolysis, which may be triggered by a number of antibiotics including septrin and penicillins. The antibiotic was withdrawn and, after lengthy deliberations, the patient was given systemic steroids. However, his general condition deteriorated rapidly and he died 3 days later.

Review the literature on toxic epidermal necrolysis and its treatment with systemic steroids. What conclusions can you draw?

Case 13.2

This history is a very classic presentation of infectious mononucleosis (glandular fever). A young adult presents with general malaise and a sore throat for which penicillin is prescribed, and 4–7 days later a morbilliform eruption develops. The student had a positive monospot test. She slowly returned to normal energy levels over the next 3 months.

Can she be given penicillins in the future?

Special study module project

- Review the current literature on the use of mycophenolate mofetil and of intravenous immunoglobulins in dermatological problems. Consider the benefit/hazard ratio. Try to see patients on either of these treatments. Review their case sheets and diagnoses, and note their previous treatments and its effect.

Further reading

Litt, J.Z. (2001) *Pocketbook of drug eruption and interactions*, 2nd edn. Parthenon Publishing, New York.

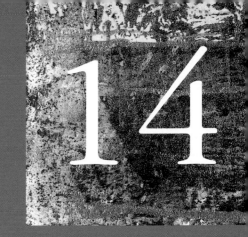

14

Cutaneous medicine

Cutaneous medicine

Problem cases

Case 14.1

A 43-year-old female patient consults you about non-painful red lesions, present on her shins for about 4 months. What would be the differential diagnosis in this case, what aspects of her medical history might be of relevance, and what treatments might be appropriate?

Case 14.2

A 38-year-old businessman who has recently lost his job comes to see you because of blisters that have developed on his face during a recent spell of warm, sunny weather. He has been very depressed because of both family problems and the inability to find employment, and he admits to drinking heavily. What is the differential diagnosis, what investigations might be appropriate, and what treatment is available?

Case 14.3

A healthy young woman whose only medication is the oral contraceptive comes to see you because of tender, red lumps on her lower legs, which have been present for 5 days. What does this presentation suggest what are the possible causes and what investigations are indicated?

Case 14.4

A 14-year-old girl is brought to you by her mother for treatment of periungual warts. The girl attends a school for those with learning difficulties and, during the consultation, the mother who is very supportive asks also for help with acne-like lesions around the girl's nose. On examination, the periungual lesions do not look like typical warts. What is the likely diagnosis in this case?

Introduction

In many systemic diseases the first signs are in the skin, and thus they may alert the physician to a developing and possibly life-threatening condition. These diseases come under the general term of 'cutaneous medicine', an important 'link area' between dermatology and other medical specialties in which an alert dermatologist can, by careful history-taking and examination, make a very valuable contribution.

Tables 14.1–14.3 list some of the commoner or more important diseases covered in this chapter. Inevitably, this is not exhaustive and the reader is referred the major dermatological textbooks for a more comprehensive account.

Table 14.1 Cutaneous manifestations of endocrine disease

Diabetes	Necrobiosis lipoidica (diabeticorum)
	Pruritus
	Fungal and bacterial skin infections
	Granuloma annulare
	Atherosclerosis and diabetic ischaemia
Hypothyroidism	Diffuse hair loss, coarse hair, broken hair
	Puffy oedema, xeroderma, pruritus
Hyperthyroidism	Hyperhidrosis
	Fine hair + hair loss, pruritus
	Pretibial myxoedema (usually associated with exophthalmos)
Cushing's syndrome	Acne vulgaris, hirsutism
	Cutaneous striae
	'Buffalo hump' obesity
Acromegaly	Soft tissue hypertrophy
	Seborrhoea
Addison's disease	Increased cutaneous pigmentation, especially intra-oral

Table 14.2 Commoner dermatological associations with gastrointestinal disease

Dermatitis herpetiformis	Gluten-sensitive enteropathy
Flexural eczematous eruptions	Malabsorption, mild zinc deficiency states
Acrodermatitis enteropathica	Defective zinc absorption
Peutz–Jeghers syndrome	Polyps of small intestine
Gardner's syndrome	Polyps of large intestine
Pyoderma gangrenosum	Ulcerative colitis, Crohn's disease, rheumatoid arthritis
Perineal ulceration and skin tags; sinus formation	Crohn's disease

Dermatological problems associated with endocrine disease

Diabetes

Patients with diabetes are at risk of a wide range of dermatological problems. Occasionally, the skin manifestations may be the first sign of diabetes, but more often they complicate pre-existing diabetes. Table 14.1 lists the commoner dermatological problems, which may complicate diabetes.

Necrobiosis lipoidica diabeticorum (Fig. 14.1), is usually seen on the shins and may predate frank development of diabetes by several years. A proportion of

Key points

Necrobiosis lipoidica on the shins may precede development of overt diabetes.

Table 14.3 Cutaneous features of other systemic disease

Porphyria	Photosensitivity, skin fragility, blister formation, hypertrichosis, pigmentation
Sarcoidosis	Blue-red subcutaneous nodules, Lupus pernio, 'Scar' sarcoid
Hyperlipidaemias	Xanthomata—tendinous, tuberous, and eruptive
Neurofibromatosis	Multiple cutaneous neurofibromata, freckling and *café au lait* spots
Tuberous sclerosis	'Adenoma sebaceum' (perifollicular fibromata), periungual fibro mata, shagreen patches
Pellagra (nicotinic acid deficiency)	'Diarrhoea, dermatitis and dementia', erythema after sunlight exposure
Scurvy (vitamin C deficiency)	Bleeding gums, purpura, poor wound healing

patients with the problem never develop frank diabetes. The individual lesions are shiny, atrophic, red or yellowish plaques with marked telangiectasia over their surface and a tendency to ulcerate. These ulcers may be very slow to heal. The severity of necrobiosis lipoidica is not directly related to the severity of the diabetes, nor does it improve with careful diabetic control.

Treatment is unsatisfactory, but protection from trauma and resultant skin damage are important. Intra-lesional injections of a steroid such as triamcinolone acetonide may be initially beneficial in some cases. Reports of response to PUVA therapy are encouraging, but larger numbers of treated patients and a longer follow-up time are needed.

Many patients with diabetes complain of **pruritus**. This is sometimes, but not always related to poor control of diabetes. **Pruritus vulvae** is relatively common in female diabetics and urine should always be checked for glycosuria in a patient first presenting with this problem. Those with diabetes are particularly prone to bacterial and fungal skin infections, and again diabetes should be excluded in any stubborn or unusually florid infection of this type.

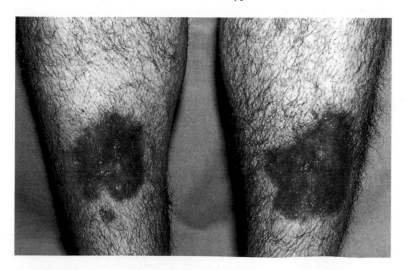

Fig. 14.1 Necrobiosis lipoidica. Firm, reddish-yellow plaques are seen on the shins.

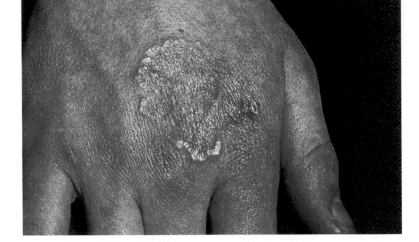

Fig. 14.2 Granuloma annulare on a typical site, the dorsum of the hand.

Granuloma annulare is found more commonly on the skin of diabetics than by chance (Fig. 14.2). The condition is commoner in children than in adults and it would appear to be more frequently associated with diabetes when it occurs in adults. The lesions are erythematous and circular with a well- marked, raised, palpable lateral border. The hands and feet are most commonly affected. The lesions are frequently multiple and tend to clear spontaneously after 3–6 months or longer. Occasionally, trauma, such as a diagnostic biopsy, appears to stimulate spontaneous clearance in the remainder of the lesion.

Secondary trophic skin change from diabetic ischaemia and atherosclerosis is a less specific, but common finding. The epidermis is thin, fragile, and has a glazed appearance, particularly on the lower legs. If these changes are present, diabetic gangrene is a very real hazard of inexpert chiropody or minor trauma.

Thyroid dysfunction

Abnormal hair growth is common in thyroid disease. Classically, in myxoedema the scalp hair is sparse, coarse, and brittle, and the outer part of the eyebrows is lost, while in **hyperthyroidism** there is fine scalp hair and sometimes associated alopecia.

Pretibial myxoedema is seen mainly after successful treatment of hyperthyroidism, especially when there are also ophthalmological complications. Clinically, there are asymptomatic, raised, red nodules and, although the name suggests that they are found chiefly on the shins (Fig. 14.3), they are also seen around the ankle and on the dorsum of the foot. Histological examination shows oedema and mucin. These patients have high levels of long-acting thyroid-stimulating hormone (LATS).

Topical corticosteroid preparations may be of some benefit, but in general these lesions are resistant to any type of treatment.

Adrenal cortical hyperfunction — Cushing's disease

This may present with acne vulgaris, seborrhoea, and hirsutism. Cutaneous striae may develop with great rapidity and be associated with 'buffalo hump' type of

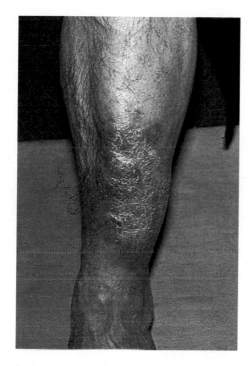

Fig. 14.3 Pretibial myxoedema. Raised, reddish plaques and nodules are seen on the shins.

obesity. If due to endogenous steroids, a search for enlarged adrenals, excessive production from the adrenals, or an adrenal tumour should be carried out. However, a high proportion of patients with cutaneous lesions suggestive of Cushing's disease have these as a secondary phenomenon due to oral steroid administration for another disease and it may be necessary to continue oral steroid therapy.

Adrenal cortical hypofunction — Addison's disease

Adrenal cortical hypofunction may be associated with a striking increase in melanin pigmentation, particularly on mucous membranes (Fig. 14.4) and sites of friction. This is a result of melanocyte stimulation by raised circulating levels of ACTH.

Acromegaly

This condition is associated with acne, seborrhoea, and soft tissue hypertrophy (Fig. 14.5). It is can easily be confused initially with adrenal hyperfunction.

Dermatological problems associated with gastrointestinal disease

Gluten-sensitive enteropathy

Gluten-sensitive enteropathy is common in dermatitis herpetiformis and has already been discussed (p. 277). Few patients with dermatitis herpetiformis will complain of clinical features of frank malabsorption, but jejunal biopsy will reveal

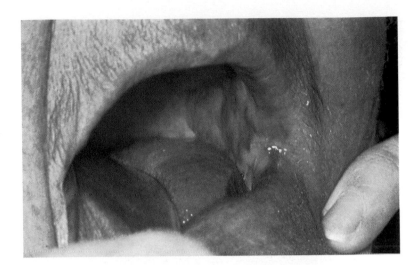

Fig. 14.4 Intra-oral melanin pigmentation seen in Addison's disease.

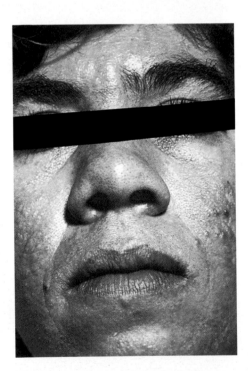

Fig. 14.5 Acromegaly. Note soft tissue hypertrophy, acne, and seborrhoea.

subtotal villous atrophy in the majority and many patients with DH will find that there skin lesions improve if they adopt a gluten free diet.

Malabsorption syndromes

These may lead to a secondary dermatosis in which there are moist, eczematous skin lesions, chiefly in the flexures. These may have a psoriasiform appearance and a small proportion of patients may have a remediable zinc deficiency.

Acrodermatitis enteropathica

Acrodermatitis enteropathica is a genetically determined disorder due to grossly defective zinc absorption. It is frequently first seen when the infant is being weaned off breast milk, and presents as erythematous, raw, and pustular areas around the mouth, anus, fingers, and toes. Severe diarrhoea is common, and if the condition is not recognized and treated, hair and nails will be shed. Oral zinc supplements bring about dramatic and rapid improvement, and must be continued for many years, possibly for life.

A similar condition is seen in patients receiving total parenteral nutrition or elemental diets in which zinc is lacking. Onset can be very rapid, but once the diagnosis is made and zinc supplements administered, the lesions clear equally rapidly.

Peutz–Jeghers syndrome

The Peutz–Jeghers syndrome (periorificial lentiginosis) consists of freckle-like pigmentation on and around the lips (Fig. 14.6) and polyposis of the gastrointestinal tract, particularly the small bowel. It is inherited as an autosomal dominant trait and the gene responsible is a serine threonine kinase LKB1 on chromosome 19p13.1 Intussusception may develop, but the polyps are rarely premalignant.

Gardner's Syndrome

This is an autosomally dominantly inherited syndrome and the gene has been mapped to chromosome 5q21–22. Affected family members have sebaceous or epidermoid cysts, lipomas, leiomyomas, and polyposis coli which progresses to gastrointestinal malignancy in 40% of affected individuals

Pyoderma gangrenosum

Pyoderma gangrenosum (p. 216) may precede the development of frank gastrointestinal symptoms in both ulcerative colitis and Crohn's disease. Patients with Crohn's disease also tend to have multiple perianal skin tags, ulcers, and fistulae,

> ### *Key points*
> Patients with Peutz–Jegher syndrome may develop intussusception.

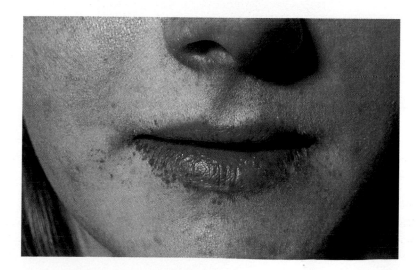

Fig. 14.6 Peutz–Jeghers syndrome. Macular melanin pigmentation is seen on and around the lips

and occasionally severe oral ulceration. Pyoderma gangrenosum is also associated with rheumatoid arthritis and Still's disease.

Porphyria

The porphyrias frequently present with cutaneous signs and symptoms. **Porphyria cutanea tarda** is most likely to present to the dermatologist, and is characterized by photosensitivity, skin fragility, sub-epidermal blister formation, and hyperpigmentation and hypertrichosis of sun-exposed skin (Fig. 14.7). There is usually a history of underlying liver damage, due most commonly to excessive alcohol intake. The diagnosis can be confirmed by demonstrating grossly elevated levels of urinary uroporphyrins. Elevated levels of serum iron are a feature and venesection to reduce this will alleviate symptoms. A variety of drugs aggravate the condition and the patient should be given written instructions on avoidance of these.

Other much rarer forms of porphyria may present to dermatologists. In **erythropoietic protoporphyria** very brief exposure to sunlight may cause itch, pain, and oedema. Pitted scars tend to develop on facial skin. Elevated erythrocyte and plasma protoporphyrin levels confirm the diagnosis. Topical sun-screens, particularly preparations that give physical protection with titanium dioxide, will give symptomatic relief.

Sunscreens can be divided into those that give physical protection, by deflecting UV rays, and chemical protection, which absorbs UV. Physical sunscreens contain zinc or titanium dioxide, and although perhaps less cosmetically acceptable they are very effective.

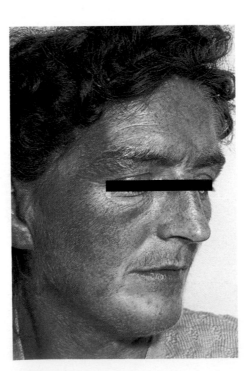

Fig. 14.7 Cutaneous hepatic porphyria. Hyperpigmentation and hypertrichosis are present.

Sarcoidosis

Sarcoidosis frequently presents with cutaneous lesions.

The cause is not yet known, but it may be significant that sarcoidosis is much commoner in countries where tuberculosis has been well controlled. The commonest dermatological presentation of sarcoidosis is **erythema nodosum** and an appearance on chest X-ray of hilar lymphadenopathy. Other cutaneous signs of sarcoid are **lupus pernio** (Fig. 14.8)—blue-red nodules on the nose, face, and hands—and **scar sarcoid**—the development of sarcoid granulomas in scars.

The basic pathological process is non-caseating granuloma formation in a variety of sites.

Most patients with sarcoid have elevated levels of angiotensin converting enzyme, but this is not a finding specific to sarcoid. Treatment of sarcoid is unsatisfactory. Patients with erythema nodosum and hilar adenopathy usually have a self-limiting condition, but lupus pernio tends to persist and can be very disfiguring. Low dose, alternate day systemic steroids may be helpful.

Hyperlipidaemias

The hyperlipidaemias may present or be associated with **xanthelasmata** and **xanthomata**. Xanthelasmata are white or yellow plaques of lipid deposited in the peri-orbital skin. The majority of these are not associated with hyperlipaemic states and are of cosmetic importance only, but in 10–20% of cases fasting lipids

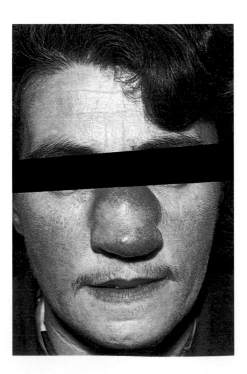

Fig. 14.8 Lupus pernio seen in sarcoidosis.

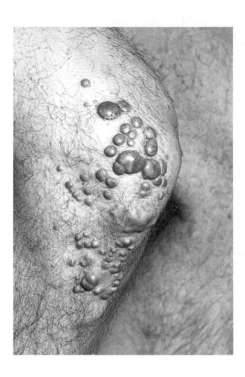

Fig. 14.9 Tuberous xanthomata. This patient had a normal lipoprotein profile.

will be elevated. An arcus senilis may also be seen. Simple xanthelasma should be treated, if necessary, by excision or destruction with trichloracetic acid.

Most **cutaneous xanthomata** are eruptive, tendinous, or tuberous (Fig. 14.9). The rare variant of **plane xanthoma** may resemble plane warts and may be associated with paraproteinaemia. Eruptive lesions occur on any body site and have an inflammatory halo. Tendinous lesions are most commonly seen over the Achilles tendon or on the dorsa of the hands, and tuberous lesions, which may be very large and bizarre in shape, tend to be prominent around knees and elbows. Xanthomata may be a pointer either to a primary hyperlipaemic state due to a genetic abnormality or to a secondary hyperlipaemic state due to renal, hepatic, endocrine, or pancreatic disease. The hyperlipaemias are classified according to relative proportions on serum electrophoresis of a-lipoprotein, pre-b-lipoprotein, b-lipoprotein, and chylomicrons.

Treatment will vary according to the type of hyperlipoproteinaemia identified, and may include dietary restriction of fat and carbohydrate, possibly with additional systemic therapy, such as bezafibrate or pravastatin.

Multiple neurofibromatosis (von Recklinghausen's disease)

This genodermatosis is inherited as an autosomal dominant trait, so a positive family history is usually present. The majority of patients who have cutaneous features of neurofibromatosis have neurofibromatosis type 1(NF1). The *NF1* gene has been identified and is a very large gene on chromosome 17q11.2.

The cutaneous features include macular hyperpigmentation (*café au lait* patches), neurofibromata, and multiple skin tags (**molluscum fibrosum**). These are soft, sessile, pink lesions, which may be extremely numerous and disfiguring (Fig. 14.10). The pigmentary changes may be relatively mild, but the presence of even a few macular pigmented lesions in the axillary vaults is regarded by some workers as pathognomonic.

Forty per cent of sufferers may develop neurological complications, such as acoustic neuroma or optic nerve glioma, and careful neurological examination at presentation and thereafter is therefore important. Sarcomatous change within such a tumour is reported.

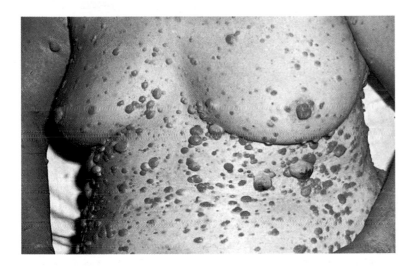

Fig. 14.10 Multiple molluscum fibrosum of von Recklinghausen's disease.

Behçet's syndrome

Patients with Behcet's syndrome have severe and persistent oral and genital ulceration, iritis, and arthropathy (Fig. 14.11). A viral aetiology is postulated.

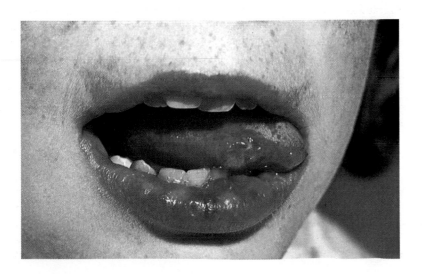

Fig. 14.11 Behçet's syndrome. Severe oral ulcers are seen. Genital ulcers and iritis were also present.

Involvement of the central nervous system may result in clinical features very similar to disseminated sclerosis. An interesting dermatological feature is 'hyperergy', i.e. the tendency of sterile blisters to develop at venepuncture sites. Behçet's syndrome will come into the differential diagnosis of severe persistent blistering on mucosal surfaces. The diagnosis will be confirmed by excluding other causes and by identifying non-cutaneous features of Behçet's. Treatment is difficult. Systemic steroids or cyclosporin may help some cases.

Tuberous sclerosis (epiloia, Bourneville's disease)

Tuberous sclerosis is inherited by autosomal dominant transmission, but may not first present until puberty or later. The gene is situated on chromosome 9q34.

Tuberous sclerosis comprises the triad of cutaneous abnormalities, mental retardation, and seizures. There are four main types of skin lesions:

- periungual fibromata—multiple, hypertrophic nodules around the nails, which may look rather like viral warts (Fig. 14.12);

- **shagreen patches**—normal-coloured plaques on the trunk, which have a firmer texture than normal skin;

- **adenoma sebaceum**—this term is pathologically incorrect as these lesions are, in fact, **perivascular fibromata** and are raised, red papules on the face, mainly around the nose (Fig. 14.13);

- **ash-leaf hypopigmentation**—this is well demonstrated under Wood's light as multiple, oval areas of hypopigmentation and may be the earliest sign of the disorder.

The individual prognosis varies with the degree of mental retardation and neurological involvement.

Treatment of the perivascular fibromata with diathermy surgery or laser therapy will produce a considerable cosmetic improvement.

> **Key points**
>
> It is possible to mistake adenoma sebaceum of tuberous sclerosis for acne.

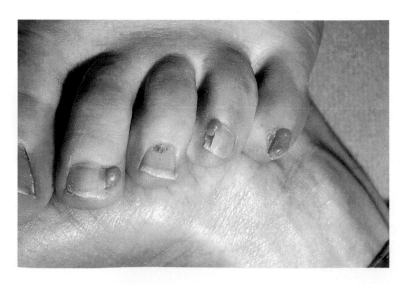

Fig. 14.12 Periungual fibroma in a child with tuberous sclerosis. Note wart-like lesions between nail and nail fold.

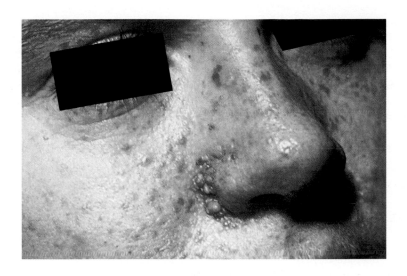

Fig. 14.13 Adenoma sebaceum (perifollicular fibroma) of tuberous sclerosis.

Nutritional deficiency disorders

A variety of relative nutritional disorders may present with skin lesions in the absence of frank malnutrition.

Scurvy

Hypovitaminosis C, even frank scurvy, is seen in elderly people with a low vitamin C intake. Their bleeding gums, easy bruising, and even frank purpura may all be dismissed as 'age changes'. Low levels of leucocyte ascorbic acid will confirm the diagnosis and oral vitamin C supplements will be curative.

Pellagra

This is due to nicotinic acid deficiency. It is rare, and presents with the triad of dermatitis, diarrhoea, and dementia. The dermatitis affects sun-exposed sites and consists of scaly erythema with a clear-cut, raised lateral margin, and subsequent hyperpigmentation. This is sometimes called Casal's collar or Casal's necklace.

The anti-tuberculous drug INAH can cause the same syndrome. Nicotinic acid replacement is rapidly curative.

Kwashiorkor

In kwashiorkor (protein malnutrition) the affected infant's skin is dry, with a glazed erythematous eruption, and the hair is dry, brittle, and hypopigmented. Oedema and ascites may also be present.

Dermatitis artefacta (factitial dermatitis), dermatological Munchausen's disease

This term describes bizarre lesions on any body site deliberately initiated or aggravated by the patient.

> ### Key points
>
> Dermatitis artefacta is rare, but should be considered in bizarre lesions, particularly on an exposed site.

Incidence and aetiology

This condition is rare and commoner in women than in men. In some cases, 'dermatological malingering' or self-induced aggravation of pre-existing lesions may be related to claims for industrial compensation, but in the majority no obvious motive is identified. Many patients are withdrawn, solitary individuals and consultation with medical attendants is one of their few social contacts. Clearly, complicated psychological motives and, at times, frank psychoses, are involved in the aetiology of this group of disorders, but recognition of this and appropriate referral is not always accompanied by disappearance of lesions.

Clinical features

These are very varied. The condition should be considered in any bizarre skin lesion, particularly if it is on an exposed site, and is an unusual angular or geometric shape (Fig. 14.14). Application of caustic liquids to the skin will cause erythema to develop on the site of drips or splashes from the applicator. Material may be injected into the skin, and finger-nails and hair may be damaged or even removed. Important pointers are an inappropriate interest in the lesions with relative lack of real concern and persistence or extension of the lesions if treated as an out-patient. In contrast, hospital admission, if it is an option, is often accompanied by rapid healing of the lesions.

Treatment is difficult. Direct confrontation will usually result in angry denial and failure to keep return appointments. A complicated degree of collusion may exist between the patient and the patient's relatives so that they too may react in this manner to a direct statement that the lesions are self-provoked. Similarly,

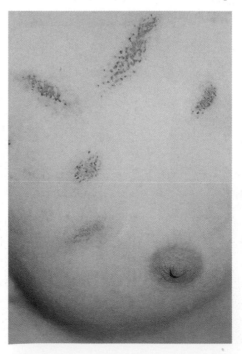

Fig. 14.14 Dermatitis artefacta. Note striking bizarre lesions on patient's trunk.

referral for psychiatric consultation may result in the signal for the patient moving to another dermatologist.

In general, treatment and, on occasion, cessation of self-mutilation becomes possible when the dermatologist establishes a degree of rapport with the patient, and it is understood, but not frankly stated, that both parties know how the lesions are produced. Collaborative treatment with a sympathetic psychiatrist may help, but much can be achieved by emotional support. The lesions will clear speedily if occlusive dressings and bandaging are used, but tend to recur on other body sites.

Cutaneous graft-versus-host disease

Acute and severe forms of graft versus host disease are now rare as a result of pre-conditioning of bone marrow prior to infusion into the recipient. Mild forms of the disease are associated with satisfactory engraftment.

Although there is some overlap, graft-versus-host disease has two relatively distinct clinical presentations. These are early onset graft versus host disease appearing within 100 days of marrow transplant, and late or chronic graft-versus-host disease appearing after the 100 day period.

Acute graft-versus-host disease

Affected patients usually have fever, diarrhoea, and a skin rash. This is commonly seen 7–10 days after the marrow graft at a time when the patient has been on multiple drug therapy. Because of this, the rash, which may be transient, may be confused with a drug eruption. The rash of graft-versus-host disease at this stage is maculopapular and tends to involve the trunk, palms (Fig. 14.15), soles, and oral mucous membranes. This distribution may be of some value in differentiating the rash from a drug eruption.

A skin biopsy taken at this point in time will show a lichenoid tissue reaction in the skin with liquefaction degeneration of the basement membrane and will frequently show the histological sign of 'satellite cell necrosis'. This describes the

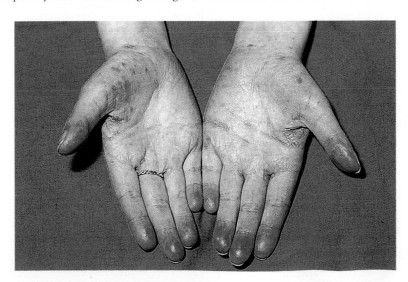

Fig. 14.15 Acute graft versus host disease. Note palmar erythema.

pattern within the epidermis of a lymphocyte in contact with an apparently necrotic keratinocyte. It is not totally specific for graft-versus-host disease, but its presence will help the pathologist suggest the diagnosis.

Chronic graft-versus-host disease

The onset of this form of graft-versus-host disease is usually more insidious. Patients may first notice a darkening of their normal skin colour, followed by a tightening and sclerosis of the skin causing immobility and contractures around the joints. Hair and nails may be shed, and the overall picture resembles that of systemic sclerosis. A skin biopsy taken from this type of graft-versus-host disease will show very gross thickening of the dermal collagen.

Treatment

Treatment of either type of graft-versus-host disease is difficult, but the acute phase may respond to high-dose oral steroid therapy. PUVA and high dose UVA alone have been reported to be helpful in sclerotic graft versus host disease.

Photosensitivity

Unusual cutaneous reactions to natural sunlight may be part of a systemic disease, such as systemic lupus erythematosus and porphyria, or an isolated finding as in rosacea. A number of drugs may also cause a photosensitive eruption. These include non-steroid anti-inflammatories, thiazide diuretics, antibiotics, and anti-arrhythmics such as amiodarone. It is particularly important to warn elderly patients taking such medication of possible photosensitivity provoked by a sunny holiday.

All patients with photosensitivity should have a careful drug history taken and bloods checked for anti-nuclear antibody. The possibility of porphyria should be considered and appropriate screening carried out if the clinical features are suggestive.

Polymorphic light eruption is a common photosensitive disorder, seen most often in young females. Patients are particularly sensitive to long wave UV in the 320–360-nm range of the spectrum (UVA), and typically present in the early spring with itchy papules on the face and hands (Fig. 14.16). There appears to be some hardening and desensitization of the skin as the season advances. Photosensitivity testing will confirm the diagnosis. The condition can easily be clinically confused with lupus erythermatosus and about 10% of patients have low levels of circulating anti-nuclear antibody.

Patients can be treated by slow desensitization, using a UVA source, or can be advised to use a broad spectrum sunscreen.

The investigation of pruritus

A number of systemic disease states may present with persistent and severe pruritus of clinically normal skin. Patients are usually elderly and may complain bitterly of sleep loss due to itch. However, great the temptation to dismiss the condition as 'senile pruritus' or even 'neurotic excoriation', it is important to take

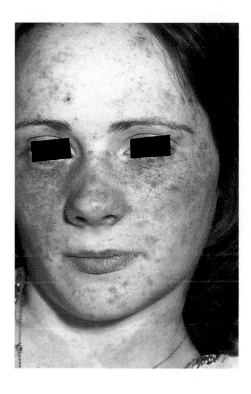

Fig. 14.16 Polymorphic light eruptions. Typical appearance in early spring of acute facial eruption on 13-year-old girl.

a careful history and carry out appropriate investigations to exclude both simple remediable causes and more serious precipitating factors.

History-taking must include details of occupational exposure to possible causative agents, for example, irritant dermatitis due to fibreglass found in loft insulation material, and also details of recreational and domestic agents. Take a careful family and contact history, and remember that scabies can be very atypical in patients who bathe regularly. A careful history of topical and systemic medication used currently and in the recent past is also essential. Well-demarcated, localized pruritus may be exogenous, but generalized itch is more likely to be due to a systemic cause.

A list of the commoner systemic associations of severe, generalized pruritus is given in Table 14.4. Diabetes, primary biliary cirrhosis, and polycythaemia are associations that should be excluded in a patient with persistent severe itch.

After obtaining a full history, appropriate investigations should include a full blood count, chest X-ray, serum urea, electrolytes and cholesterol, serum iron and TIBC levels, liver enzymes, thyroid function studies, and an auto-antibody screen. More specialized, subsequent investigation will depend on the history and results of this screening procedure.

If all results are negative, a diagnosis of idiopathic or 'senile' pruritus may be justified. Relief from pruritus in this condition may be obtained by vigorously treating dry scaly skin. The prescription of lubricant bath oils and substitution of emulsifying ointment BP or liquid paraffin 50% in white soft paraffin in place of soap may be curative.

Table 14.4 Some of the commoner systemic disease associations with cutaneous pruritus

Diabetes mellitus

Thyroid dysfunction (hypo- and hyperthyroidism)

Hepatic disease

Primary biliary cirrhosis

Chronic renal failure: itch may be present despite regular dialysis and normal blood urea

Polycythaemia

Haemochromatosis

Lymphoma

Hodgkin's disease

Neurological disorders, e.g. tabes dorsalis

Parasitosis

Drug addiction and abuse

Systemic antihistamines may give some relief, but tend to cause confusion in the elderly and should therefore be used with caution.

In **pruritus ani** and **pruritus vulvae** it is important to exclude easily remediable infections such as candidosis, trichomonal vaginitis, and threadworms. Women should be examined carefully for the presence of lichen sclerosis et atrophicus (p. 194), although here both itch and pain are the usual symptoms. The urine should be tested for sugar to exclude diabetes. In a high proportion, however, no obvious precipitating cause will be identified. Many of these patients are relatively obsessional, rather tense individuals whose symptoms flare at times of domestic or occupational stress. Both psychosomatic and psychosexual explanations have been offered for their symptoms.

Many large dermatological centres nowadays have vulvar clinics run by a multi-disciplinary team of dermatologists and gynaecologists who may be able to help these individuals.

Treatment should include advice on the avoidance of proprietary local anaesthetic preparations, which can cause allergic contact dermatitis. Patch testing to an appropriate battery of possible allergens may both identify causative agents and exclude others. Weak topical steroid/antibiotic combinations may offer some relief. Systemic antihistamines and anti-depressants may be of some value, but the condition tends to be resistant to therapy.

Cutaneous manifestations of systemic malignancy

An interesting group of cutaneous lesions are those associated with internal malignancy. Skin lesions may be the first indication of a malignancy, which has not yet been diagnosed, and is therefore an important area of collaboration between the dermatologist and the general physician, internist, and oncologist. The list of skin conditions that, on occasion, have been proven to be seen in association with a systemic malignancy in this category can be very long, indeed, and it is important to remember that in many cases solid statistical evidence of the association is lacking. Many of these cutaneous problems are seen predominantly in the elderly who have a higher incidence of many types of malignancy. Nevertheless, the conditions listed below should prompt the thought that there may also be an occult and possibly curable malignancy present, and initiate appropriate investigations.

Acanthosis nigricans

This rare condition, which may be associated either with malignancy or gross obesity, is characterized by hyperpigmentation and hyperkeratosis, most marked in the body flexures (Fig. 14.17). The commonest association is with gastrointestinal malignancies.

Dermatomyositis

This condition has already been discussed (p. 195). Ten to twenty five per cent of adult-onset dermatomyositis have been reported to be associated with an occult malignancy involving any body site. The dermatomyositis may precede the development of the malignancy by months or even years. Removal of the tumour may result in clearance of the dermatomyositis.

Glucagonoma (necrolytic migratory erythema)

These patients present with a raw, painful tongue, and superficial erosions and blisters on the face, buttocks, thighs, and abdomen. Diabetes is present and the malignancy is generally a glucagon-secreting tumour of the pancreatic islet cells. Removal of the tumour will result in dramatic clearance of the skin lesions.

Acquired ichthyosis

The development of excessively dry and scaly skin in elderly patients may herald the development of Hodgkin's disease, non-Hodgkin's lymphoma, or a solid tumour.

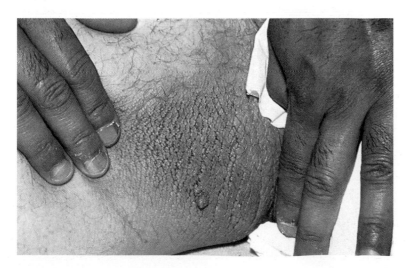

Fig. 14.17 Acanthosis nigricans of the inner thigh. This patient had a carcinoma of stomach.

Bowen's disease

A small proportion of patients with Bowen's carcinoma *in situ* of the skin (p. 339) will also have an unrelated systemic neoplasm.

Cowden's disease (multiple hamartoma syndrome)

This condition is a marker for breast and thyroid malignancies. Although rare, it is important, as the association with malignancy is so strong. The *Pten* gene on chromosome 10q.23 is mutated in a high proportion of patients. Patients develop multiple papules and papillomata on the face, hands, and forearms, and also have papules and a cobblestone appearance on the mucous membranes. Neural abnormalities may also be present.

Paraneoplastic acrokeratosis (Bazex syndrome)

Patients with this rare condition develop psoriasiform plaques on the hands, feet, and face. There is thickening of the palmar and plantar skin, and the nails may become dystrophic and break easily. All reported cases of the condition to date have had a malignancy of the pharynx or larynx.

Other associations

Other rare associations between cutaneous lesions and systemic malignancy include severe herpes zoster and erythema gyratum repens (a pattern of cutaneous erythema resembling wood grain that rapidly changes shape on the skin), and the sudden appearance of profuse growth of lanugo hair or of multiple basal cell papillomata. Individual case reports associate severe bullous pemphigoid with concomitant systemic malignancy, but this may be a chance association of two conditions both commoner in elderly people.

Discussion of problem cases

Case 14.1

Red areas on the shins alone suggests erythema nodosum, pretibial myxoedema, or necrobiosis lipoidica. In this case, the duration and lack of pain do not make erythema nodosum likely. A careful history should be taken of symptoms or past treatment related to either thyroid problems or diabetes. The patient had no thyroid related problems, but did have a strong family history of insulin dependent diabetes. A biopsy confirmed the presence of palisading granulomas typical of necrobiosis lipoidica. The lesions responded slightly to topical steroid application, and three years later the patient developed frank diabetes.

This case illustrates the fact that necrobiosis lipoidica can precede development of diabetes.

Case 14.2

The differential diagnosis of blisters in an adult include a bullous adverse drug reaction, bullous pemphigoid, and problems associated with systemic disease

Discussion of problem cases continued

including porphyria. The patient was on no possibly relevant drugs, and the distribution of the blisters was not typical of pemphigoid. The history of excess alcohol and the fact that the blisters are all on sun-exposed sites suggests cutaneous hepatic porphyria. Blood porphyrin levels confirmed this clinical diagnosis, and it was also noted that the patient had a very high serum iron. Other cutaneous feature noted were hypertrichosis around the temples and poor healing after minor trauma.

The patient was counselled on restricting alcohol intake and had a pint of blood removed weekly for 6 weeks. The blisters cleared on this routine and did not recur.

Case 14.3

The rapid onset of painful nodules confined only to the shins suggests a diagnosis of erythema nodosum. A biopsy will confirm this. Erythema nodosum is, however, a tissue reaction pattern that may be caused by a wide range of precipitating agents, which will need to be sought in this case. Drugs are a common cause of erythema nodosum and the oral contraceptive could be responsible, but other causes should first be excluded.

On chest X-ray, the young woman was found to have hilar adenopathy. The combination of hilar adenopathy and erythema nodosum is the commonest pattern of presentation of sarcoidosis. She also had a raised serum angiotensin converting enzyme level and on this basis a diagnosis of sarcoidosis was made.

With no treatment other than rest, the lesions of erythema nodosum resolved over the following 6 weeks and 6 months later her chest X-ray was normal.

Case 14.4

Unusual periungual lesions, learning difficulties, and a facial eruption around the nasolabial folds should alert you to the possibility of tuberous sclerosis. It is not unusual for the diagnosis to be made after the periungual fibromata have been mistaken for warts, but have not responded to treatment. A large proportion of patients with tuberous sclerosis appear to have spontaneous mutations of the *TS* gene as there is a negative family history.

In this girl's case the diagnosis was confirmed by cerebral CT. She also had shagreen patches on her trunk. Her parents were informed of the diagnosis, counselled on the likely progression, and given information about the Tuberous Sclerosis Association.

Further reading

Braverman, I. (1998) *Skin signs of systemic disease*, 3rd edn. WB Saunders, Philadelphia.

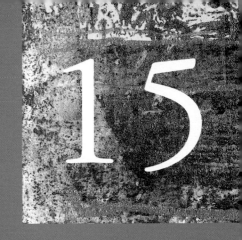

15

Skin tumours-benign and malignant

Skin tumours-benign and malignant

Problem cases

Case 15.1

An elderly male consults you about a solitary, scaling, crusting lesion over his left scapula. He has no idea how long it has been present. He is also receiving treatment for prostate cancer. What is the differential diagnosis here, what is the most likely diagnosis, and what action do you take?

Case 15.2

A female missionary in her fifties consults you about diffuse hair loss. In the course of the consultation you notice a translucent, nodule about 1 cm across below her left eye. What action do you take?

Case 15.3

The professional at the local golf club consults you about irritable, crusting lesions on his scalp. He has extensive male pattern baldness, but when younger was red haired. What is the likely diagnosis here and what is an appropriate management plan?

Case 15.4

Last week there was a 40-minute television documentary from Australia on a young man dying of melanoma, which has aroused a lot of additional publicity. This week three patients attend tour surgery who have seen the documentary and who are concerned.

The first is an elderly lady who lives alone and who is very worried about several fairly large pale brown lesions on her back. She does not know how long they have been there, but tells you that from time to time parts of the lesions crumble off.

The second is a young man brought to you by his wife. He has had a congenital melanocytic naevus, 5 cm in largest diameter, on his thigh since birth, but over the past 2 years it has developed several central areas of dark brown to black pigmentation.

The third is a woman in her late twenties who is concerned about an irregular pigmented lesion on her upper arm present and growing for 6 months. It has an irregular outline, and has areas of tan and blue-black colour.

What action do you take in each of these three situations?

Introduction

Benign epidermal tumours and naevi arising from either keratinocytes or melanocytes are extremely common and increase in prevalence with age, particularly on white skin. Benign tumours arising from the melanocyte, melanocytic naevi, have already been described (p. 230)

Benign tumours arising from the Langerhans cell or Merkel cell have not yet been recognized.

There is also a wide range of benign lesions arising from dermal cells, and a very wide, but relatively rare, range of benign or only locally expansile tumours arising from cells involved in the skin appendages. It is extremely useful to be able to identify clinically at least the commoner of these benign cutaneous lesions, as many need no treatment other than to reassure the patient.

There is a smaller range of benign tumours or naevi, which have the capacity for malignant transformation and, here again, clinical recognition is useful, but often surgical removal is needed to confirm a clinical diagnosis. If not, surveillance may be necessary.

Malignant tumours arising from the epidermal keratinocyte—the basal and squamous cell carcinomas—are the commonest malignancies of all on a world scale, but are often omitted from cancer registration returns because of the belief that they are very rarely fatal. While this is in general true, the workload generated in removing these non-melanomas skin cancers is considerable, especially in a country such as Australia where a high proportion of white skinned individuals are exposed to long hours of natural sunlight.

The cutaneous malignancy responsible for the majority of skin cancer related deaths is the malignant melanoma, arising from the epidermal melanocyte. Malignant melanoma is of particular current interest because of its rapidly increasing incidence in all parts of the world, and because of the fact that it affects relatively young adults in the third and fourth decades, thus resulting in a high number of years of potential lost life for every melanoma death.

Malignant tumours also arise in the dermis. Kaposi's sarcoma, arises from the dermal vasculature. A subset of patients who develop Kaposi's sarcoma have AIDS, but there are also other at risk groups.

Cutaneous lymphoma is relatively rare, but may at times come into the differential diagnosis of psoriasis.

Finally, it should be remembered that the epidermis, and more often the dermis, can be the site of metastatic spread from primary tumours arising in other parts of the body.

Factors predisposing to cutaneous malignancy

Both genetic and environmental factors influence the development of cutaneous malignancy.

Two major genodermatoses predisposing to cutaneous malignancy are xeroderma pigmentosum (p. 341), associated with defective, post UV exposure unscheduled DNA repair, which predisposes to all types of cutaneous malignancy, but especially squamous cell carcinoma, and Gorlin's syndrome or the basal cell naevus syndrome, which predisposes to basal cell carcinoma (p. 343).

The major environmental factor currently recognized as predisposing to skin cancer is excessive exposure of pale skin to natural ultraviolet radiation. Excessive exposure to ultraviolet radiation in the UVB (280–320 nm) part of the spectrum is carcinogenic in man, and a clear quantitative, linear relationship exists between UVB exposure of Caucasian skin and the incidence of squamous carcinoma. The evidence for sunlight in general and UVB in particular influencing the incidence of cutaneous malignant melanoma is also strong, but case control studies suggest that short episodes of intense burning sun exposure are more important than cumulative sun exposure. The highest incidence of melanoma recorded in the world is among the white population of Queensland, Australia, a tropical state of Australia with a high proportion of pale skinned red haired immigrants of Scottish or Irish descent.

Incidence figures for both malignant melanoma and squamous carcinoma in black- and white-skinned populations in the same geographic area show a very much lower figure for black populations, suggesting that melanin plays a significant role in protecting against ultraviolet-induced carcinogenesis.

Case control studies from many parts of the world in the past decade have clearly indicated that for both melanoma and non-melanoma skin cancer, early childhood excessive sun exposure is an important risk factor for the development of skin cancer two or three decades later. This observation emphasizes the point that the development of cutaneous malignancy is a multi-step process, and that one or more of the initial steps may occur very early in life. This clearly has implications for skin cancer prevention campaigns.

Exposure to ionizing radiation is an additional factor, which predisposes to cutaneous malignancy, but modern methods of limiting such exposure makes this a relatively rare cause by comparison with exposure to ultraviolet radiation.

Similarly, although chemical carcinogens have been used traditionally in studies of cutaneous carcinogenesis using animal models, their role in the current epidemic of skin cancer in man appears small.

Benign cutaneous tumours

The differential diagnosis of a lump or bump on the skin will include a variety of benign skin tumours. In general, these are very much commoner than the malignant lesions and it is, therefore, important to be able to recognize these lesions in order to reassure patients and then make a decision as to whether or not excision is necessary.

Seborrhoeic keratoses (Basal cell papilloma, seborrhoeic wart)

Definition

A benign proliferation of epidermal keratinocytes of unknown aetiology, which does not progress to epidermal malignancy.

Seborrhoeic keratoses are extremely common and become commoner with increasing age. Their aetiology is unknown, and despite the term seborrhoeic wart, the human papilloma virus does not appear to be a causative factor. Clinically, they present as raised, frequently multiple lesions, mainly on covered body sites (Figs 15.1 and 15.2). Many are brown due to benign and incidental

Key points

If a lump or bump on the skin is worth removing in the surgery, it is worth sending for pathological reporting. In this way you will not make the tragic mistake of curetting off an early melanoma and arranging no further treatment.

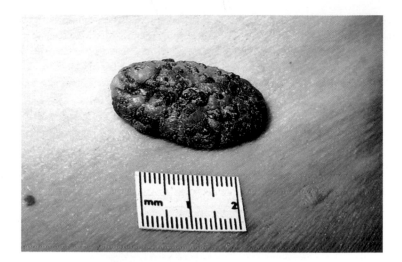

Fig. 15.1 Classic basal cell papilloma. Note greasy warty surface and superficial stuck-on appearance in relation to the underlying skin.

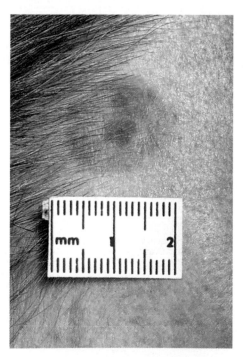

Fig. 15.2 Flat type of seborrhoeic keratosis or basal cell papilloma on facial skin. This type of lesion can be confused with a lentigo maligna melanoma (p. 348).

melanocytic activity within the lesion, and may therefore be mistaken for more serious problems such as malignant melanoma. The very superficial 'stuck on' appearance is a helpful differential point as the lesion grows out of, rather than infiltrates down into the epidermis. The keratin cysts are also useful when making a clinical diagnosis. Facial seborrhoeic keratoses may be relatively flat and difficult to differentiate from lentigo maligna or lentigo maligna melanoma (see p. 348).

If the diagnosis of seborrhoeic keratosis is clinically obvious, removal is not essential. If removal is requested for cosmetic reasons, cryotherapy or curettage and diathermy are effective, but the lesions are multiple and tend to recur.

Epidermal naevi

Definition

A raised, often linear, plaque arising from a localized, benign proliferation of epidermal keratinocytes.

It is suggested that epidermal naevi arise as a result of an aberrant clone of keratinocytes. Epidermal naevi are relatively common, and range from a small raised area, often mistaken for a viral wart, to a very large and disfiguring pigmented area of hyperkeratosis covering 30% of the body surface and associated with neurological problems. This is known as the epidermal naevus syndrome.

Epidermal naevi are not usually visible at birth, but develop during childhood. Initially, there may just be an area of hyperpigmentation, but over a period of months or years this becomes rough and hyperkeratotic. In flexural areas, this may result in bacterial colonization and secondary infection leading to odour and discomfort. Many of these naevi are linear (Figs 15.3 and 15.4). Patients with the epidermal naevus syndrome have large epidermal naevi and commonly also have neurological problems.

A variant of the epidermal naevus is the so-called **Becker's naevus** (Fig. 15.5), which is an area of faint hyperpigmentation and associated hypertrichosis. It is most commonly seen on the skin over the shoulder area, and may develop after sunburn. It is associated with benign proliferation of smooth muscle cells in the underlying dermis.

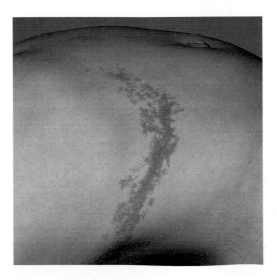

Fig. 15.3 Linear warty epidermal naevus on the trunk of a young man.

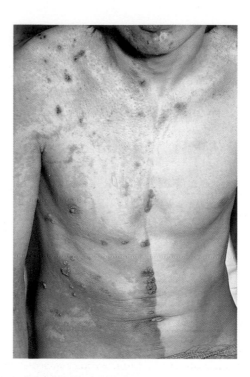

Fig. 15.4 Extensive epidermal naevus covering a large part of one half of the body in an older boy.

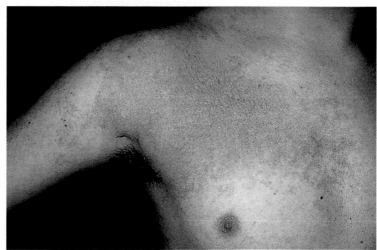

Fig. 15.5 Becker's naevus. Note subtle pigmentation and some increase in hair growth over the shoulder area.

Treatment

With small lesions no treatment may be necessary. For larger lesions, abrasion and keratolytics may reduce the hyperkeratosis. In some cases, laser surgery or scalpel excision is the most acceptable option.

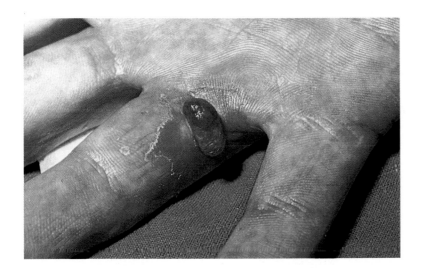

Fig. 15.6 Pyogenic granuloma. Tender raised lesions develop over a period of 1–2 weeks.

Pyogenic granuloma

Definition

A rapidly growing, benign tumour arising from the cutaneous vasculature.

Classically, these lesions develop after trauma, commonly on the fingers of keen gardeners after pruning roses (Fig. 15.6). Over a period of 2–3 weeks a raised, oozing, pedunculated lesion develops, and frequently becomes secondarily infected. The rapidity of growth may give rise to concern about a malignant lesion, but the natural history is of spontaneous regression over a period of weeks or months. The histological appearance is of a network of capillaries embedded in an oedematous stroma.

Surgical excision or diathermy is recommended, as the lesions can be painful and inconvenient.

Histiocytoma (dermatofibroma, sclerosing angioma)

Definition

A firm flesh coloured yellow or brown nodule, most commonly on the lower leg.

This lesion appears most commonly as a firm, elevated yellow/brown nodule on the leg (Fig. 15.7). In some cases there is a history of trauma, such as an insect bite, to the site. The nodule is often brown and this pigmentation, together with a history of fairly rapid enlargement, may cause concern that the lesion is a malignant melanoma. In fact, however, the pigment is chiefly iron, rather than melanin and the lesion is quite benign. The so-called dimple sign is useful. If the area around the lesion is squeezed and puckered, a dimple develops in the middle of the histiocytoma because of the firm tethering of epidermis to dermis. This is not seen in a tumour arising from melanocytes.

Local excision may be necessary to obtain histological confirmation of the clinical diagnosis.

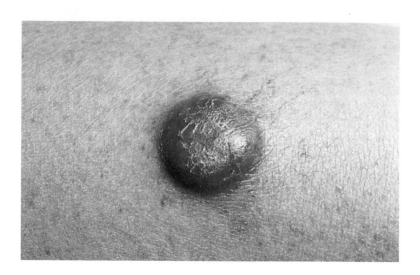

Fig. 15.7 Histiocytoma. The pigment seen in these benign lesions is both iron and melanin.

Skin appendage tumours

Definition

A wide range of benign tumours arising from cells comprising the hair follicle, sebaceous glands, eccrine, and apocrine sweat glands. Local extension of these tumours may occur, but malignant skin appendage tumours giving rise to metastatic spread are rare.

There is a very large range of rare tumours in this group, many of which will never be recognized clinically, but only by the pathologist after excision of a non-specific nodule. The suggested clinical diagnosis is often a cyst or a basal cell carcinoma. Skin appendage tumours arise most commonly on the head and neck area. The three skin appendage tumours most likely to be encountered in non-specialist practice are the **organoid** or **sebaceous naevus**, the **pilomatricoma** or **calcifying epithelioma of Malherbe**, and the **eccrine poroma**.

The **organoid** or **sebaceous naevus** is a localized area of excessive quantity of sebaceous glands and hair follicles (Fig. 15.8). Clinically, they are raised, irregular, yellow nodules most commonly on the scalp, and are often first seen in the first and second decades of life. Their importance lies in the fact that basal cell carcinoma may develop at an early age in between 10 and 25% of organoid naevi. For this reason, prophylactic surgical removal with a narrow margin of normal skin is recommended.

The **pilomatricoma** is a relatively common, benign tumour of childhood arising from hair follicle components. It presents often in the first decade as a raised nodule on any part of the body surface. They are usually excised to obtain a histological diagnosis.

The **eccrine poroma** arises from the eccrine sweat gland apparatus and is usually seen on older adults on the foot, presenting as a raised, red, moist nodule.

Some skin appendage tumours have malignant counterparts, but these are excessively rare. Local excision of the benign skin appendage tumours is usually necessary both to obtain a diagnosis and as a cure.

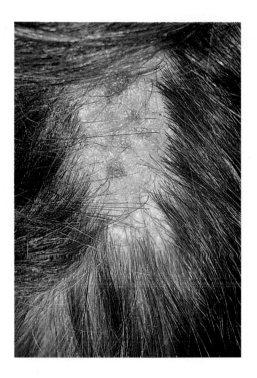

Fig. 15.8 Organoid naevus on scalp. Note large yellowish papillomatous lesion.

Premalignant lesions and carcinoma *in situ*
Actinic keratoses
Definition

Actinic keratoses are scaly, erythematous, crusting lesions, seen most often on the scalp, face, and back of the hands (Figs 15.9 and 15.10). They are extremely

> ## *Key points*
> Premalignant lesions and carcinoma *in situ* should be identified, and treated to prevent malignant change.

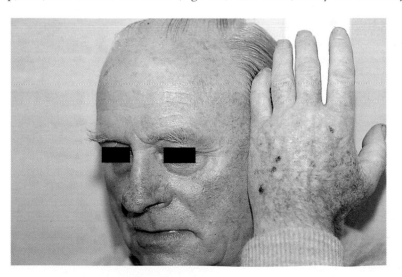

Fig. 15.9 Actinic keratosis on the face and hands of a male who has spent some time in the Tropics.

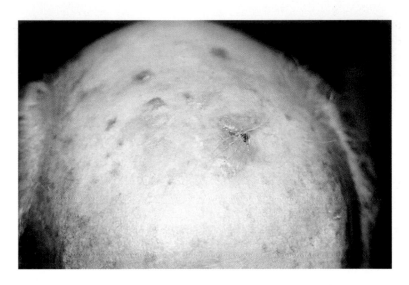

Fig. 15.10 Higher power view of multiple actinic keratoses on a male scalp.

common and usually multiple on the skin of fair skinned individuals who have an outdoor occupation or recreation. In the UK they are unusual before the age of 40, but in countries such as Australia they may be seen on fair-skinned individuals at a much earlier age.

Actinic keratoses were commonest in the past on outdoor workers. Nowadays, however, recreational rather than occupational sun exposure is likely to be an important factor. Genetic factors are also important, and the fair- or red-haired, blue-eyed, freckled individual who tans poorly and burns easily is particularly at risk. Actinic keratoses have the potential for transformation into metastasizing squamous carcinoma. One Australian study has suggested that the rate of malignant transformation is around 1% per year. However, most individuals have not one, but 10–20 actinic keratoses and thus the risk of malignant change over time is higher.

In practice, actinic keratoses should be treated because of the risk of malignant change, and patients should be given advice about sunscreen and hat use to reduce further sun exposure, as there is now good evidence that if such advice is taken that some of these actinic keratoses will regress.

The striking histological changes in the epidermis are a loss of the normal keratinocyte maturation pattern, with some epidermal cells showing individual cell keratinization, and the appearance in the dermis of a dense area of 'elastic' tissue replacing the collagen of the papillary dermis—the so-called senile or actinic elastosis

Treatment

Treatment of existing actinic keratoses can be by cryotherapy or topical application of the cytotoxic preparation 5-fluorouracil (Efudix). This preparation has the interesting property of 'seeking out' and stimulating an inflammatory response in 'preactinic' lesions that are not yet clinically visible. It is applied topically to the affected areas daily, carefully avoiding the eyes. After 2–3 weeks a brisk inflammatory reaction develops and the skin looks temporarily very much worse. After this, the lesions slowly clear with a good end-result. Topical diclofenac (Solaraze) is a relatively new topical non-steroidal preparation, which appears to clear actinic keratoses effectively with regular application. Photodynamic therapy (PDT) involves applying a topical photosensitising cream to the actinic keratosis for about 4 hours, and then irradiating the area with long wavelength light at 630 nm for around 30–40 minutes. Malignant cells are destroyed, but normal cells are not damaged by this approach. PDT is particularly useful for treating multiple lesions and has the advantage of being virtually pain free.

Bowen's carcinoma *in situ* (Bowen's disease)

Definition

A form of intra-epidermal carcinoma *in situ*, which on rare occasions progresses to invasive squamous carcinoma.

Clinical features

Clinically, Bowen's disease presents as an isolated, scaling, erythematous plaque, generally on the trunk (Fig. 15.11). It may look like an isolated patch of psoriasis and is frequently initially treated as psoriasis. If untreated, the lesions slowly expand laterally over a period of years. A proportion of lesions of Bowen's disease develop into invasive squamous carcinomas.

Pathology

The histological features include thickening of the epidermis (acanthosis), and lack of normal organization and maturation of the keratinocytes within the epidermis.

Treatment

It is wise to confirm the clinical diagnosis with an incisional biopsy. Cryotherapy is a common and acceptable form of therapy thereafter. At present, there are ongoing trials of photodynamic therapy to establish the efficiency and recurrence rate.

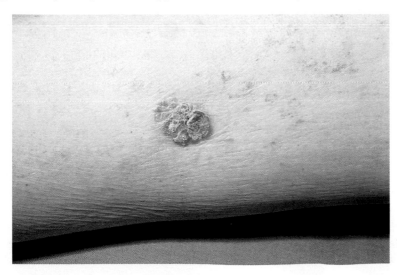

Fig. 15.11 Scaling lesions of Bowen's disease on lower leg of elderly female.

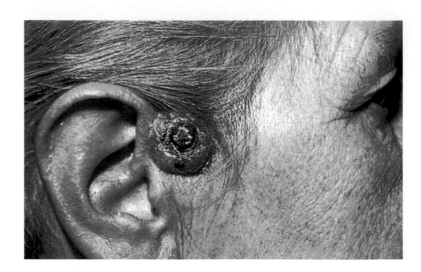

Fig. 15.12 Keratoacanthoma. This lesion had grown to the size seen in a period of 3–4 weeks.

Keratoacanthoma

Definition and clinical features

A rapidly developing and subsequently self-healing epidermal nodule with pathological features indistinguishable from early squamous cell carcinoma.

Keratoacanthomas usually develop as raised solitary lesions on the face and may grow over 2–3 weeks to a size of 2–3 cm in diameter (Fig. 15.12). Thereafter, the nodule develops a necrotic, crusted centre, and clears spontaneously often leaving an unsightly pitted scar.

Treatment

Currently, some pathologists are very reluctant to report a lesion as a keratoacanthoma because of the very real difficulty in differentiating it from a squamous cell carcinoma. It is therefore current practice to excise these lesions with a narrow margin of surrounding normal skin.

Cutaneous malignancies

Squamous cell carcinoma

Definition

A malignant tumour derived from keratinocytes.

The great majority of squamous carcinomas arise on sun-damaged skin. A few may develop in scar tissue. Squamous cell carcinomas are commoner on the sun exposed skin of transplant recipients and the risk of developing squamous cell carcinoma increases with duration of transplant.

Clinical features

Clinically, the lesions present as hyperkeratotic, ulcerated, expanding nodules (Fig. 15.13). On palpation, there is obvious depth to the lesions, compared with

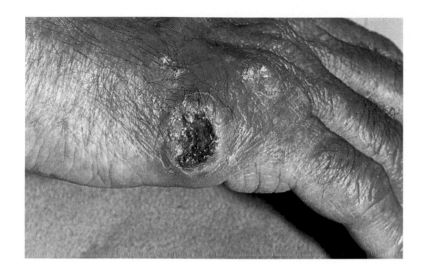

Fig. 15.13 Invasive squamous carcinoma.

actinic keratoses. They are relatively common on the backs of the hands and the face, and may also develop on the edge of scars such as burns scars.

On the skin of immunosuppressed transplant patients they may clinically be subtle, although the pathology will be that of a deep invasive squamous cell carcinoma. Always be suspicious of a lesion on the skin of a transplant recipient and biopsy such lesions sooner, rather than later.

Metastatic spread to the local draining lymph nodes and beyond can occur from squamous cell carcinoma. Tumours arising on sites such as the lip and ears appear to have a higher rate of metastatic spread than from other body sites.

Pathology

The striking histological features are gross disorganization of the epidermis with invasion of tongues of epidermal tissue and isolated discrete foci of malignant keratinocytes into the underlying dermis. Mitotic figures, both normal and abnormal, are seen in these malignant keratinocytes.

Treatment

Once a histological diagnosis has been established by biopsy, the tumour can be treated by excision or radiotherapy. In most centres, surgical excision with an adequate margin of normal tissue is the preferred option. Patients should be on regular follow-up thereafter to detect either recurrence or the appearance of a second primary squamous cell carcinoma.

Xeroderma pigmentosum (XP)

Definition

A group of genetically determined disorders associated with defective or virtually absent levels of unscheduled DNA repair after exposure to ultraviolet radiation, and associated with a very high incidence of all types of cutaneous malignancy, particularly squamous cell carcinoma.

> ### *Key points*
> Remember that skin malignancy is common in transplant recipients.

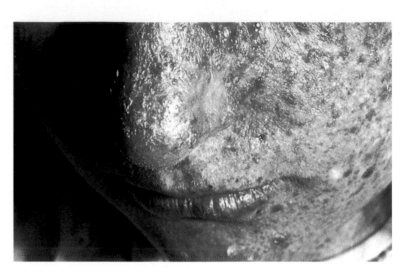

Fig. 15.14 Xeroderma pigmentosum. Gross sun damage is seen on the facial skin of this 12-year-old girl.

At present, eight subsets (XP types A to G plus pigmented xerodermoid) of xeroderma pigmentosum (XP) are recognized. Those in group A have virtually no unscheduled DNA repair capacity after UV radiation and the gene for this variant has been localized to chromosome 9q34. The least severely affected are those in group G in which the gene lies on chromosome 13q33.

XP is inherited by autosomal recessive transmission, and the two commonest groups are A and C. Children in affected families show very prolonged UV induced erythema in the first year of life and this is quickly followed by grossly accelerated photo-ageing changes if the child is not protected from further sunlight exposure. Mothers will tell their family doctors or dermatologists of their child's tendency to hate the sun and to sunburn after literally minutes of sun exposure during the first year of life. Exposed skin becomes freckled, telangiectatic, and atrophic (Fig. 15.14), and before the age of 5 years the child will have actinic keratoses and squamous cell carcinoma. They are also at risk of developing basal cell carcinoma and malignant melanoma. Patients with XP groups A and B also have central nervous system degenerative problems.

Treatment

If a regime of total sun avoidance is practised, these children can grow to adult life with signs of accelerated skin ageing, but without frank cutaneous malignancy. In practice, this means having clothing that totally covers the body and sunscreen applied 365 days a year. It also means avoiding any direct sunlight, and rescheduling exercise and sporting activities for dusk or after dark.

Even with this stringent antisocial regime, regular dermatological supervision is essential to detect and treat early skin cancers.

Basal cell carcinoma (rodent ulcer)

Definition

A common, slowly growing, and locally destructive tumour thought to arise from a subset of the basal cells in the epidermis.

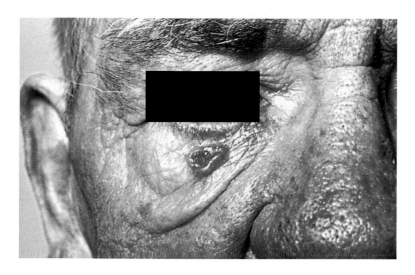

Fig. 15.15 Basal cell carcinoma.

This tumour is by far the commonest form of cutaneous malignancy.

Pathology

A mass of basophilic keratinocytes is seen pushing down into the dermis, but retaining its contact with the overlying epidermis. Mitotic figures are plentiful, but the turnover time is slow.

Clinical features

Basal cell carcinomas are seen predominantly on exposed sites, commonly around the nose and inner canthus. Initially, the lesion is a reddish, dome-shaped nodule with a translucent surface and visible, dilated surface capillaries. As it expands, the central area may show necrosis and ulceration, leaving the characteristic rolled edge (Fig. 15.15). The lesion has frequently been growing for 1–2 years before the patient seeks advice, and further slow growth will continue if the lesion is not treated. Although these lesions do not metastasize, they may cause extensive and mutilating local destruction of soft tissue, cartilage, and even bone (Fig. 15.16).

Morphoeic basal cell carcinoma is a rare variant in which the tumour may appear like a firm scar despite the lack of prior local trauma. Morphoeic basal cell carcinomas are particularly prone to recur locally.

Treatment

Basal cell carcinoma can be treated either by surgery or by radiotherapy. In frail and elderly patients, curettage or cryotherapy may be acceptable therapy, but follow-up is essential. Trials of photodynamic therapy suggest a high clearance rate in superficial basal cell carcinomas, but a high recurrence rate of thicker basal cell carcinomas.

The prognosis for basal cell carcinoma is excellent and follow-up should be aimed at early detection of local recurrence, more common in certain sites, such as the nasolabial fold, and with certain morphoeic histological variants. In the very rare instances when a basal cell carcinoma is thought to metastasize the histology should be carefully reviewed.

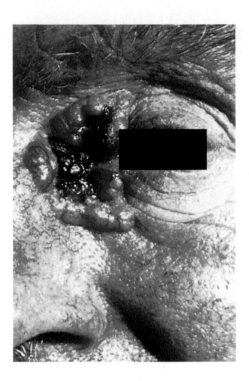

Fig. 15.16 Basal cell carcinoma.

In rare cases of recurrent basal cell carcinoma or morphoeic basal cell carcinoma, the tissue sparing technique of **Mohs surgery** can be very useful, particularly if the lesion is close to vital structures such as the eye. The principle behind this technique is to remove every single tumour cell, but as little normal tissue as is necessary. Basically, the tumour is pared away in thin slices parallel to the skin surface and carefully orientated pathological examination is carried out on each slice until no tumour cells are seen in the specimen.

Gorlin's Syndrome (basal cell naevus syndrome)

Gorlin's syndrome is characterized by the combination of multiple basal cell carcinomas, jaw cysts, palmoplantar cutaneous pits, and skeletal abnormalities. Inheritance is by an autosomal dominant gene, on chromosome 9q22, identified as the human homologue of the patched gene (*ptch*). This gene is important in developmental biology, and plays a role in limb bud patterning and positioning in foetal life.

Affected families develop basal cell carcinomas in childhood. The basal cell carcinomas are very numerous and may be clinically atypical small skin tag- like lesions. These basal cell carcinomas should be treated by surgery and not by radiotherapy, as if radiation is used there may be an explosion of small basal carcinomas on the area of irradiated skin. Photodynamic therapy is also useful in the management of these lesions.

Cutaneous malignant melanoma

Definition

A malignant tumour arising from the epidermal melanocyte

Incidence and aetiology

At present there are about 10 new cases of melanoma per 100,000 of the population per year in Europe and the United States, but much higher numbers in Australia and New Zealand, where the incidence is the highest in the world. The lifetime risk of developing melanoma in the UK at present is around one in 100, but as the incidence is doubling in each decade, this figure is likely to become higher. In 2002 over 53,000 people will develop invasive malignant melanoma in USA

Numbers of melanoma cases are highest among the white-skinned individuals in countries with long hours of strong sunshine and case control studies strongly suggest that intermittent exposure of unacclimatized white skin to intense sunlight is a major risk factor for melanoma. Emigrant studies looking at populations who emigrate from, for example, Europe to Australia or Israel as young children show that early childhood sun exposure is an important risk factor for melanoma in later life. Although these emigrants have a greater risk of developing melanoma than their relatives who remain in Europe, they never acquire as high a melanoma risk as the native born Australians.

Exposure to long-wave artificial UV (UVA) from sunbeds appears from case control studies to be an additional risk factor.

Genetics

An active search is in progress for melanoma susceptibility melanoma genes. Around 2% of melanomas are familial and, in a third of these familial melanoma cases, mutations in the CDKN2A gene on chromosome 9p21have been detected. The wild type form of this gene is a tumour suppressor gene and controls entry into the cell cycle, whereas mutated forms lose this function, and thus permit cells with damaged DNA enter into the cell cycle and replicate. The fact that only one-third of known familial melanoma cases have this mutation clearly indicates that other melanoma susceptibility genes remain to be discovered.

Clinical features

Malignant melanoma is most commonly seen on the leg in females and the back in younger male adults, and on the face in older adults of both sexes. At present, more females than males develop melanoma in the UK, but in most parts of the world the sex incidence is equal. Melanoma presents as a growing, changing area of brown or black coloured skin.

The **seven-point checklist** may be useful in identifying early melanoma and differentiating it from other pigmented lesions.

The seven-point checklist comprises three major signs:

- change in shape of a new or pre-existing pigmented lesion;
- change in size;
- change in colour;

and four minor signs:

- over 5 mm in diameter;
- inflammation;
- crusting or bleeding;
- symptoms of minor itch or irritation.

Patients with lesions with one major and one or more minor signs should be considered for a diagnostic excision biopsy. The seven-point checklist is sensitive, but not specific, so that conditions other than cutaneous malignant melanoma may be included, but true melanoma is unlikely to be excluded.

Four subdivisions of melanoma can be recognized if both clinical and pathological features are combined. The commonest of these is the **superficial spreading malignant melanoma** (Figs 15.17–15.19), which comprises around 80% of

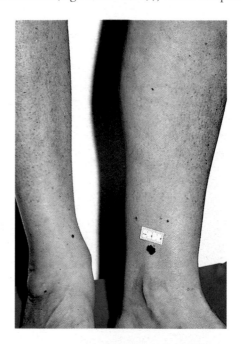

Fig. 15.17 Superficial spreading melanoma on inner malleolus area of female leg.

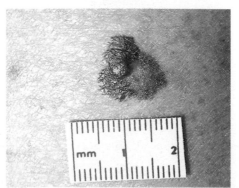

Fig. 15.18 High power view of superficial spreading melanoma showing irregularity in pigmentation.

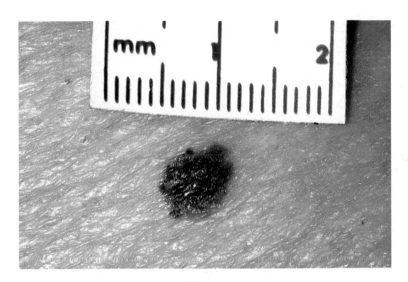

Fig. 15.19 High power view of superficial spreading melanoma showing irregular margin.

all melanomas in Caucasians. It is relatively easy to recognize as an irregularly shaped, expanding, pigmented lesion with more than one colour. Shades of brown, blue, or black are present. A rarer, but more aggressive type is the **nodular melanoma** (Fig. 15.20), which is a rapidly growing red or black nodule on the skin with no surrounding pigmentation. Early bleeding is frequent. In older patients, the **lentigo maligna melanoma** variant is seen most often. This is the most slowly growing variety, and is usually seen on the face as a gradually expand-

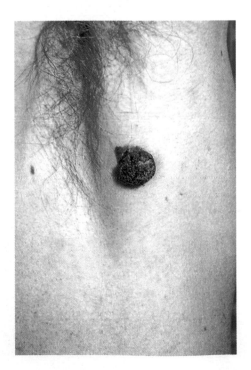

Fig. 15.20 Nodular melanoma.

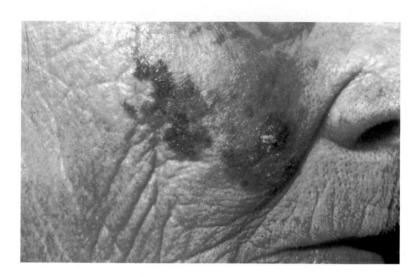

Fig. 15.21 Lentigo maligna melanoma.

ing flat lesion on the cheek (Fig. 15.21), which, if not treated, will develop, raised central nodules over time. The rarest type of melanoma on Caucasian skin, but the commonest on Asian skin, is the **acral melanoma** found on the palms and soles (Fig. 15.22). This again is a slowly expanding, irregularly shaped area of pigmentation.

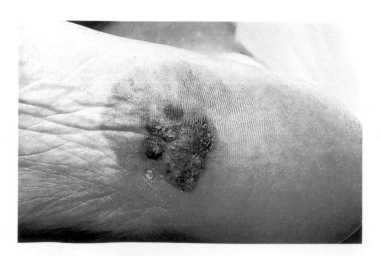

Fig. 15.22 Acral melanoma.

A variant of the acral melanoma is the **subungual melanoma**, found around the nail bed apparatus. This may present as an area of pigmentation on the nail or around the nail fold, but is frequently not recognized until it has partially destroyed the nail (Fig. 15.23).

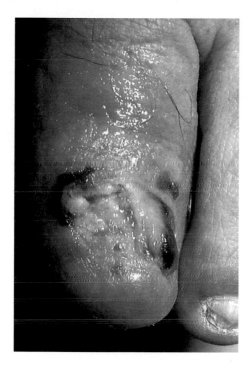

Fig. 15.23 Subungual melanoma.

Early melanoma is generally pain free, and the only symptom which patients complain of, if any, is of mild irritation or itch.

Pathology

Malignant melanocytes are seen to develop from melanocytes in the basal area of the epidermis and invade the underlying dermis. The depth to which these malignant cells have invaded is the most important prognostic factor for patients with primary melanoma. This measurement, which is made in millimetres, is called the tumour or **Breslow thickness** (Fig. 15.24, see overleaf). It is essential that the pathologist reporting melanoma includes this in his report, as it is vital for prognosis for the individual patient. For example, if an invasive malignant melanoma is less than 1 mm thick, there is an over 90% chance that the patient will be alive and disease-free at the end of 5 years, whereas if the tumour is thicker than 3 mm the likelihood of disease free survival falls to only 50%.

Differential diagnosis

The lesions to be included in the differential diagnosis of malignant melanoma include all types of benign melanocytic naevi and other non-melanocytic, but pigmented lesions, such as seborrhoeic keratoses or even angiomas.

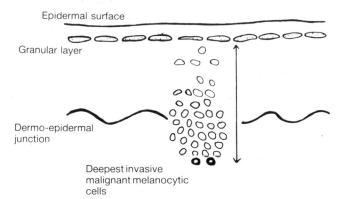

Fig. 15.24 Diagrammatic representation of tumour thickness measured by the Breslow method. The distance between the granular layer and the deepest tumour cell (arrowed) is the Breslow thickness in millimetres.

For superficial spreading malignant melanomas, the commonest differential diagnosis lies between superficial spreading malignant melanoma and melanocytic naevi. The history of growth, the irregular outline, and the colour variation all suggest the lesion is likely to be melanoma, rather than a naevus, as benign naevi do not usually enlarge in an adult, have a regular lateral outline, and are composed of one shade of brown or black. For nodular malignant melanoma, the differential diagnosis may be between a vascular tumour or histiocytoma. This is a difficult clinical differential diagnosis and an excision biopsy is recommended if there is any clinical doubt.

For lentigo maligna melanoma differential diagnosis is most commonly from the flat type of seborrhoeic keratosis or basal cell papilloma.

Dermatoscopy

The technique of dermatoscopy has become very popular as a clinical aid to melanoma diagnosis in some countries in the past 5 years. The technique involves applying a light oil to the skin surface, which makes the stratum corneum more translucent, and then using a hand held microscope on the skin surface usually at a magnification of ×10. This allows structures to be seen that are common in melanoma, but rare in benign skin lesions. It should be noted, however, that the technique is not totally sensitive or totally specific. Features that suggest melanoma include an irregular network of melanin pigmentation, irregular black dots within the lesion, and the presence of a blue/white veil-like structure in the lesion. Training is needed before the dermatoscope can be used with accuracy and, even then, it will usually be necessary to excise a worrying pigmented lesion to obtain a pathological diagnosis, which remains the gold standard.

Treatment

If malignant melanoma is suspected, a diagnostic excision biopsy with a narrow margin of 2–5 mm of normal skin should be performed without delay. The specimen must be sent for pathological examination. The pathologist reporting the lesion should include tumour thickness in the report as this will determine the need for and extent of any further surgery. If invasive malignant melanoma is diagnosed, the patient should be referred to the local expert centre for advice on further management. In general, melanomas thinner than 1 mm require a lateral excision margin of 1 cm, those 1–2 mm thick require a margin of 2 cm of normal skin, and those thicker than 2 mm require a maximum margin of 3 cm of normal skin. These margins may allow the definitive surgical procedure to be performed without a skin graft.

The technique of **sentinel lymph node biopsy** is currently being carried out on a trial basis in many parts of the world for patients with melanomas thicker than 1 mm. The assumption behind this technique is that in nodal basins, such as the groin and axilla, there is a so-called sentinel node, which is the most distal node, and that if a patient has a melanoma on the leg or arm this node will be the first to show evidence of melanoma cells metastasizing. The surgeon therefore identifies by lymphoscintigraphy, radiolabelled colloid, and injection of blue dye into the primary melanoma site the likely sentinel node, and removes only this node for pathological examination. If this node is free of tumour, no further surgery is carried out, but if melanoma cells are present, the patient has a full dissection of the affected lymph node basin. Over the next year or two results of trials in progress will establish whether or not this improves the patient's survival prospects.

There is no proven effective non-surgical treatment for patients with melanoma that has spread beyond the primary site, but there are trials in progress to establish whether or not interferon treatment improves survival prospects.

Histiocytosis X

This is a rare proliferative disorder of the epidermal Langerhans cell. Opinion is divided as to whether it is a true malignancy or a hyper-proliferative condition. Patients usually present as infants with a greasy rash on the scalp and in the flexures. This can look like severe seborrrhoeic dermatitis, but there is also hepatosplemomegaly. A skin biopsy will confirm the clinical suspicion, as large atypical Langerhans cells will be seen.

Merkel cell carcinoma

Malignancies arising from the Merkel cell are also rare. They are usually found on the head and neck area of older people, and present as non-specific nodules. The treatment is surgery, but the prognosis is poor and about 50% of patients develop metastatic spread.

Kaposi's sarcoma

This malignancy arising from the dermal endothelial cells, and may be seen both in HIV positive and HIV negative individuals. In HIV negative individuals it is seen more commonly in those of Mediterranean origin and in patients after chemotherapy.

Cutaneous lymphoma

A small number of lymphomas may actually arise in the skin or preferentially involve it. Most of these originate from T lymphocytes. Cutaneous lymphomas include a wide range of very rare lymphomas. The commonest is mycosis fungoides or primary cutaneous T cell lymphoma, but even this is a rare disorder.

Key points

Cutaneous lymphoma could be confused initially with psoriasis.

Mycosis fungoides

Definition

A slowly evolving T cell lymphoma initially involving only the skin.

Clinical features

The condition is seen mainly in middle-aged or elderly individuals who present with pruritic, cutaneous plaques (Fig. 15.25). They may clear spontaneously,

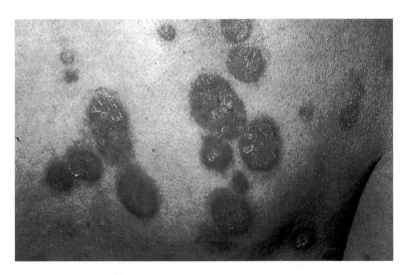

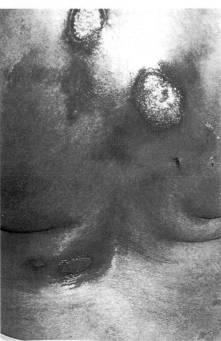

Figs 15.25 and 15.26 Cutaneous lymphoma of mycosis of fungoides type.

remain relatively unchanged, or progress to frank nodules and ulceration (Fig. 15.26). A small number of patients present with nodular lesions from the start and others present with poikiloderma (dappled skin)—a macular pigmentary change with alternating increased and decreased pigmentation developing on thin dry epidermis.

The lesions are usually associated with severe and persistent itch.

Pathology

Large numbers of morphologically atypical T lymphocytes are seen in both the dermis and epidermis. They may gather in small clusters within the epidermis, a pattern called a Pautrier abscess.

Gene rearrangement studies show that this is a monoclonal T lymphocyte proliferation.

Treatment

Treatment is aimed at control, rather than cure, of the disease. Topical steroids, conventional ultraviolet light (UVB), and photochemotherapy (PUVA) all improve symptoms; the latter may cause dramatic regression of lesions, but maintenance therapy is generally required. A course of electron beam therapy or low-penetration superficial X-rays may alleviate symptoms for long periods of time. Topical nitrogen mustard may also relieve symptoms. Trials of the systemic retinoid bexarotene in patients with advanced T cell lymphoma are encouraging, but longer periods of follow-up are required.

Metastases to the skin from tumours arising in other organs

Patients with advanced malignancy of any type may develop metastases to the skin and, occasionally, cutaneous metastases may be the first sign of such a malignancy. For example, breast tumours may metastasize to the scalp, causing painful nodules and hair loss. The diagnosis is made by biopsying the cutaneous nodule and then initiating a careful search for the primary site. Secondary deposits from many other tumour types, such as lung and prostate, may also appear in the skin. Skin nodules in patients with known malignancy elsewhere should always be regarded with suspicion and biopsied to obtain a diagnosis.

Prevention of cutaneous malignancy

Skin cancer is the commonest of all malignancies on a world-scale. It is likely that the numbers of affected patients will increase still further in developed countries with an ageing population, and the tendency of white-skinned populations living in cold northern countries to spend long periods of time in Mediterranean or warmer climates during the winter months. Skin cancers should be at least partially preventable by encouraging sensible sun exposure. This involves avoiding direct Mediterranean summer sun during the hours around noon, using clothing such as wide-brimmed hats, long-sleeved shirts, and long cotton trousers as sun screens, and applying high SPF broad spectrum sunscreens to exposed skin in an adequate quantity. These recommendations are particularly important for children.

Discussion of problem cases

Case 15.1

This description suggests an area of Bowen's intra-epidermal carcinoma *in situ*, an extra-facial basal cell carcinoma, or even an isolated patch of psoriasis, although solitary patches of psoriasis are extremely rare. The fact that he also has prostatic cancer is probably not relevant to this lesion, as although cutaneous metastases from prostate cancer do occur, they are commonly multiple nodules.

An excisional biopsy into the edge of the lesion confirmed that the plaque was an extra-facial basal cell carcinoma, and thereafter the entire plaque was excised with a narrow margin of surrounding normal skin and the wound closed directly.

Case 15.2

This patient clearly needs appropriate investigation to exclude remediable causes of hair loss including haematological and thyroid function assessment. The nodule below her eye should be examined carefully. It is raised, translucent, and has visible capillaries on the surface. This picture strongly suggests basal cell carcinoma. An excision biopsy was therefore arranged and pathological examination confirmed that the diagnosis was basal cell carcinoma, and that the lesion was completely excised. What follow-up plans would be appropriate?

Case 15.3

This description and the outdoor occupation of the patient strongly suggests that the lesions are actinic keratoses. The fact that he is a fair-skinned redhead makes this even more likely. Multiple actinic keratoses can be treated by several methods including cryotherapy, or by the use of topical 5 fluorouracil (Efudix), or topical diclofenac (Solaraze). This patient had three sessions of cryotherapy with obvious improvement. He was also advised to use a high SPF broad spectrum sunscreen throughout the year and to wear a hat in sunny weather.

Case 15.4

While programmes such as the one described are useful in encouraging self-awareness about skin lesions and prompting earlier self-referral with true skin malignancy, they also result in a large number of consultations from the 'worried well', who require reassurance. It is very useful to be able to triage these patients into those who have no serious problem, and require only reassurance and an explanation of the nature of their lesion, those who have a possibly more serious problem, and who require an excisional or incisional biopsy to obtain a tissue diagnosis, and those who do appear to have true cutaneous malignancy and require definitive treatment.

The description of the first patient suggests that she has several seborrhoeic keratoses or basal cell papillomas on her back. They are very common on the trunk of older, white-skinned individuals, and have no premalignant potential. They frequently crumble or lose some substance after minor trauma, but tend to regrow and may become quite large. No definitive treatment is necessary, unless a lesion is being irritated by clothing. Removal by curettage and cautery is a reasonable approach to treatment if the diagnosis is clear on clinical examination.

The second patient illustrates a relatively common problem with congenital melanocytic naevi. There is a very small risk of malignant change, but minor,

Discussion of problem cases continued

non-malignant, degenerative changes are much commoner. However, it is not usually possible to confidently differentiate between the two on clinical grounds and pathological examination is needed. The young man had an excision biopsy with a margin of 2 mm of normal skin around the naevus. Pathological examination confirmed that there was no evidence of malignant change.

The third patient is the most worrying. Growing, changing, pigmented lesions in adults should be regarded with suspicion as this is the usual way in which cutaneous malignant melanoma presents. The irregular outline and the fact that the lesion is multi-coloured are additional worrying points. This lesion was excised with a margin of 5 mm of surrounding normal skin and pathological examination confirmed that it was a superficial, spreading, malignant melanoma, which was 0.48 mm thick and non-ulcerated, a good prognosis lesion. The scar was re-excised with 1 cm of normal skin in all directions, including in depth. Three years later she is well with no evidence of recurrence.

What would you examine this patient for at follow up visits? For how long would you follow her up?

Special study module projects

Arrange to follow-up and see as many skin cancer patients as possible. This may involve attending a rapid referral skin cancer clinic, skin biopsy sessions, plastic surgery clinics, or outpatient oncology clinics. Try to see the pathology of all the lesions from the patients you have identified. Review the relative numbers of each type of skin cancer and the treatments available for each type.

Further reading

Burg, G. and Braun-Falco, O. (1983) *Cutaneous lymphomas*. Springer-Verlag, Berlin.

MacKie, R.M. (1995) *Skin cancer*, 2nd edn. Martin Dunitz, London.

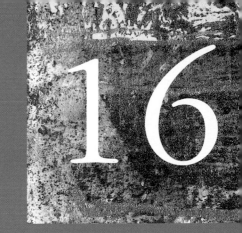

16

Brief notes on dermatological therapy

- Introduction
- Vehicles (bases)
- Emollients
- Sunscreens
- Topical steroid preparations
- Dressings

Brief notes on dermatological therapy

Introduction

Therapy for skin disease can be broadly divided into topical preparations, physical therapy such as ultraviolet light or laser treatment, and systemic therapy. In the past 5 years the use of potent systemic agents in chronic or severe psoriasis, acne, and eczema has become much commoner. Oral retinoids and a wide range of immunosuppressive agents are now used fairly routinely in hospital departments of dermatology, and the use of cytokine modulating therapy, such as anti TNF alpha agents is becoming commoner for patients with severe psoriasis. While use of these drugs has revolutionized the control of severe dermatological problems for many patients, they all have toxicity profiles, and must be used with appropriate monitoring. Oral retinoid use in acne without absolute contraception has led to tragic foetal malformations. Regular haematological monitoring is an absolute requirement for all patients on immunosuppressive drugs, and careful follow-up is needed for those on the cytokine modulating agents to identify new side effects or toxicity. For example, at the present time there is concern that the TNF-alpha blocking agent etanercept or enbrel may unmask tuberculosis. The size of this problem is not yet established, but careful patient supervision is essential.

Dermatologists and others who prescribe and apply topical treatments need to have some understanding of the types of preparation available. Very few dermatologists or departments now compound their own topical preparations, but some understanding of which type of topical preparation to use for different conditions is required.

Vehicles (bases)

A vehicle is defined as the (usually) inert carrier of the active ingredient. Vehicles are made up of liquids, greases, and powders in varying proportions according to the final consistency required. Thus, liquids alone may be used as **wet dressings** or **tinctures**, liquids and powders result in a shake **lotion**, which is cooling and drying due to evaporation, grease alone is an **ointment**, and a grease and powder mixture results in a **paste**.

Lotions are used in acutely inflamed weeping conditions. A useful preparation is ichthyol 1% in calamine lotion BP. Lotions may be applied directly to the skin or on swabs or dressings that have been soaked in the lotion. In either case, frequent changing of dressings (for example, every 4 hours) is necessary as otherwise the lotion will crust and cake.

Liniments are lotions with some additional oil, which tends to prevent this crusting, and it is therefore possible to change dressings less frequently. The advantage of rapid evaporation and cooling is, however, lost.

Creams

These are either oil-in-water or water-in-oil emulsions, and contain preservatives to prevent bacterial and fungal growth. The commonest preservatives are chlorocresol and parabens. Either may cause sensitization and subsequent allergic contact dermatitis. Oil-in-water emulsions rub into the skin and are easily washed off. They are, therefore, very suitable for use on the face, but may have a drying effect on the skin. Water-in-oil emulsions are greasier. Less evaporation of water from the skin surface is possible through these preparations, and they are therefore useful in conditions characterized by dryness and flaking. Water-in-oil emulsions are based either on petrolatum or on lanolin, which is a potential sensitizing agent.

Ointments

Ointments contain no water, but are greases with the permissible addition of up to 40% of powder by weight. A higher concentration of powder would change the consistency of the preparation to such an extent that it would be a paste. The lack of water in ointments makes the use of preservatives unnecessary, but emulsifying agents are frequently added to facilitate spreading. Ointments are useful in any condition characterized by dry skin (for example, atopic dermatitis, chronic hand dermatitis). They are less easily washed off than creams.

Pastes

These are greases containing more than 40% powder by weight. They are useful for dry surfaces, but are very difficult to remove.

Gels

These are semi-colloids, which liquefy in contact with the skin. They are commonly used in anti-acne preparations and also in scalp preparations.

Modern dermatopharmacology is a large and important section of the pharmaceutical industry. The current trend is to devise totally synthetic vehicles with a high degree of cosmetic acceptability and many preparations are now available, which are neither ointments nor creams, but have some of the advantages (and possibly disadvantages) of both. The tendency to use lanolin less and to avoid preservatives where possible should, in time, lead to a decrease in the incidence of medicament-induced allergic contact dermatitis. There are tables available in all prescribers' journals giving details of the content of preservatives, fragrances, etc., in a very wide range of topical preparations. These should be consulted.

Emollients

Emollients are now available in many different forms, as bath additives, soap substitutes, and creams and ointment. They are of great value in the regular care of ageing skin and of all dry skin conditions, particularly the ichthyoses and atopic dermatitis. The pruritus that frequently accompanies dry skin conditions can be significantly relieved by emollients and the need for topical steroids can be greatly reduced. This is of particular value in the management of paediatric problems.

Key points

Dry skin needs emollients not topical steroids.

Patients differ in their response to emollient preparations and, for this reason, it is good practice to initially offer a range of five or six preparations, so that the patient can select those most effective and acceptable. It is common to find that one preparation is preferred for the body and another for the face.

Useful emollients include:

- **Soap substitutes**: liquid paraffin 50% in white soft paraffin, E45 wash cream emulsifying ointment BP, unguentum M.
- **Bath additives**: alpha-keri, Oilatum emollient, Balneum, Dermalo Emulsiderm, Hydromol.
- **General purpose preparations**: aqueous cream BP, Oilatum cream, Diprobase, Doublebase.

Sunscreens

Sunscreens contain both chemical and physical sunscreens. In general, the physical agents, such as microfine titanium dioxide, are appropriate when sun protection is needed for photosensitive skin disease, such as lupus erythematosus. A preparation with a minimum SPF of 20 should be chosen and should also offer broad-spectrum protection. The SPF figure gives an indication of the anti-UVB protection and the broad-spectrum star rating system will give some indication of the anti-UVA protection.

Effective preparations include Piz Buin SPF 30, Roc total sun block, and Spectraban Ultra.

Topical steroid preparations

Topical steroid therapy has already been discussed in the relevant treatment sections and their undesirable side effects in Chapter 13. Prescribers' journals give comprehensive tables listing steroid preparations by potency, and also giving details of additives such as preservatives and fragrances. These details change regularly as new preparations are marketed and current tables should be consulted. Most dermatologists make themselves familiar with a small selection of varying potency preparations and are aware of the additives in each.

Dressings

The need for frequent renewal of topical preparations is reduced by the use of appropriate dressings. For trunk and limbs expandable stockinet dressings can be made into neatly fitting 'body suits', which are very useful in mild, but extensive eczema or psoriasis, and can be worn under normal clothing. Smaller areas can be covered with narrower dressings of similar material. When pastes are used, it best to spread the paste on to a dressing, then apply the dressing to the area, and bandage it in position. Large raw areas should be covered with a dressing such as sterile paraffin gauze, which does not stick to the granulating surface.

In chronic dermatitis the use of occlusive tar or ichthyol impregnated bandages may help to break the itch-scratch-itch cycle and allow the skin to heal. These bandages (for example, Coltapaste, Tarband, Ichthopaste) can be covered with a stockinet dressing and left in position for up to a week.

Occlusive dressings of this type are also extremely useful in the out-patient management of stasis ulcers. A dry gauze swab can be used to cover the ulcerated area and an Ichthopaste or Viscopaste bandage applied from the ankle to below the knee and covered with an elastocrepe bandage. This can be changed by the district nurse at weekly intervals or even less frequently. The Viscopaste bandages have the advantage of being easily unwound from the leg, even after 2–3 weeks in position.

Trained dermatology nurses are invaluable in demonstrating to patients how to apply their topical preparations. Newly-diagnosed patients with psoriasis or eczema should always have a practical hands on demonstration with a dermatology nurse. This will help compliance and give the patient confidence.

Further reading

Bickers, D.R., Hazen, P.G., and Lynch, W.S. (1984) *Clinical pharmacology of skin disease*, Monographs in Clinical Pharmacology, Vol. 7. Churchill Livingstone, New York.

Seville, R. and Martin, E. (1981) *Dermatological nursing and therapy*. Blackwell Scientific Publications, Oxford. (A useful, inexpensive paperback.)

Stone, L.A., Lindfield, E.M., and Robertson, S. (1989) A *colour atlas of nursing procedures in skin disorders*. Wolfe Medical Publications, London.

Reference sources

Two major English language textbooks on adult dermatology are:

Fitzpatrick, T.B., Eisen, A.Z., Wolff, K., Freedberg, I.M., and Austen, K.F. (eds) (1999) *Dermatology in general medicine*, 5th edn. McGraw-Hill, New York.

Rook, A., Wilkinson, D.S., and Ebling, F.G.J. (eds) (1997) *Textbook of dermatology*, (4 vols), 6th edn. Blackwell Scientific Publications, Oxford. [7th edition in preparation.]

A new excellent paediatric dermatology text is:

Harper, J., Oranje, A., and Prose, N. (2000) *Textbook of paediatric dermatology*. Blackwell Science, Oxford.

Useful journals include:

Journal of the American Academy of Dermatology

British Journal of Dermatology

American Archives of Dermatology

Journal of Investigative Dermatology

Clinical and Experimental Dermatology

Increasingly websites are the most up to date source of current information. The list below will be useful.

BMJ Clinical Evidence, evidence-based therapy updated 6-monthly: www.clinicalevidence.org

The website of the British Association of Dermatologists: www.bad.org.uk

Information on guidelines, meetings, patient associations, etc.

The website of the American Academy of Dermatology, another very comprehensive source of information. www.aad.org

Patient associations and support groups-many with excellent information on their diseases

National Eczema Society: www.eczema.org

Psoriasis association: mail@psoriasis.demon.co.uk

Neurofibromatosis: www.nfa-uk.org.uk

Pemphigus: www.pemphigus.org

Pseudoxanthoma elasticum: www.pxe.org.uk

Raynauds disease: www.raynauds.demon.co.uk

Herpes: www.herpes.org.uk

Tuberous sclerosis: www.tuberous-sclerosus.org

Vitiligo: www.vitiligosociety.org.uk

Lupus erythematosus: www.lupus.org

Rosacea: www.rosacea.org

Dariers: www.dariers.8m.com

Epidermolysis bullosa: www.debra.org.uk

Ehlers Danlos disease: www.ehlers-danlos.org

Alopecia: www.hairlineinternational.co.uk

Index

Note to index: *learning scenarios* include problem cases with discussion and treatment plans